WHERE DID YOU GO TO, MY LOVELY?

Dementia Days – A Reflection.

Keith Brocklehurst

Grosvenor House
Publishing Limited

This book is published by
Grosvenor House Publishing Ltd
Link House
140 The Broadway, Tolworth, Surrey, KT6 7HT.
www.grosvenorhousepublishing.co.uk

A CIP record for this book
is available from the British Library

ISBN 978-1-83975-795-2

Preface

"Where Did You Go To, My Lovely?" recalls the final 5 years of my mother's 91 years on this earth. Sadly, they were marked by the dreaded Dementia.

The 'Introduction' sets the general scene for those recollections, and 'Where Did You Come From, My Lovely?' offers the reader a brief background to her generally robust and healthy constitution and life prior to the late onset of the Dementia.

Via relevant incidents, from around 2012-2013, 'The Gathering Storm' and 'Incidentally' describe the onset, creep and build of both Mum's Dementia and of the 'medicalisation' that quickly accompanied it.

'The Beginning Of The End' jumps the story forward to 2016, with both the Dementia and the medicalisation well established; but still without the real help that we had hoped for.

'The Dementia Diaries' make up a significant and central part of the book, and take the form of my reproduction of relevant, hands-on, and dated, content lifted from the hand-written day-to-day log-books (with relevant explanation where appropriate), that my two siblings and I kept for our own benefit and, to some degree, sanity, as we effectively took on the role of sole carers for Mum between 2012 and 2016 and tried to honour her previously compos mentis wishes to 'never be put in a home'.

'(Care) Home From Home' documents our eventual failure to keep that promise, and her arrival and 10-month residency IN a Care Home from the summer of 2016.

'Am I Going To Be Alright?' was an oft-recurring question that a deteriorating Mum asked as she picked up further 'health issues' both prior to, and *in* the Home, and was sadly forced to experience a trio of not-exactly-restorative Hospital stays... the final time, in Aug. 2017, resulting in her 'not getting out alive'.

To complete the experience, I have included 'Wish You Were Here (Letting Go)'. This brings a *sort* of 'closure' to the whole sorry saga, by describing her sad demise, *in* hospital, (first and foremost *from* Dementia according to her death certificate), and how I personally coped with the immediate aftermath, the funeral and its arrangements, and the inevitably lengthy period of pain and loss that accompanied Mum's passing.

Acknowledgements

The original 'Dementia Diaries' (log-books) were as much the work of my elder brother, Trevor, (T), and my younger sister, Lorraine, (L), as of myself. Together, we made up the triumvirate of Mum's committed offspring, and, (essentially), sole carers, for all of their writing. Without their vital contributions this work would probably have remained unwritten. So, to them, a special "Thank You".

In memory of Nellie Brocklehurst, a most lovely Mum.

Contents

Introduction

In November 2016, the BBC (amongst other respected institutions) announced that Dementia had, for the first time, overtaken heart disease as the biggest single cause of death in the UK.

Official Government figures ('Office for National Statistics' website), for that year confirm this, with 70,354 Dementia-related deaths being registered; compared to 65,824 related to heart disease. And that trend, sadly, was still evident in the Government's later (ONS) figures for 2017 and 2018; one of the many and impersonal statistics for 2017, even more sadly, accounting for the *very* personal loss of my much-loved and dearly-missed Mum.

So it appears, and somewhat ironically, that more and more of us may have become potential, if not inevitable, *victims* of our society's continued medical and social services progress, and that the old biblical (psalm 90),'3 score years and 10' description of a human lifespan is now so often a thing of the past for so many; because, on the whole, and with potential access to better diets, medications, housing, heating, environments, and social care, etcetera, so many more of us are physically living much longer... alas, and regrettably, we are all still aging during that longevity; and in *mental* health terms, at least, so many of us are *not* necessarily enjoying the sort of *cognitive* longevity that is commensurate with the extended physical one.

Dementia is what is accompanying more and more of us into our increased *physical* longevity. Indeed, it is estimated that there are currently approaching 1 million Dementia sufferers in the UK.

Dementia is essentially about loss of memory, and associated cognitive (thinking) skills, and, for all those that it touches, (as victims, but also as their carers and loving relatives), it is a particularly cruel and teasing disease.

According to the Alzheimer's Society, Dementia "is used to describe a group of symptoms – these include a decline in judgement and understanding, memory loss, confusion, and mood changes". Where these symptoms apply, it is usually taken as a sign of reduced blood flow to certain parts of the brain.

Dementia is thought to start in the cortex, the area where it is thought memories are formed, and that it may sometimes involve a series of 'mini-strokes'. Again, as the Alzheimer's Society puts it, and for whatever reason, "brain cells stop working properly inside specific areas of the brain, which can affect how you think, remember and communicate".

We all forget things occasionally, as we age, don't we? How many of us more mature folk can recall instances when we've set off upstairs with a purpose, only to find that we have completely forgotten that very purpose by the time we reach the top. Dementia, however, is not just about forgetting *occasionally*. Although it's a disease that usually does develop gradually, and people can often find ways of coping with it in the early stages, once it takes hold, it usually, alas, leads to a slow, but permanent, mental decline, and a corresponding loss of independence and of control over mood, thought, and action, in the long term. In what becomes eventually, if progressively, a fundamentally 'uncontrollable' circumstance, the ability to remember, (especially in the short-term), and thereby to understand, to rationalise and to reason things out, and in consequence to communicate, and to take appropriate action, and, in short, to function normally, is severely compromised henceforth until, alas, the slow progressive worsening of the disease invariably affects the brain's ability to either fight infection, (by failing to properly trigger the body's own immune system), or, and often in tandem, to keep *vital organs* functioning; and brings about the sufferer's demise.

Within that broad description, however, Dementia, like a finger or DNA-print, is also likely to be unique to the person suffering it, and to progress in many different ways and at very different rates. Indeed, it can even take different forms; of which perhaps the most common are Alzheimer's itself, and *Vascular* Dementia.

What actually causes these brain cells to stop working is still uncertain although age appears to be the single biggest factor, and the disease is apparently rare, (though certainly not unknown), in those under 60.

So, sadly, with the *cause* of Dementia still largely unknown, it is not too surprising that no-one has yet found either a preventative, a 'holding' or a curative *treatment* for the disease; and, of course, it has obvious, and increasingly acute, (personal, financial and social) implications for civilised social care, and for appropriate resources, as we nonetheless *exist* for longer.

What follows is my personal (and where possible sociological) perspective on my mother's decline, from her mid-to-late 80s, and on towards the end of her life; and reflects on the slow but definite decline in both her physical, but particularly her mental, capacity, (and in relation to that latter, apparently through a combination of both 'late onset' Alzheimer's Disease *and* Vascular Dementia), and through the interconnection of both, to the sad yet steady and unstoppable decline in *her* independent functioning and the unavoidable need for her to, eventually, leave the home that had been hers for over 6 decades, to be 'looked after', in residential care until her further, and then final, hospitalisation, and her passing, just 10 months later.

It is also a personal (and again where possible sociological) perspective on the consequent and equally unavoidable interactions with this well-off society's (supposedly 'helping', but too often, alas, in my experience, underfunded, understaffed, over-used, over-stretched, and therefore *acutely frustrating*) medical, public legal, social, local government and residential and caring *agencies*, (each usually defending their own inherent, and typically uncoordinated, procedures, bureaucracies, and especially budgets) that her steady decline necessitated.

In particular too, and throughout, I return regularly to my lay person's 'deep suspicion' of the role that *prescribed medication* may have played, (in my *Mum's* Dementia at least), and that it was not an entirely 'innocent party' in proceedings. Indeed, whilst in the throes of my scribblings, I came across plenty of authoritative publications to support my 'suspicions'. Take, for example, "Too Many Pills", which I stumbled across in 2019, and written by retired GP and journalist, James Le Fanu. At one early point, he refers to a "classic medical textbook on pharmacology", which long ago stated that, "Any drug that is worth using can cause harm". At another he refers to what "doctors" call, "The Prescribing Cascade", whereby a patient "experiences bad side-effects from one drug, so the doctor prescribes another to deal with them. Yet another is prescribed to deal with the side-effects of the second drug, and so on". Obviously, such texts gave me plenty of 'food for (further) thought'.

PS My Mum was born in the same year as, (and just 81 days before), her Majesty Queen Elizabeth II; but the sceptic in me leads me to suspect that the latter might well qualify for quite a different level of service accessibility and support in old age than the former.

PPS At the time of final preparation for publication of my work, (Winter 2020) the dreadful, hitherto unknown, Covid 19 Coronavirus pandemic had been sweeping not just the country, but the World - for many months - triggering unprecedented 'lockdowns' of varying degrees, and (also) claiming more than 70,000 recorded deaths (related to the virus) in the UK in a single year. It is likely that a significant number of these registrations will have included elderly and vulnerable individuals who succumbed due to 'underlying' issues such as Dementia. However, there is now real hope on the horizon, in the form of the fully tested vaccines being rolled out for Covid 19. Alas, there is no such hope in the offing for tackling Dementia; and, when Covid is 'history', there is every likelihood that Dementia will *still* be wreaking its havoc as the newfound No.1 cause of death here.

CHAPTER 1

Where Did You Come From My Lovely?

As I say, my mother was born just 81 days before Her Majesty, Queen Elizabeth II; and in the same month and year (1926) that John Logie Baird gave his very first public (and apparently *mechanical*) demonstration of television. Yes, *that* long ago!

Accordingly, on the last day of January 2017, my mother saw in her *91st* birthday. Well done Ma'am.

Despite a life of both real and relative poverty, of relentless 'scrimping and saving', of poor and very limited education, and of a subsequent lack of wider opportunity, and experience, (she'd never been abroad, unless you count North Wales, never flown anywhere, never learned to swim or ride a bike, and certainly not to drive, or how to deal with anything other than basic *domestic* finances, or the fast-moving modern challenges associated with technology, computers and the like; and, despite having a vote, had still to adequately understand how much of this society is structured and works at a commercial, social and political level, for example), she had, nonetheless, managed to survive pretty-well intact, both physically and mentally, for all but the very last few of her 91 years; and as a kindly, compliant, generally good-natured, and thoroughly decent person, mother and member of her society for even the latter. Very well done, Mum.

Born on the very last day of the very first month of 1926, her childhood and early life had been lived (both happily and healthily, if her fond reminiscences are anything to go by), as the third-youngest child of a poverty-stricken, Catholic, working-class, twelve-some, in a northern mill-town in the UK.

With her siblings, she walked nearly a mile each way, each day, to her 'one-and-only' school; a sturdy, single-storey, stone-built, 'Catholic' educational structure, (with a similarly-built

1

companion *church* close by), on the edge of town. She left that school at the tender young age of 14; and, as I've intimated, she left it with the very minimum of education, (she insisted that she was taught exclusively, and quite strictly, by nuns, but apparently no less enjoyably for that), essentially to work as mill fodder, and more specifically, as a 'winder' in one of the many clattering local cotton mills; and thereby to contribute a few hard-earned pennies to the family's always-empty coffers. However, despite rarely attending church once married, (age 23), and especially once she'd had her first child, (age 24), and was living a little further afield, she never managed to shake off the more *general* constraints of the initial and subsequently (and arguably lifelong for her) far-reaching influences (not to mention some very real *fears*) of the wider Catholic church and religion. On the other hand, like many who hold onto their religious beliefs, she also continued to find a significant degree of comfort in them ("He'll take me when he's ready", being a typical, presumably consolatory, presumably preparatory, but most of all presumably *belief-based*, saying of hers in later life) right up until 'the end'.

Any early income that she (and her siblings) contributed to those hard-pressed family coffers, by the way, became all the more vital when her father (who, incidentally, and according to his obituary, had, in his younger role as a Grenadier Guard, been, "a member of the military escort at the funeral of Queen Victoria"), died suddenly in the autumn of 1944, aged 65, and when Mum herself was just 18.

Luckily her own mother seemed to be the one supplying Mum with most of her 'healthy and resilient' genes, as, despite going through the childbirth experience herself on a dozen occasions, *she* went on to support Mum well into both adulthood and motherhood, (I recall her visiting often), and until she herself only gave in to the ravages of time, and actually died in 1979, on the very day before Mum's 53rd birthday, (so Mum was never likely to forget that anniversary, was she?), also at the ripe old age of 91.

At some point in her early twenties, Mum obviously met my (equally local, and barely better-off, working-class, but Methodist) Dad, and they married in 1949; 're-visiting' her familiar 'old'

Catholic church and religion for the ceremonials. Alas, and perhaps predictably, given her (and his) generally conforming personality, deprived background, circumstances and milieu, Mum fared little better in improving her social and economic prospects in her adult/ later life; and that despite my father's life of honest endeavour, 'hard-labour' and working-class toil on behalf of both her and their offspring. *He* too was a decent human being, and a decent man, and father, who, having done his bit as a young man conscripted into the 2nd World War, (partly in India, but mostly, we have learned posthumously, as a Prisoner of War in Burma; and probably put to work on constructing the infamous Burma railway, as most were), had then spent most of his working life, (in a 'glutton for punishment' sort of way), employed in lowly, labour-intensive, work as a 'lengthman' and 'platelayer', helping to maintain the local rail-track for the then British Railways; and thereby managing to just about 'bring home the family bacon'.

Unfortunately, despite its' very physical, and out-in-all-weathers, hardship, (like much of the heavy industry work available to the masses of the day), it was very poorly paid work, and offered equally poor prospects, and Mum's (and Dad's) limited life-chances in adulthood were inevitably, and very directly, a reflection of Dad's equally limited education, and therefore (like so many of his working-class peers), opportunities to improve his earning capacity, and thence lifestyle. (Though both my parents were of at least average intelligence and could probably have made more of their abilities had they *had* the education, and therefore gained both the necessary knowledge and confidence, to pursue the available opportunities).

Nonetheless, nature, as I've said, appears to have compensated Mum (and indeed Dad), through a generally robust constitution, and despite her near-destitute beginnings, she appears to have enjoyed a relatively trouble-free childhood, both physically and mentally, and to have been able to carry that healthy constitution through into her teen years, and then on into adult/parenthood. And from such apparently resilient underpinnings, she was able to give birth to, and raise, 3 equally healthy offspring, and to live all

3

but the very last few years of her own *adult* life in remarkably 'fit and well' fashion. So, whilst Mum's life might have been financially poor, for the most part, I like to think it was happy and enriched in most other respects. My over-riding image of her is as a kindly, loving, child-centred, (in an instinctive sort of way, rather than via any formal, *greatly-researched,* parental knowledge), strong, generally fine-looking, morally good, able-bodied, (she was always busy about the house, walked everywhere if at all possible, and could bend down to pick up a coin without bother at 80 better than I could at 60!), naturally caring, (I couldn't have wished for a better or more caring Mum; nor Dad a wife; whilst, for instance, in her late 50s, she willingly looked after even the most basic elements of an elderly next-door neighbour's needs for many weeks, and for absolutely no reward, after his wife died, before the local social services finally 'got their act together'), if anxiety-prone, and (sometimes over?) sensitive, (especially if out of her 'comfort zone' and/or beyond the borough boundaries), industrious, but scrimping, yet 'always there', home-maker of a Mum. She also managed to neatly underpin all that with a ready, mischievous, but equally healthy, sense of humour. Moreover, she managed to garner that agreeable image, and all those aptitudes and qualities, almost entirely provincially, (though again not noticeably resentfully or unhappily), whilst living in a basic, and basically-updated wherever and whenever limited funds permitted, 2-up-2-down stone-built, end-terraced house in one of her home borough's satellite *village*, (and therefore pleasantly bucolic), settings; and a setting in which I recall both a generally healthy, and generally happy, free-to-roam, almost idyllic, yet far from well-off, 1950/60s village life and childhood myself. (Domestic features that we now just take for granted, such as TVs, fridges, washing-machines, central heating, holidays, and even indoor bathrooms and toilets, remained non-existent well beyond my, and indeed most of my peers, primary-school years; and the radio, newspapers and coal were still king, for example).

So, for Mum, it was an adult/ parenting life spent (largely, and like so many working class others around her in the 1950s, 60s & 70s), as a 'make-do-and-mend', stay-at-home, (in our case *village-based)*, mother of her (3) children; and latterly, as those three now morally-endowed offspring (eventually) matured, and could be safely left for a while in their teens, it was also spent toiling part-time back in the *paid* labour market; variously, as a factory shift-worker, and latterly office, school, and domestic 'hygiene technician' (yes, that's a cleaner); before those children eventually left home, (but never strayed *too* far, and always kept regular contact), and *she* had no alternative (like Dad; and indeed like us all) but to face and embrace the unsolicited spectre of aging; and that of the equally limited income and lifestyle that came with 'state-pensionable' retirement.

That said, the arrival of her 2 grandchildren, in quick succession, in the autumns of 1988 and 1989, when Mum was in her early 60s, certainly put a bit of a spring back into her retirement step. She always enjoyed having *them* round, and looked forward to taking them out and treating them; which included most Saturdays during their primary school years; with regular contact thereafter. (Mum even stayed alive just long enough to meet her first *great* grandchild, in the Spring of 2017).

Following Dad's passing, in 1996, and for 20 of the final 21 years of her life she lived alone, (and for all but the final few 'Dementia years' quite contentedly), in that same, simple, secure, bucolic home and setting that had been hers for over 60 years; and she did remarkably well to self-maintain both her home, and her independence, for so long; albeit with our regular, and in the end daily, support... until, alas, the dreaded Dementia took its unforgiving hold and eventually necessitated first her hospitalisation for a few weeks, then her final 10 months being 'looked after' in a care home, and finally what would end as another spell, but this time culminating in a terminal 'last stand', at the hospital.

It's perhaps pertinent to note here that both of my Mum's parents, and all of her 11 siblings, (2 others of whom also made it to 91, and 6 of the other 8 making it well into their 80s) are now deceased but that not a single one of them are known to have died from Dementia-related causes. That is to say, there was no known history of Dementia in Mum's family prior to her own diagnosis.

CHAPTER 2

The Gathering Storm

January 2016 marked not only Mum's 90th birthday, but also the 20th anniversary of the passing of my father, (aged just 76). He died in 1996, and at relatively 'short notice', from the undetected return and spread of prostate-cancer-related issues and complications; and he and Mum had been married, lived in the self-same house, and been rarely apart, for over 40 years.

As that 'passing anniversary', and her 90th birthday, came and went, in quick succession, and for the 20 years past, Mum was *still*, (albeit with our regular, lengthening, and latterly *daily*, support visits) living, and (especially) sleeping alone, and still, ostensibly, living independently, in that 2-up-2-down terraced home, in that same village, that had, by then, as I say, been her adult life's focus and abode (and the family home), for well over 60 years.

Despite her earlier domestic hardships and privations, (or perhaps because of having to *overcome* them), in general, Mum had remained both physically and mentally robust until the 'Dementia years', and had had no serious, certainly no life-threatening, illnesses during her core adult life as our mother. In truth, I cannot recall a single instance of her abandoning her parenting duties, and taking to her bed with extended sickness, nor needing any significant in-patient, let alone serious, hospitalisation, during her motherhood. What I do vaguely recall is her requiring a very brief stop-over and minor surgery for the 'stripping' of the rather unsightly varicose veins that had developed in both her lowers legs. A glance at her GP's medical records shows this as occurring early in 1974; and just prior to her 48th birthday; with *only* a solitary (1971) entry for a 'psoriasis' consultation preceding it. (By 1974, of course, I was in my early

6

20s, and, like the rest of her offspring, I was relatively self-sufficient).

The next entry in her medical records is as far into the future as 1996, and logged as a 'bereavement reaction', and that, of course, relates to Dad's passing. It is not clear from my limited access to her medical records what, if any, (short-term) medication or treatment followed this diagnosis.

What *is* clear though, is that this 'bereavement reaction' was to prove the forerunner for a more active series of post-Dad, and on the face of it unrelated and minor, health issues between its' supposed identification and moment in time and the autumn of 2002.

So, next up, in September 1998, and age 72, was a diagnosis of 'Ischaemic heart disease'; or, as both the hospital 'specialist' and latterly the GP told it to her, a 'touch of angina'. Whether it was in any way related to the 'bereavement reaction' was never actively raised with either her (as their patient) or with us (as Mum's next-of-kin) by either medic, but it followed an isolated "funny turn", and an accompanying degree of mild upper-left-arm pain, whilst out walking in a local country lane one day with my sister. This never actually required any in-patient/hospital treatment, and could probably have passed almost unnoticed as a significant, let alone a major, health issue, save for the fact that, after a single, standard, 'precautionary' outpatient visit to the 'specialist', following 'precautionary', surgery-organised, blood tests and the like, the safety-first, 'doctor's union', diagnosis-cum-advice was that Mum be treated with a 'precautionary' course of what would turn out, (with due hind- sight), to be a *'landmark'* prescription of 2 different *'long-term'* pills; as initially recommended by the 'specialist', and thereafter endorsed and freely prescribed by her GP... for the rest of her life.

Then, the following year, and in relatively quick succession, came her two, separate, day-long, outpatient attendances, (one at each end of the *summer* of 1999), for pretty regulation eye operations for 'cataracts'; (age 73).

Whilst, on the upside, these minor 'eye-lights' further improved her occasionally 'clouding' sight a little, on the downside, the *process* inevitably brought with it plenty of attendant worries and anxieties for someone of Mum's age and background.

Perhaps unsurprisingly then, just a couple of months later, in the *September* of that year, (yes, you've guessed it), she was prescribed more *pills*; this time a short course of 'azepams', (probably Valium, but, alas, my perusal of her medical records revealed nothing more specific), as treatment for an unexplained "anxiety state" that appeared to accompany her short-range post-cataract recuperation; and which, once again, we'd felt obliged to consult her GP about.

Next, in November 2001, came her inaugural complaint of an initially manageable and intermittent pain in the upper right part of her tummy. This had resulted in a further GP referral, followed by a short period of monitoring. However, its persistence eventually led to Mum's most significant 'surgical' *inpatient* status so far. It took the form of a very brief admission for what was then contemporary *keyhole* surgery, after she'd been beset by a sudden, more painful, and even more persistent bout of 'acute cholecystitis'; otherwise known as 'gallstones'. The condition had refused to bow to non-invasive prescriptions, and the eventual resolution for the matter was the removal of her entire gallbladder, in the May of 2002; age 75.

Then, in a busy 2002, and just a couple of months after the loss of her gall bladder, came her initial complaint of a lower-left-leg 'ache' that also stubbornly refused to respond to non-prescriptive, over-the-counter, remedies, settled in as bearable but *chronic*, and eventually lead to another 'precautionary' referral to the GP, in the *July* of that year. That brought a diagnosis of Peripheral Arterial Disease (PAD) or Atheroma, (known more colloquially as 'hardening of the arteries'), and the first prescription of yet another pill which would become (her third), *long-term* medication.

The foregoing minor matters notwithstanding, she had actually continued to remain remarkably fit and healthy, certainly 'everyday active', and generally well throughout her 70s and her early 80s; busying herself with a full quota of household tasks and upkeeps, mile-each-way walks to the nearest shops and post office, (the latter to independently collect her pension, and pay bills), a weekly solo shopping trip over to the town on the local village bus, enthusiastically accompanying her offspring on various walks and days out, and often looking after, including exercising, my own family's Cavalier King Charles Spaniel, for up to 2 weeks at a time, whilst my family and I holidayed abroad, for example.

So, after the inevitable early months of grieving, and that inaugural fresh logging on her medical records (of that 'bereavement reaction'), and with those regular home visits and that general support from her offspring, she had, to all intents and purposes, actually come to cope better than I could ever have hoped following Dad's sad passing. Or had she?

For surviving the latter may have been more anxiety-provoking and stressful than we offspring had fully realised, and, unbeknown to either she or we, may not have been without its more long-term emotional costs and consequences for her. Indeed, I would not have been surprised to learn that Dad's death, and the inevitable strain that accompanied it, had been a contributory factor to any of the minor medical 'conditions' aforementioned, or the eventual onset of the Dementia, (perhaps even *via* some sort of mini-stroke), a little further down the line.

I suppose the 'stress' and 'anxiety' clues were already there if only we'd looked hard enough...in the bereavement reaction itself, and in the symptoms that lead to the claimed Ischaemic heart disease, for example.

With regard to the latter diagnosis, however, and from a position of taking *no* prescribed medication whatsoever, at age 72, (and, like me, a life-long avoider of *any* long-term chemical medication if at all possible), Mum was suddenly being 'sold' a course of supposedly 'essential' medication that was (intentionally or otherwise) destined to be retained *long-term*, in response to this 'Disease'. (See under 'Medicalising Mum'). It would start her on an initially resistant, then reluctant, but in the end passive and subservient, late 'career' of prescribed pill-popping, and therefore dependence, that she would never again be entirely free of; and

9

this despite the condition never being definitively proven, nor the original, one-off, 'funny turn', or indeed any further heart-related problem for that matter, ever again rearing its head. (I suppose the medics would claim that this was *because* the medication was working). Yet, despite some significant, indeed, ultimately irredeemable, deterioration elsewhere, (again see later), her heart was probably the *last* organ to fail her, and just kept on pumping away until the very end; even in the face of the many and confusing pressures and stresses that she, and it, must have been put under latterly, by the deadly Dementia, and its menagerie of related medical and 'living' issues.

Then, there was that more blatant 'anxiety state', and the subsequent course of 'azepams' in 1999. Because it followed so closely after the last cataract operation, we had presumed the 'eyely' optical manoeuvrings had provided the trigger and sole reason for it, but perhaps it was actually a more general (re) awakening of a broader 'anxiety'; a 'state' that had probably been lying dormant in Mum's personality to some degree, anyway; especially given her desperately poor education and limited confidence-building experiences in both child and adult-hood, and her consequent, and relative, 'out-of-domestic-comfort-zone', dependency on my father throughout much of their married life. Regardless, once (re)awakened here, and given a fresh foothold, it was a 'state' (of anxiety) that would, sadly, raise its' head much more regularly in the coming future, as a key factor in, and reaction to, her poorer, Dementia-contaminated, mental workings and associated poorer functioning, as the disease staked its unforgiving claim.

Then again, that painful and unanticipated attack of 'cholecystitis' and its treatment also caused her a great deal of stress and anxiety; both before and after the removal of the gall bladder, in 2002. Of course, its presence bore no obvious connection to Dad's passing; but, once again, having to adjust to living alone probably didn't help. (Any connection here, between her long-standing ingestion of prescription pills, some since 1998, and the onset of the cholecystitis, or indeed any other state, remained unexplored in medical circles; though the latent cynic in *me* certainly ensured that the thought spent more than a moment or two pausing, if not *yet* taking up a more active residence, in *my* mind).

That said, *post*-cholecystitis, post-gallbladder and post-2002, and for the next few years, we saw a return to relatively stable, if marginally more age-expected, health for Mum; with just the well-established trio of different prescription pills for her to manage and imbibe on a daily basis, her self-medication of everyday aches and pains with over-the-counter remedies as necessary, that generally manageable susceptibility to occasional bouts of anxiety, the inevitable seasonal cold, and just the standard 'preventative' check-ups and jabs at the GP's. Indeed, in that vein, and with those limited 'qualifications', she returned to (relatively) rude health, and went the best part of a decade without either fresh concerns of note, or the further need for any significant *reactive* medical intervention or additional pills.

Then came the first significant 'turning point' in terms of the Dementia; not that we saw it as such at the time. With no history of Dementia in Mum's birth family to cloud our initial perspective, we simply presumed that we were witnessing the onset of some occasional 'senior moments'.

It would have been around 2009, and Mum would have been around 83, I guess, when we first began to witness the sporadic instances of 'forgetfulness'; such as where she had mislaid everyday items like her reading glasses, her pension book, her 'paper' money, or the TV remote; and, just occasionally, what day it was; though, in relation to the latter, and in the absence of a weekday newspaper or similar, many of those days had little to distinguish them anyway. (Perhaps more poignantly, as the situation deteriorated later on, and long after she had been introduced to *more* prescription medication, she had sometimes failed to *take* some of it, whilst vigorously claiming that she had, and had also occasionally seemed temporarily unsure of how to complete certain relatively complex, but hitherto familiar, tasks, such as how to, independently, collect her pension).

These 'forgetful' incidences also seemed to coincide with some later signs of her *physical* aging; in particular with some more frequent back/left-hip pain, and the advent of occasional bouts of painful osteoarthritis in a couple of finger joints; all of which was also beginning to slow her down by then, and frustrate her somewhat, in her much-preferred keep-busy, keep-clean, domesticity; and we initially supposed that time was just catching up with her a little...as of course, it was, to a certain degree.

At first, then, we just acknowledged and accommodated these 'forgetfulness' factors as best we could, and as a matter of (aging) course; simply playing them down, offering her calm reassurance, suggestions on where best to keep things so that they *didn't* 'go missing', additional support as she requested it, or we deemed it necessary, (for example, by providing her with a prominent wall calendar on which to tick off each day, and its prescribed breakfast-time ingestion of tablets, or actively *accompanying* her to the Post Office for her pension), visiting more frequently, dropping in 'on spec' more often, and each adding a daily reassuring telephone call on our technical 'days off'; (so that she either spoke to, or saw, *each* of us *every* day).

However, when her 'forgetfulness' began to crop up a little too frequently for our comfort, and sometimes persisted for more than a moment or two, and that despite our extra input, we decided, again as an intended 'precautionary' measure, to consult with, and seek what we hoped would be appropriate help and advice from, the 'professionals'. Accordingly, my sister, in her accepted role of 'female lead support' with regard to most of Mum's personal health and medical issues, agreed to make a further appointment with Mum's GP.

That was the second significant 'turning point'; for it was from here, and from Mum's early-to-mid- 80s, that, for better or (arguably) for worse, the Dementia was both 'formalised' and indeed 'institutionalised'.

The GP's initial response was to 'monitor' Mum, and, in particular, to try and establish some sort of 'benchmark' for doing so, by arranging for her to be seen by the local hospital 'specialist'.

A referral was duly made, and after several weeks of waiting, an initial appointment was at last received, and attended upon early in 2010. There then followed any number of further call-backs and time-consuming, (but not obviously productive), outpatient visits (transport and 'escort service', of course, to be provided by us), to this (not always 'top man', but sometimes stand-in, presumably experience-gathering underling) 'specialist', interspersed with a series of subsequent appointments at the hospital's 'memory clinic'; and these spread over many months, indeed probably in excess of 2 years, before we were (eventually) able to prise from the GP the verbal advice that Mum had, finally, and officially, been diagnosed with early-stage *vascular* Dementia. That, by then, would have been around the summer of 2012. (Oddly, my more recent access to the GP's medical records, in 2016, has Mum's original referral logged as *"Alzheimer's* disease with late onset", and is dated all the way back to the initial referral, in Oct. 2009; but none of us have even the *faintest* recollection of being advised of this confusingly different, pre-assessment, version being added at the time). Interestingly, even after the lengthy period of (so-called) assessment, any sign of an official, *written*, confirmation of the definitive diagnosis, or even better, of some kind of welcome treatment plan, proved all too frustratingly elusive from *any* source, despite my request for both on at least two occasions; but, at least and at last, by the autumn of 2012 we had that *verbal* confirmation, from the GP, of the existence of the degenerative Dementia that, by then, we'd not only started to presume on, and to glimpse more frequently, but also to fear.

Just to reiterate, the initial referral to the GP on the matter, in late 2009, had only been meant as a *precautionary* action on our part; for, at the time of that referral, Mum was *still* pretty 'compos mentis', and, with our regular but discreet supervision, she was still living and sleeping alone by preference, and inhabiting a more or less independent, and passably normal life. For example, she was still making her own (appropriate) shopping choices, (albeit whilst doing so in the company of one of us more often), at the supermarket, and as I've said, still managing her own hygiene, food preparation, money, and general finances, running her own home, self-medicating well enough, (for example, choosing appropriate over-the-counter cold remedies, paracetamol for headaches, or muscle-rub to ease the pain in her sore or swollen finger joints), taking the *prescribed* medicine appropriately for the most part, and making normal, still ostensibly rational, and age-appropriate, conversation, and decisions; and, indeed, was still remembering *most* things. It was only really *occasionally* that she was exhibiting those more conspicuous instances of that 'forgetfulness'. In short, at this early stage, it was still the relative infrequency and therefore novelty of these occurrences that made them stand out so but, unbeknown to us, we (she) had started a rather large and powerful 'ball' rolling.

That said, finally hearing *confirmation* of the delayed diagnosis (of *vascular* Dementia) still came as a bit of a shock to all 3 of we offspring; and that *despite*, (or again perhaps *because* of) the apparent 'no rush', long wait for it, from the supposed experts and professionals in this specialism. In practice, though, with no obvious support/treatment plan from the medics to back up their diagnosis, and with Mum still performing relatively well at an 'independence' level, the initial jolt from that one-off *verbal* confirmation of her condition soon began to dissipate, and, in truth, after the initial impact, made relatively little *actual* difference to either Mum's or our established daily living patterns in the short term.

Eventually though, as the weeks passed, and as the incidences of 'forgetfulness' had refused to go away, and indeed were suspected of becoming a *little* more frequent than hitherto, (and particularly in the *continued* absence of any *regular* involvement, let alone any confidence-boosting or practical 'initiatives', from either the social or medical services), and to formally acknowledge, and to sort of 'mark', the Dementia diagnosis, as a new baseline, I suggested that we instigate a more structured and more regular visiting pattern/rota ourselves, by way of yet more watchful supervision. To that end, I also suggested the introduction of a 'Log Book'.

Both ideas were likely to impinge the more on our own lives, and time, and implied quite a bit more work on all our parts with Mum, but were (eventually) agreed as worthwhile, at least as a 'trial'; and duly implemented.

As luck had had it, and with my worries about Mum's possible Dementia just starting to prey on my mind, up had cropped the very timely option of taking early retirement from my stressful, inner-city, 'frontline', social work employment; in the summer of 2010. Due to quirks in the benefits system, my wife had already been able to retire, officially, the previous year, (age just 60) with full access to both her work and her statutory pensions, and even though *I* would only qualify for a single, and reduced, 'works' pension until my statutory pension kicked in some 6 years hence, (but with our own mortgage recently matured and paid off), I'd grabbed the offer with both hands; at least in part, so that I *would* be well positioned to put in any increasingly likely 'extra time' with my very dear, but inevitably aging, Mum. That being so, I *was* then pretty well placed to respond to my proposed new supervision structure, and, although working from a base some 17 miles away, to me being allocated each subsequent Tuesday, Thursday, and Saturday, from lunch-time onwards, as MY ascribed visiting/supervision days/'shifts'; (along with that continued daily phone call which, by custom and practice, eventually settled in at around 4pm, on *my* 'days off'; and, of course, with our open-ended offers for Mum to ring 'at any time'). And, (though not without some occasional domestic umbrage taken by my own partner, as the novelty of my thrice-weekly neglect of matters on my own 'home front' took on a more or less 'permanent' status), I'd soon adjusted my own household routines to fit; and with it being my idea, I was 'nominated' to both provide the actual Log-Book, and to make the inaugural entry in it.

Accordingly, it made its debut, and accepted its first entry, during the late afternoon of Tuesday, the 14th of August 2012.

As a new venture, and picking up on the popular Star Trek theme of the time, I quite spontaneously, and unilaterally, decided to christen it 'Captain's Log, Star-date Aug. 2012', and wrote this *boldly* on the front cover for a bit of light-hearted levity; but, in truth, it was just a bog-standard, lined, A4-sized writing pad from the local newsagent; which would henceforth be kept at Mum's house, in the far corner of the 'front room', on the shelf, beneath the telephone table; and, in due course, would be added to by subsequent 'volumes', (diaries) as the (Dementia) years unfolded.

From now on, it was to be here that we 3 siblings would record our initially short (but gradually lengthening), summaries of what we individually judged to be the vital/valid/relevant content of our respective dealings with Mum. Here, we would be able to formally report back, and to keep each other 'up to speed with' any significant developments, incidents, mental lapses, 'good', as well as 'bad', days, 'news' and 'facts' appertaining to our respective visits/ 'shifts' /contacts with Mum. The idea was that such 'Logs' (diaries) would provide us with both a useful timeline and a reminder/ history of *past* dates and events; and each arrivee with an up-to-date awareness of Mum's *current* situation every time that arrivee 'landed' there; regardless of whether Mum remembered to tell us or not. (Mum never wrote anything in it herself; nor requested to; and indeed, I cannot recall her ever reading it; or asking to; even at the very beginning. Of course, as the Dementia made its play, and her mental condition worsened, she eventually lost the essential 'wit', cognition, and therefore ability to do so...let alone to *understand* it's sometimes rushed, often scribbled, and therefore barely legible, content).

For what it's worth, that inaugural entry must have felt somewhat lonely. It was not in any way a controversial entry, and merely reported positively on our enjoyable trip over to town, to shop at her (then) much favoured (Coop) supermarket, and on how Mum met and laughed (appropriately) with a neighbour that she met there, how we bought some nice mixed flowers, how we called in at the 5-minute-drive-away cemetery to put them on Dad's grave and say 'hello' to him, and on what we'd had for tea. And things must have remained just as uncontroversial at the beginning, because it was the *only* entry that the Log-Book received for the rest of that (August) month. It certainly wouldn't stay lonely, but for the *next* few months other entries did *remain* uncontroversial, and, therefore, somewhat intermittent, as, ironically, Mum seemed to hit a quite settled 'patch'.

Physically, too, and I still presume by coincidence, (occurring only a short time before the official 'Dementia' confirmation), aggravating issues were beginning to crop up. In particular, and following a worsening of her left-lower-leg Atheroma, (which was not only steadfastly refusing to respond to muscle-rub, paracetamol, or any other over-the-counter remedies, but now also to the current dose of *prescribed* stuff), we had again reached a point where we felt obliged to consult the GP. From *that* consultation sprung a 'revamped' diagnosis and confirmation *of* a more aggravated 'hardening of the arteries'. Yet despite re-consulting the GP thus, and despite the subsequent and permanent 'upping' of her prescription dosage here, (supposedly to further 'thin' the blood and help it flow even easier in the relevant arterial locale), this stubbornly resistant ache never really left her again during any significant outdoor mobility; and indeed, *in* its' worsened state, it caused Mum's hitherto strong, fit, gait to first falter *sometimes*, and then quite quickly burden her with the legacy of a slight left-side limp, as she tried to cope with the recurrent bouts of nagging pain whenever she put too much pressure on that foot, or walked too far.

Despite not smoking for decades, or drinking alcohol barely at all, (she might perhaps be persuaded to imbibe the odd Christmas 'snowball' or rare tot of birthday sherry), and whilst getting plenty of 'natural' (walking/ domestic / housework-type) exercise that kept her at an ideal healthy weight for just about all of her adult life, (though she did have a highish *fat and sugar* diet that included 2 full teaspoonfuls of processed white sugar in her frequent cups of tea, a less than perfect intake of 'greens' and fresh fruit, and an avid attraction to chocolate and cake), the medical/GP advice was that she was continuing to experience a *common*, 'age-related blood-flow' problem, as the walls of the arteries in that particular part of the lower leg narrowed further, due to a long-term, probably life-time, build-up of cholesterol and other 'fatty' deposits...apparently called "plaques" in the trade.

Alas, despite no obvious *improvement* from the increased dosage, Mum was still left to deal with any respective 'upping' of any accompanying *side-effects*. In particular, both she and we would still be left to deal with some protracted additional difficulties associated with trying to stem the flow of this 'thin' blood, whenever she cut herself!

i. Medicalising Mum – Round 1. At Home.

At this point, and given its increasing later-life presence and influence, it seems pertinent to make particular, and indeed more precise, mention of Mum's prescribed, active, and 'baseline', intake of medication. For it was a topic that had become, and would remain, an ever-present factor post-Dad, and on through Mum's own slow Dementia-ridden aging, decline and eventual 'departure'.

As I say, for most of her adult life, Mum's (physical and mental) health had remained remarkably robust, and she had barely needed to 'touch base' at all with either her GP or any other medical service; and certainly not with regard to prescription medication; yet barely more so with regard to any freely-available, 'over-the counter', *chemist* stuff like aspirin or a cough-bottle. I guess you could say that Mum's genetic 'inheritance', and her tough early life and upbringing, (her nature and nurture), had made for a generally *resilient* sort of soul.

Of course, after sharing such a close life, of over 40 years, with Dad, there was bound to be some sort of, almost obligatory, 'bereavement reaction', following his passing, and we saw traces of that as 1996 progressed; but, with our support, and her own resilience, she seemed to have rallied by the year's end, and to have been left with no *obviously* negative long-term legacy; certainly not one that required ongoing medication.

Then, in that September of 1998, age 72, and just that couple of years after Dad's demise, came that unexpected diagnosis of 'Ischaemic Heart Disease'. As I say, it followed Mum's reporting of a 'funny turn'; that is, of both feeling 'dizzy' and of experiencing an unusual ache/pain in her upper–left arm, whilst out walking with my sister. As a precautionary measure, my sister had, of course, taken her straightway to the GP's practice, and following some standard surgery-based, observational, blood- pressure and stethoscope 'tests', and the like, he had found *nothing significant*, or immediate, to treat. Even so, he had not wanted to discount the possibility of a rogue/ indiscriminate attack of 'angina', so he too had erred on the side of safety and had recommended his own 'precautionary' referral to the area, hospital-based, 'specialist', 7 miles away, in the next town; and, with the GP's appropriate assurances that her medical needs were not pressing, and his advice to simply take some paracetamol for the arm ache, as necessary, in the meantime, Mum returned readily to her normal domestic (usually quite physically busy) routines, without further ado, or reported repetition of the symptoms.

Then, and quite a few weeks later, (yet still in that autumn of 1998), Mum had received a letter from the hospital. It had contained that GP-solicited outpatient appointment, and it was for the following week. This, not unnaturally, had raised her anxieties a little, but (in the reassuring company of my sister), she had nevertheless made it to her appointed slot; and, after waiting for an hour or so, and then seeing the 'main man' for but a few minutes, she had indeed received the 'specialist's' confirmation of the 'suspicion' of the very diagnosis that the GP's referral letter had primed him for. This 'suspicion' was then formally logged on both her GP and hospital records, under the general title of 'Ischaemic Heart Disease'. (A minute searching the internet told me that it is also apparently known as 'coronary artery disease' and can encompass anything from such occasional episodes of angina to a full heart attack).

On the day, however, it was simplified (presumably to a level that the doctor thought Mum might understand, and to allay any natural angst that she might be harbouring), *to* the 'softer', more familiar, and, I guess, less anxiety-provoking, term *of* 'angina'. ('Angina', incidentally, has been described, on the NHS website, as "chest pain that occurs when the blood supply to the muscles of the heart is restricted"; and the site adds that it "can sometimes spread to the left arm, neck, jaw or back". Mum hadn't actually complained of any pain in her *chest*, or anywhere else for that matter, apart from that one-off 'mild' ache/pain in her upper left arm).

Anyway, the upshot of her brief appointment at the hospital was that she had headed home from her visit with an allegedly 'precautionary' prescription of 2 daily "Carvedilol" ('beta-blocker'),'heart' tablets (1 to be taken each morning, with breakfast, and another after her evening meal), and one daily (breakfast) 'blood pressure' tablet, going under the boxed name of 'Amlodipine'; and despite neither serious nor over-active follow-up, (beyond first 6-monthly, and eventually annual, almost token, check-ups, and invariably by different, sometimes 'placement', doctors at the practice/ hospital), nor any *obviously* repeated instances of the same (or associated) symptoms either around the time, or afterwards, (yes, you *could* argue that the pills were properly doing their job), repeat prescriptions of these tablets then flowed uninterrupted; and their imbibing never again seemed to be seriously questioned by any of the assorted medics that subsequently crossed Mum's path. Unbeknown to us at the time, though, and at the age of just 72, Mum had effectively been started on a programme of 'pills for the rest of her life'.

Accordingly, the prescriptions for these original, home-imbibed, drugs (and later for others, as they were appended) were renewed and repeated ad infinitum, and became collectable, without seeing the doctor, usually 4-weekly, by either herself or one of us, from the local chemist, as required, for the rest of her home-based life; and indeed their imbibing continued just as unhindered and/or unquestioned (as did some added along the way), throughout not only her 3 brief, late-life, periods in the next town's hospital, (during the summers of 2016 and 2017), but also throughout the subsequent and intervening 10 month stay in residential care.

So, from her early-to-mid-70s, and despite the lack of *definitive* evidence of their (certainly long-term) medicinal need, or of any serious questioning of their continued prescribing, Mum had been quietly initiated into membership of the 'pill-taking' populace, and effectively ushered onto the 'pill-taking' bandwagon; and she would never again have the chance to experience the feeling of being pill *free*.

At the outset, in 1998, of course, she was only taking her twice-daily (morning and evening) *Carvedilol* (prescribed for a supposed heart condition that was always 'suspected', but, as

20

I say, never really proven), and once-a-day *Amlodipine* (prescribed for raised blood pressure). Then, following the initial 2002 diagnosis of Atheroma, she had been prescribed a daily *Clopidogrel* tablet, (to 'thin' the blood and help it to flow better). Next up, in her early-to-*mid* 80s, and almost a decade later, she had been prescribed an *increased* dosage of her *Clopidogrel*, (supposedly to 'thin' the blood still further, and allow it to flow even better through any 'restricted' arterial areas, but, as I've said, to no noticeably improved effect; and yet bringing the adverse effect of making it much more difficult for her blood to actually clot, and therefore for her/us to stem the steady trickle of blood whenever it broke through the skin!), plus a *Bendrofluazide* ('water') tablet, or diuretic, (this one, we were told, would reduce the amount of water/fluid, and therefore weight, that Mum's body was carrying, and give the heart a little less work to do), and a *Simvastatin* tablet, (as the name suggests, a statin; and usually prescribed for cholesterol/fat related conditions; and the benefits (not to mention side effects) of which are still argued about today, in medical circles. (On the latter, let me again cite retired GP, James Le Fanu, for instance, in a national newspaper article from 2019, where he draws attention to an active 'cyclist and hill walker' patient told by his GP that, "his cholesterol was high and needed to take statins". The patient then described his "stamina disappearing", and developing "severe muscle cramps in my neck every night at about 1am". Then, when he decided to stop taking the statins, and in his own words, "Bingo, no cramps").

Anyway, from around her mid-80s, certainly by the age of 85, and just as the Dementia was threatening to take a more serious hold, Mum was blithely, and for the most part uncritically, self-organising and ingesting this daily cocktail of 6 prescription tablets, as requested, i.e. for at least the 5 years prior to her 90th birthday; and, of course, she still had completely 'open' access to optional/occasional over-the-counter medicines, (including pain-killing back-up from the likes of paracetamol or aspirin), with the GP's blessing.

So, as a minimum, all 6 of these prescription tablets, (each with its own, and presumably interactive and *combined*, side-effects) had been well-established and active, in her bloodstream, prior to the introduction of the Log-book, and had had to be borne by her increasingly vulnerable, and inevitably weakening, old (mind and) body from well before our recording came 'on stream'.

End of Round 1.

CHAPTER 3

Incidentally...

If you've followed the story so far, you may not be surprised, given my somewhat frustrated and sceptical tone on the matter, to learn that, in truth, I had *frequently* wondered whether *all*, or indeed any, of Mum's medication was still *absolutely* necessary. (And whether any or all had made any significant contribution to Mum's worsening Dementia). I had also remained suspicious that, at their respective *commencements* in particular, many of these tablets' side-effects were indeed 'active', and, in that sense at least, contra-indicatory. (Regular instances of nausea, sleepiness, light-headedness, dry mouth, occasional vision and breathing disturbance, and, latterly, frequent bouts of constipation being amongst the diverse symptoms that Mum made intermittent, but usually stoic, mention of. Needless to say, I'd *noted* that most 'chimed' with the acknowledged side-effects, detailed in the literature that accompanied each new pack of her prescribed drugs; indeed, many of these, and others, appear to be pretty *common* side-effects across *many* prescribed drugs; and, as my later research tended to confirm, *all* prescribed drugs carry *some* sort of side-effect, so the benefits of taking *any* drug needs to be weighed *against* the likely side-effects, not to mention the potential for more *acute* adverse reactions. That would seem especially poignant later on, when applied to someone battling the already confusing and disturbing effects of Dementia).

Equally though, I had done little, thus far, to get past my own inherent reverence, and therefore deference, for the title of Dr., and a presumption that he/she 'knew best'; and so, for many years, I had been *complicit* in asking Mum to take the prescribed medication, and lax in allowing my 'wonderment' (suspicions) to remain just that, and therefore unresolved.

As fate, and circumstances, would have it, though, (and luckily with my 'arguments' much better marshalled and my deference already receding accordingly), I was about to finally confront the problem.

The trigger was a particularly unique, indeed, deeply disturbing, home-based 'incident' that lasted for only a few, but quite scary, minutes. It was an 'incident' that I *physically* logged, of course, but also one so noteworthy-cum-traumatic, that I involuntarily 'filed' it, mentally, and carried it round in my head, thereafter, as Mum's first and (by far) worst, "Don't know where I am, Keith" moment...and it occurred in the late afternoon of Saturday the 6th of April 2013.

As the rather dramatic quote suggests, it centred on her temporary, though no less frightening, loss of awareness, (though not of consciousness - see later; and under 'Dementia Diaries' for that date), and (rightly or wrongly) immediately had me jumping to the ready suspicion that the attendant side-effects from her medication *might* just lie behind its weird-cum-bizarre occurrence.

With a little more time on my hands, after retiring early from my long, and often *very* stressful, front-line social work career, and in the Spring of 2013, (with the Dementia making its' play), the sheer, always-on-my-mind, niggling, persistence of that previous 'wonderment' had already started to get the better of me. For, by then, 'wonderment' had morphed into a more uneasy *worry;* and spurred on by the timely arrival of my first home computer I had stumbled across an invaluable means of accessing independent information regarding the very side-effects of the various pills that Mum was hooked on.

Armed thus, and with the inaugural and incredible, "I don't know where I am, Keith" incident still firmly imprinted on my consciousness, I had arrived at the optimum moment, with the optimum combination of reason, motivation, impetus, confidence and information, to politely, but firmly, challenge that medical 'aura' and to see if my suspicions had 'legs'.

And when I did so, I actually seemed to make quite swift and unexpected headway! Indeed, the supposed necessity of *some* of

Mum's long-prescribed medications was shown to be patently *un*necessary, when they were readily, and *immediately,* deemed discardable and summarily withdrawn!

My first, and most unexpected, opportunity to behold this phenomenon was provided by a visiting, surgery-attached, 'practice nurse'; and just a few days after the inaugural 'don't know where I am' incident.

I wasn't actually present at this nurse's 'short-notice' descent on Mum, but my sister, who had wasted no time in contacting the GP, to express our general worries (and make mention of *my* 'medicinal' thoughts), about the likely causes of the 'incident', *had* been in attendance, and had quickly made my brother and I fully aware, (both in person, and, for posterity, in her log), of the pretty surprising outcome from that 'audience'.

The central, and unanticipated, upshot of that (on this occasion commendably speedy) home visit had been that this 'practice nurse', (presumably with the GP's explicit prior agreement), and in the *presence* of my sister, had simply *cancelled* both the Bendrofluazide *and* the Simvastatin on the spot; despite Mum having been 'on' each of them for a good 3 years! And I had been so surprised, to hear thus, that I had felt obliged to make specific reference to, and quite critical consideration of, the suitability of such an apparently unplanned and 'immediate' withdrawal, in my log of Sat. the 13th of April. (See also under 'Dementia Diaries' for that date).

Incredibly, though, more of the same was about to follow. For, just a few weeks later, at a follow-up *family* 'house meeting' that *I'd* sought for the 21st of May, 2013, and in the presence of the latest 'allocated GP', (again not the one with whom Mum was registered, but yet another 'placement' doctor/ 'stand-in' from the practice), we met with further unexpected 'success'. By the time *he* left, and despite Mum having been prescribed it since 1998 (fully 14 years!) the evening Carvedilol tablet had also been cancelled; and simply because I provided anecdotal 'evidence' to suggest that this 'lone ranger' of a pill might be making Mum more confused and upset just before going to bed, and by posing the real possibility, indeed suspicion, that she might not be taking it consistently anyway. Most surprising of all was that, once again, the pill's cancellation was immediate!

So, in the space of just a few weeks, 3 of her 6 well-established prescription pills (the Bendrofluazide the Simvastatin, and the early-evening Carvedilol), were no more! Despite entering Mum's blood-stream every day for at least 3 years, (the Carvedilol for 14!), they had, surprisingly, suddenly, unceremoniously, and with minimal ado, been rendered redundant. Confined to history. 'Dropped', *instantly;* and simply because we'd respectfully, if a tad repeatedly, raised our qualms and concerns.

(I don't think that I was expecting to secure more than a *cautious* withdrawal from perhaps *one*, if any, of these well-established dosages, but 'hey presto', by the end of the month of May, *three* were *gone completely!* Goodness knows if any of her subsequent symptoms and 'off' days had passed unrecognised as side-effects from such stark withdrawals, but thankfully, with our customary perseverance all round, and suitably repeated reassurances to Mum, both she and we had managed to cope and carry on, and their loss seemed to be absorbed without any *noticeably lasting* effect!)

Looking back, 2013 could probably be described as quite a *pivotal*, game-changing, year; probably *the* single most significant 'turning point' year in the signalling of Mum's move from independent cognition to more *de*pendent and age-related, Dementia-induced, decline, and to slow but chronic and inexorable submission to the attendant medical (and social) 'conditions' that began to plague her; and we had sought the latest medical contacts (with what turned out to be the 'practice nurse', and the 'stand-in' GP, respectively) in order to clarify not only the position regarding her medication, but also a *number* of accompanying, and newly-associated, (emotional and social) worries relating to the creeping effects of the Dementia.

Primarily, though, we (with myself as the sceptical instigator-in-chief), had sought the meetings because we feared that Mum might be getting a little *more* forgetful; both in general, and most recently in the (scary) particular; and we presumed her doctor would be the best and most logical first point of contact for advice.

As I say, the crucial trigger for those meetings was that extraordinarily upsetting 'incident' lasting no more than about 15-minutes. *During* those few desperate minutes, though, Mum had presented me with an acutely disturbing, hitherto unseen, instance of an oddly 'distant', noticeably 'vacant', sort of behaviour; and the episode had stayed etched in my memory *because* I had never seen the like of it before from her, nor heard the pitiful single ("I don't know where I am, Keith") utterance that brought 'the incident' to its worrisome head before I was able to guide her gently back to something resembling cognitional normality.

This, I guess, was the first time that I'd had a *true* glimpse of the untrodden, one-way, rock-strewn, path to purgatory that the Dementia might *really* be leading us (her) down.

She had clearly been distressed to the point of traumatised by the apparent failure of her usual mental faculties and resources to come to her aid during those few bewildering minutes; and by the accompanying, and hitherto alien, mental state and experience that she had obviously found herself having to confront. And by how she had then struggled to gather her thoughts and her composure, and to make sense of her feelings, back in the 'present'.

With her words still resonating, so affectingly, in my brain, I'd just shuffled, instinctively, along the sofa towards her, leaned over, took her hand, squeezed it gently, and asked her to try and describe her feelings to me. By degrees, and between prolonged pauses to wipe away tears and to reset the security of her own tight grip of my hand, she'd attempted to do so.

The overriding theme had been that sensation of "fear" (a word and description that she would return to regularly as the Dementia progressed), accompanied by a "sort of fog", that had gradually engulfed her, following an inability to "think straight" and "make proper sense of things".

As I listened attentively, and struggled to hold back my own tears, I fell back, equally instinctively, (not to mention gratefully), on some fairly formulaic words of quiet *reassurance* that I had often relied upon in my long social work career. So, I was able to reassure her, for example, that 'the incident' was 'just a blip', that it was 'over now', that we *all* have such mental blips, and that 'everything would be OK'.

At that point I'd no real reason *not* to have faith in either my assessment of the situation, or my attempted words of comfort; nor to assume that she *hadn't* just experienced a singular, *one-off*, upset. And so I'd *continued* down that path of quiet support and calm 'reassurance' until, but a few minutes later, she did seem to have become calmer, and to have collected herself again.

Twenty minutes more, suitably rested, and with her faculties effectively restored, she seemed to have actually *forgotten* the specifics of 'the incident'. Yes, she still felt very tired, and she still knew that something had drained her so, but, incredibly, she could no longer recall just what; nor could she recall the sense of alarm and anxiety that had accompanied it. Thankfully, she did seem to have returned to something akin to normality once more, and had readily accepted my suggestion that she'd simply been 'lost in deep thought'; and just minutes later, she was pottering off into the kitchen to make us both a cup of tea. (Ironically, her failure to remember other 'negative' incidents for too long would become a very useable bi-product in our overseeing and management of the Dementia, as she slowly succumbed to the steady creep of its effect).

Even though it had shocked me to the core to see her so terribly, and so extraordinarily, 'lost' and disturbed, and to hear her speaking of 'not knowing where she was', I *had* managed to avoid getting sucked into panic and anxiety mode myself. Instead, and falling back on my years of negotiating my way through so many emotionally-charged social work situations, I'd somehow managed to conjure up just the right level of apparent calm and unruffled *composure* needed to keep the situation in check; and to deliver the sort of gentle reassurance that *did* seem to aid her steady recovery.

Thankfully, and barely an hour later, a calm normality had descended again. My early supportive touch and quietly repeated reassurances seemed to have paid dividends. (For both her sake and mine). For by then she seemed to have no active recollection of the incident *at all*, and was sitting at ease in her chair, and talking normally; about things on the telly, or the highlights of her week ahead, for example. To my abiding relief, she appeared to 'be herself' again; so much so that, by the time her (7-30pm) bedtime arrived, and whilst writing up the episode in the 'Logbook' for my siblings to read in their turn, I had watched her go through her usual nightly preparations for bed without any sign of a problem.

It was around 7-45pm, then, that I finally accepted that she was "very tired" and ready to "head up", and bowed to her insistence that I should "for goodness sake go". With the usual appeal for her to ring me if she had even the slightest concern, and feeling sufficiently confident that she would now be OK, I left her to her usual home-alone devices, and headed for my own abode.

Once there, I rang my siblings and made them aware of the incident that I'd witnessed; in case of any emergency or back-up need during the night; but, thankfully, neither I nor they heard a peep out of her again that evening and when I rang her early on the following day, she made no mention of 'the incident', was actually quite cheerful, and was awaiting my brother's usual Sunday-morning visit in apparent good spirits. Normal service did indeed seem to have been resumed for now.

Alas, though it may have *presented* as a one-off, particularly unique, certainly traumatic, if relatively short-lived 'incident' on that particular Saturday, it *wouldn't* be the only time that we would be party to such heart-breaking states of confusion; nor to the mutually upsetting moments of "fear", anxiety, frustration and tearfulness that invariably accompanied them. That first, worst-case, 'incident' would turn out to be but a harbinger, a horrible first-taste forerunner, of similar instances, that would become gradually, (but no less distressingly), more common-place as the ensuing months ticked slowly by. And we, (as both her distressed offspring *and* her main/ only carers), would have no option but to 'bite the bullet', and to find ways of supporting, and of coming to terms with, such episodes. Ways to just grin and bear them, manage them, (practically and emotionally), with and for her. In short, ways to just stay calm and carry on.

For Mum, of course, there was to be no such luxury; no such easy 'out', going forward. For the random re-appearance of such confusion-lead feelings, (not to mention the attendant moments of *isolation* that she undoubtedly experienced on some occasions), *would* eventually take its toll as the time passed, and the disease slowly, but inexorably, worsened.

In the long run, such emotionally-charged burdens and afflictions were always likely to bring about *changes*, I guess, to both her confidence, and, eventually, to her personality. And they did.

Not surprisingly, for instance, such feelings were prone to generating more *intense* states of anxiety sometimes...ones that bordered on panic attacks. These, in their turn, tended to reinforce that sense of "fear" on an increasing number of occasions. They were *all* upsetting. Of course, they were. (For both she and we). A few that I witnessed in the later stages of her struggle lasted for up to 20 minutes. Most were, thankfully, of much shorter duration, and, (along with any overnight, *pre-arrival* 'remnants'), usually responded quite quickly to our arrival, continued presence and quiet Reassurance. That said, and especially in the latter stages, they did also seem to nurture increasing instances of 'a place for everything, and everything in its place' OCD, (Obsessive-Compulsive Disorder), as a sort of auto-response coping strategy for both her ongoing anxiety *and* the sheer frustration involved in her efforts to try and make sense of, and retain some control over, her new and changing cognitive 'inheritance'. (And all this whilst also trying to cope with the chronic *physical* aches and pains being posed by her general aging, and the 'hardening of the arteries', and 'blood-flow', issues associated with her lower left leg and ankle... plus, in the end, those posed by her failing left hip). Yet still, (until the very late stages), she remained sufficiently (indeed remarkably) compos mentis for most day-to-day in-house routines and tasks; and also for repeatedly, and quite steadfastly, declining all thought of moving from the familiarity of her own home to the unknown, *un*familiar, but (ostensibly) *supported* world of a care home.

Despite our devotion and our commitment to supporting Mum, and our attendant concern for her obviously worsening predicament, the option to incorporate her into the household of one of we offspring proved just too impractical. None of us really had the room and set-up, in our relatively small homes, to make her special needs better supportable than in her own much-loved home. When we visited her there, of course, our time and attention was solely and entirely focused on her; and the house and locale were fully familiar; but in *our* own homes, as well as the limited space, we had lives to live, other family members making claims on our time, jobs and tasks to tackle, and unavoidable trips out to undertake, etc. We were also aware that residing with one of us would not only be potentially unfair on the one willing to give it a try, but also likely to require Mum to spend more time 'home alone'. In that circumstance we feared that she could be even more at risk, (left in such a relatively *un*familiar setting, whilst we *went about* those tasks and lives), than if we 'spread the load', and each continued to visit and support her in her own *very* familiar home, and environs, on an everyday rota basis.

Perhaps the cruellest of all the cruel ironies of Mum's predicament was that (for all but at the very end, and arguably even then) she did remain *sufficiently* compos mentis, and on sufficient occasions, to remain very much aware of 'it' all going on around her; that is, *aware* of her failing memory, and of her deteriorating cognition, of her constraining mobility issues, and of her increasingly mixed-up thoughts and concerns. Yet, *because* of this element of 'awareness', she *remained* sufficiently compos mentis to be regularly able to express her firm preference for, indeed, insistence upon, staying in her own home for so long; and, in that light, her view, of course, had to be respected.

Indeed, under the Mental Capacity Act of 1995, and for all but her final few months, (when she herself became increasingly aware of her 'home alone' vulnerabilities and started to give further, if occasional, and reluctant, thought to her options), Mum would, almost certainly, have been deemed to be making a *suitably-informed* decision to stay in her own home; and legally entitled to do so.

Over time, of course, she was always going to suffer some degree of (mental and physical) wear and tear, (much of it essentially age-related and irreversible), and again she did. Towards the end, though, and in the grip of the Dementia, she slowly seemed to be *taking on/morphing into* that generally more anxious, less confident, and more vulnerable persona; as evidenced *by* those more frequent spells of confusion and associated upset; and in consequence, as I've said, she was more easily prone to 'the fear'; *wherever* she was. (Wouldn't you be?).

The organising, managing and imbibing of her prescribed medication again provides perhaps the most enduring example of her, and our, difficulties, in policing this slowly, but inexorably, changing, and increasingly out-of-control, journey to the end of her life.

As early as 2013, her efforts to try and differentiate between her different boxes of pills, to select one from each box, to then imbibe those FIVE different 'breakfast' tablets, each day, and then to remember to take her one and only evening tablet, (until its sudden withdrawal at that late May meeting with the latest GP), had already begun to produce occasional 'hiccups'. On most occasions, a discreet inspection of the remaining pills, for example, would usually shed light on any suspicions that we held about her not taking the correct dosage. So, for example, on a couple of occasions we were pretty certain that she had taken a second *Clopidogrel* tablet, instead of the early evening *Carvedilol* version; and, on at least one other occasion, that she had repeated the same error with her *Amlodipine* tablet. Then, on a few random occasions, we became suspicious that she had not taken the evening Carvedilol tablet at all...or any other. And then there was the one late occasion when, quite by accident, my brother found some of her tablets in her dustbin. So, on at least one occasion, (knowingly or otherwise), she appeared to have gone without several of her prescribed tablets *altogether*. Of course, we then felt obliged to try and rectify these 'accidental' errors when they came to light; and to try and re-balance the dosages; if possible without her noticing; and to find appropriately reassuring explanations for doing so if she did; ones that would neither raise Mum's anxieties still further, regarding her competence, (both specifically and more generally), nor damage her increasingly brittle confidence;

especially when she was still insisting that her own home was where she wanted to remain.

And all this was regularly adding to our own sitting uncertainties, neuroses, self-doubts and worries, as her committed offspring, of course. About how best to carry out our accepted responsibilities, as her guardians and carers, how to do the 'right' thing by her, and how to deal with the various issues and dilemmas that we faced. And, of course, how to best limit the frequency, and the intensity, of Mum's own bouts of anxiety; especially post-'incident', and especially on those lucid occasions, (which were still, by far, the majority), when she herself realised that she *may* have taken the pills out of order, or erred in some other previously simple or routine task. (Whether the potential *side-effects*, of any of the prescribed medication, really *had been* a significant, or even mild, contributory factor here remained, and remains, inconclusive, and a moot point).

Such worries, then, had been both central and instrumental in our seeking out of those overdue and supplementary meetings with the medics in the Spring of 2013.

Additionally, though, there had also been a couple of strategic '*peripheral*' factors that we'd wanted to raise.

For one, we had been getting increasingly concerned about the prospect of yet more 'system' changes. The most pressing of these were the proposed changes to the local chemist's *dispensing* procedures. The GP had recently sent Mum a 'letter of notification' about certain proposed, and, for us, crucial, changes to the *organisation and delivery* of key agencies and services out there in the community; but as a fait accompli. We had not been consulted, and they were about to be forced upon us; and, in our opinion, were likely to make our 'carer' task all the harder. They were changes over which we, as end users, (Mum as patient and we as her carers) had had no say. So we'd sought the opportunity to clear the air, to 'kick back' a little, to put *our* perspective, and to at least have our voice heard; if only as a point of principle and for feedback to the 'powers that be'.

Both doctor and chemist were located almost 2 miles away, and the latest badly-thought-out proposal was that, due to supposed pressures on each, both should be blithely relieved of the initiative for renewing *ongoing* prescriptions. Almost laughably, (certainly in terms of Dementia sufferers), it was actually being proposed that the individual *patient*, (or, almost inevitably his or her representative), should monitor things, and should be given the task of ringing up the chemist, several days in advance, to trigger, and secure, future prescriptions, instead. At this point, of course, *we'd* reached a position where we feared that Mum could not be *consistently* relied upon to do so, and that, busy with our own tasks, jobs and lives, as well as continuing to support Mum in more and more areas of her life, we too might so easily let this slip from our mind and 'Hey presto', no medication! Cue panic.

For another, we remained frustrated at the lack of *continuity* in GP personnel. Mum's GP was part of a largish practice that serviced much of the area, and, as well as using the occasional 'locum', it offered regular 'training' places for would-be doctors to carry cases, and to gain GP experience in situ; and yet another had recently been assigned Mum's case. In theory, you can't argue with that, can you? They need to gain their experience somewhere; but we had already seen several *different,* short-lived, 'trainees' assigned to 'cover' my Mum's case in recent months. We feared that the practice might be placing a little too *much* emphasis on the *trainees'* 'practice and procedure' needs, and just not enough on *consistent, familiar, patient-centred,* bed-side-manner-type needs; and, in Mum's case at least, on a need for continuity, and on a trusted and recognisable face, and, therefore 'relationship', in her personal and *local* medical care. We hoped to share such concerns with whoever they dispatched.

Accordingly, for that late-May meeting on that late Tuesday morning in 2013, I had also opted for a 'put it in writing' back-up position. (See Appendix 1). I had decided to prepare, and print out, a brief, single-page, bullet-sheet, to try and concentrate the minds of all present, and to both help me remember all the issues *I* wanted to raise, and to highlight our main points of *family* concern. I was also planning to politely (and did) request that a copy of my print-out be placed on record, on Mum's medical file, to ensure that my concerns were recorded somewhere for 'posterity'. (I'm not aware that it ever was, though).

That said, of course, the *prime* issues that I wanted to raise there still related most directly to Mum's *immediate* mental, physical, medical and medicinal issues and needs.

That is, they revolved around the possible *side-effects* of all her (or indeed anyone's) medication, some recent (again I presumed unconnected) vision and possible blood-pressure issues relating to her occasionally wonky eyesight (especially the 'floater' that occasionally pestered the right), and our (my) niggling worry that she was increasingly exhibiting the sort of anxiety-based behavioural elements that bordered on OCD; in order, I suspected, to try and secure for herself a 'tighter' *Routine* and one that might compensate for her increasing instances of loss of memory.

In truth, I don't think I fully realised, at the time, just how much the latter *were* a result (arguably a *rational* result), of her creeping Dementia, and a response to those more regular, and accompanying, incidents of raised anxiety; especially when even that *Routine* element of her daily life, (and of 'the 3Rs', as I came to call them - see below), became less than certain or significantly *disrupted* at any point. As, for example, when anything she *had* come to rely on being in a 'set' place, like her glasses, her pen, her purse, or the TV remote, appeared 'lost', or when something appeared to have 'broken down', 'gone wrong' or 'stopped working' properly; which may or may not have been the case. Like the central heating, TV or kettle appearing to fail her, the kitchen curtain rail falling down, (which did actually happen once as she tugged too jerkily at it to draw it across), or her perception that *we* 'had not helped', by forgetting, or purposely 'ducking', something; say the 'mending' or 'rectifying' of one of the above, or perhaps by failing to ensure that her usual / favourite clothes, food-stuffs, toiletries or items of medication were in the 'right' place.

Somewhat ironically, we also ended up 'stealing' the 'new' GP's 'thunder' at the meeting when we had to remind him that his most constructive and enthusiastic suggestion, of using something called a 'dosette box' to better manage Mum's remaining prescription pills, was not only covered in my bullet sheet, but had already been implemented at our *own* initiative, just a few weeks earlier!; but at least we knew we had his whole-hearted support for this subtle change.

The 'dosette box' was just a slim, white, plastic organiser, available from the local chemist. It also had the seven days of the week, (Sun to Sat, left to right), clearly marked in contrasting black on the lids; and following its recent acquisition by my sister, (and now handily qualifying for a 'Doctor's Orders' validation), *we* had agreed to take ultimate charge of Mum's remaining prescription medication, and to take on the responsibility for ensuring that the correct doses were already placed inside each day's designated compartment in time for the start of each week. By doing so, we hoped to ensure Mum's more accurate imbibing of each day's remaining prescription tablets, going forward. We then agreed with Mum that the dosette box would be given the same prominent place that the egg-cup had held. That is, on the flat-top part of her wooden roll-up breadbin, in the kitchen; where she was bound to notice it whilst in the throes of making her breakfast toast. Voila! Problem solved. Or was it?

Other significant outcomes from the May meeting included, of course, this 'latest' GP's unexpected (and immediate) withdrawal of that evening Carvedilol tablet, (after 14 years), and his patently reluctant, but eventual, agreement to refer Mum for a psychiatric assessment, following my firmly-expressed OCD concerns. (Whilst expressing some sympathies, he felt there was little *he* could do, personally, to affect the coming 'organisational' and prescription-renewal changes; but he agreed to forward our feedback to the appropriate quarters). And with his departing warning to expect a long wait for the psychiatric assessment ringing in our ears, (he was to be proved right!), the meeting drew to a close, and he was gone.

Also back in early April, and following closely in the wake of the 'don't know where I am' incident, I had come up with the 'clutching at straws' idea of the '3Rs', as a home-made fall-back means of *practically* supporting Mum the more, and of managing her memory issues.

Based on my many years of front-line social work, the '3Rs' referred to ROUTINE, REASSURANCE and REPETITION. It was entirely my own 'invention', and, as I say, it soon grew into our default position for supporting Mum, practically, with her slowly-encroaching forgetfulness / Dementia; especially in relation to her *shorter-term* memory. (Once again, I had felt the need to go down the 'home-made' route as a last resort, after our efforts to garner similar useful/practical advice from the busy, oft-changing and infrequently-visiting agency representatives of the medical and/or social service professions had proved to be distinctly, and consistently, unproductive, beyond supplying a couple of nondescript pamphlets on potential support groups, that we were invited to follow up at our own convenience).

So we had 'plodded on', we 3 'musketeers'; mostly gaining our *own* 'hands-on' experience, reading snippets about Dementia where we could, and 'making it up as we went along' and as I say, mainly inventing, adapting, refining, relying on and utilising the '3Rs', as our fallback position; for about 3 years more; with Mum generally lucid enough, and coping OK much of the time at the outset, but increasingly lapsing into moments-cum-bouts of 'significant forgetfulness' as time progressed. Those, as I've said, incorporated the more frequent moments-cum-bouts of associated confusion; which, in turn, fuelled her raised sense of acute frustration, lowered her mood and confidence the more and, of course, fired up "the fear".

And so it came to pass. That unique and inaugural 'don't know where I am' incident of the early April of 2013 had indeed given birth to others of mostly lesser, yet invariably differing, degrees; and probably to the instinctive OCD reactions whenever she became aware that the workings of her mind *were* letting her down.

A belated, but weighty, consequence of that awareness, and of her (and our) subsequent worry, revolved around how she might cope if anything 'happened' whilst she was 'home alone', especially at night and might find herself unable to summon help - Mum, having rejected the sole possibility of having a warden-controlled, 'community-alarm' system fitted very early on; citing the cost, sensor-fitted complexity and over-invasiveness, and lack of effectiveness, of an available set-up where the receiving 'warden' only alerted one of *us* anyway according to *their* pamphlet.

Yet still, (until the very end), she steadfastly refused to contemplate leaving her life-long home, to consider a return to day-care, (see later), or, as she saw it, to compromise her continued quest for independence. So, apart from re-emphasising that we visited every day, were only 'at the end of a phone' the rest of the time, had stayed over whenever the situation had necessitated it before, and would do so again, and actually fitting a telephone extension by her bed, so that she might ring us the easier in the night, we fell back largely (if a little impotently) on the '3Rs'; and in particular on the *Reassurance* element.

Sadly for us all though, that particular seed of insecurity took root, and she raised the issue with us regularly, once it had 'germinated'. Equally sadly, though she had identified a very *real* issue, neither she, we, nor any members of the medical or social services ever found a definitive answer to the 'home-alone' dilemma; at least not one that left her *totally* safe yet supported in her own home, as she wanted. So it remained unresolved; and an issue that we had to address quite regularly... essentially through our ever-ready, quick-response, availability, and via plenty of extra helpings of that calm homespun Reassurance.

I'm sure, in a perfect world, she would have loved one of us to *move in* with her in the latter stages of her dementing life, but she still knew enough to know that that would mean one of us effectively giving up our own life and independence, and she never actually raised the option herself. Suspecting that it did cross her mind though, I raised it as an issue myself on a couple of pre-emptory occasions; but only to try and explain gently why it would be a far from ideal solution, anyway. (In particular, I reminded her that, even if I did live there, I would have to go out *sometimes*, and any 'risks' would still apply then). So, given that her first priority *was* still to remain in the home that had been hers for the past 60-odd years, she settled to the reality that that goal would be best achieved by having 'on tap' telephone access to us, and by us rotating our daily support to her *there*. In that event, and drawing on the tough upbringing, and life in general, that had gone before, and despite the Dementia, she clung on not only doggedly, but with a commendable degree of good-humoured stoicism and resilience; both of which, of course, involved her facing the realisation that old age was now 'knocking at the door'. Yet, even as her 90th birthday approached, she continued to try and defy those 'knockings', and to preserve both her independence, and her determination to remain living in her own home.

"I'll only leave this house in a box", she told me on more than one occasion, as she carried on her fight to 'stay put'.

So yes, for her final and most difficult 3 years, and more, as her (latterly diagnosed *vascular*) Dementia, and atheroma, combined in a sort of pitiless pincer movement, to gradually limit her independence, and therefore autonomy, we had worked together to provide our most unstinting daily support and visits; and to attend to her personal needs and dispositions, and her domestic mendings and fixings, as urgently as we were able; at least one of us visiting her for a minimum of 2 hours per day; and invariably much longer. Moreover, (and until she *was* finally, and somewhat involuntarily, prised from her own home; initially, and particularly, through a new *physical*, and quite debilitating, pain, in her left hip, in the summer of 2016; the Dementia notwithstanding), we tried our best to make our visits both 'positive' and 'active', in terms of 'social' input, purpose, interest and distraction. In an average week, they included occasional 'maintenance' visits to her GP and other standard health services, such as the optician, dentist, or chemist, and a range of carefully considered trips out into the locality chosen from a varied menu of, say, shopping, for lunch, to the garden centre, the Post Office for money and to pay bills, to visit nearby relatives and friends, to visit and maintain my father's (and her own mother's and sisters') grave at the pretty, rural, close-by, cemetery, and, (weather permitting), to drive to one of a trio of suitably accessible parks, etc.

In short, in a committed attempt to maintain a decent quality of life for her, we tried to provide not only close personal support, but also regular stimulation and distraction, and to thereby keep her in constant touch with 'normal' life, personal decision-making, and the wider community for as long as was physically, and mentally, possible.

My two siblings each lived less than 3 miles away, and so had a little more flexibility in their visiting; (on the down side they tended to pick up the unexpected or *emergency* 'gigs'), whilst, living 17 miles away, it made obvious sense to get as many as possible of my own domestic chores done before departing, and to arrive at Mum's around lunchtime, ready to spend the whole of 'my' 3 (Tues, Thurs, Sat) afternoons and early evenings with her...and latterly until she was ready for bed. A Routine that was soon set almost 'in stone'.

By the *summer* of 2013, and after a trawl of the internet, I had also introduced Mum to some easy, sit-down, NHS-recommended, breathing and relaxation exercises, (which we usually did together, whilst resting after lunch, but which she could still safely practice in my absence), to both offer a *very* light 'work- out' for her stiffening joints and muscles, and to offset any accruing anxiety from both that source, and from the creeping Dementia. And as I've said, she continued to have telephone contact 'on tap', to all or any of the 3 of us; plus, of course, the 'check-up' calls initiated by each of us on our 'non-visiting' days.

In sum, we were trying our level best to cover every angle, *short* of moving in. (She *had* once been introduced to 'day-care' through the local social services, and had attended their main 'centre', over in the town, on and off, on each Monday, for the best part of a year during 2011/12. However, she had never really been *keen*, and had mainly gone on our recommendation that it would 'do her good', and that 'a change is as good as a rest'; until she eventually reached her nadir and simply *declined* to do so; essentially because she 'found it depressing' to be surrounded all day by so many aging and disabled attendees; nearly all of whom she repeatedly described as 'much worse than her'. In short, she had expressed a definite preference to remain home-based instead, where she was comfortable, could do just as she pleased, was still, to all intents and purposes, in command of her life and faculties, and was already in a quite varied, very familiar, and well-supported Routine with *us*).

Supported thus, she was managing OK for the most part; notwithstanding those late, real and recurring anxieties *about* the possibility of things 'happening' when we weren't around, or if she couldn't get to the phone. And so, despite everything, for as long as she remained essentially compos mentis, we respected her wish not to have to 'go in a home'.

Nor (and with good reason as it turned out), was she keen to accept 'in-house' *home* 'care' from 'strangers', or those she did not know as 'family'. (From the outset, she worried that they 'didn't know her', might 'wander round her house', pass judgement on it and her struggles, or spread news of her creeping lack of independence). However, once again she had bowed to our suggestion-cum- 'recommendation', (this time between July 2014 and October 2015), and agreed to give it a try 'for an hour' - (it turned out that the agency employed could only manage *half* an hour anyway), just for an additional bit of 'social' contact, and on a couple of days where we were able to identify a 'spare window in her diary'. In truth, it was never a great success. The (private) agency identified for us by the local social services, (and therefore its workers), had, as a first and most pressing priority, brief and basic visits that targeted the *physical* well-being of their customers, (making sure they were fed, washed, etc.); whereas Mum was happy (nay keen) to occupy *herself* in these areas, and we were simply wanting to pay for their worker to provide some further socio-psychological support and mental stimulation for her by just calling in regularly for a friendly chat and a shared cuppa.

They gave it a try, to be fair; but it wasn't really their forte; and, (not least because of the sheer pressure of their workload), the worker often arrived significantly late, (on occasion almost an hour so) or was off ill, or left, and either an (unsolicited) unknown worker, or (as we'd pre-agreed in such circumstances), no-one at all arrived; but *not* always with the agreed forewarning; so no real 'relationship' between worker and Mum evolved long-term. In the end, we felt that these inconsistencies and 'no-shows', were actually making Mum even *more* anxious, and (with her unequivocal agreement) we cancelled the service when a second, (reasonably-well-established), worker left.

41

So, despite the gradual deterioration in Mum's performance, in all aspects of her life, (especially over the latter months), with only the same fall-back old yardstick of the '3Rs' to guide us, and whilst she was still (both physically, but especially mentally) able to request that option, we never wavered from our commitment to try and accommodate her deterioration 'in-house'; with only minimal further involvement from the community medical or social services, and certainly minimal *initiative* from them.

Along the way, and practically, the likes of *meal preparation, and appetite,* which had long provided us with a broad, unofficial, but pretty useful, 'indicator' of Mum's general health, mood and level of functioning post-diagnosis (with Dementia), had already begun to take on more of a vital daily 'bell-weather' role for us as the Dementia took greater hold. For example, she'd remained generally keen and able to feed herself and others pre the 'incident' of the 6th of April 2013. (It gave her everyday purpose, and she was good at it). However, the very *next* Saturday (by coincidence or not) had seen the first time that any of us could remember Mum failing to prepare the usual 'roast-beef dinner, with appropriate simple (usually home-made rice pudding) dessert' lunch for me because she had suddenly, (if only temporarily) "forgotten" both the lateness of the hour and (seemingly) some key elements of the process involved; and we had settled for the more immediate option of the beans on toast that she apologetically prepared, once she had stopped weeping; and I had Reassured her that that option was absolutely fine.

That first occasion, then, had set yet another sad precedent. Mum's previous ability to prepare a more complicated meal, (*such as* a roast dinner with some sort of 'pudding'), varied greatly thereafter; particularly as time went on. Some Saturdays she would still manage to do so, without problem, and some she wouldn't. Most often, the 'norm' saw her managing a 'partial' effort, with maybe just one item, (such as the gravy or roast potatoes), 'missing'. Sometimes, especially later, she had clearly realised that she couldn't remember the process, and had already gone for one of the simpler 'week-day' eating options that she *could* remember, such as beans on toast, a ham & tomato sandwich, soup or fish fingers. At worst, (especially towards the very end), and even on weekdays, there were occasions where she had not remembered to make *anything*, (indeed, we started to wonder if she was still capable of feeding *herself* properly in our absence), and, on those occasions, I would simply suggest that we make something together; giving me the chance to tactfully *'re-introduce'* her to some of what she *had* 'forgotten', in a hopeful attempt to re-build her confidence there. Each time though, (and hardly surprising), she became upset and frustrated at not having been able to recall a hitherto lifelong, and second-nature, recipe, and *process*, for making a particular kind of meal; and, for her last few months at home, we increasingly *settled* for (I ended up expressing a definite *preference* for) that 'simpler', soup, sandwich, beans or fish-finger-type sustenance, which she would still have the best chance of preparing, (alone if necessary), and without too much pre-planning on her part.

CHAPTER 4

The Beginning of the End – Hospital Daze.

Fast-forward to 2016; and the Spring of *that* year, alas, saw the 'mountain' finally begin to 'crumble'. The disruption, destabilisation and ultimately *removal*, of her familiar, home-based, Routine would be at the heart of this 'crumbling'. For once Mum was removed from it, (never to return to it), the deadly Dementia had very few barriers to prevent it spreading its tentacles and reeling in its prey. Portentous *change* was afoot.

Ironically, it was further *physical* change that would provide the trigger. Nevertheless, the beginning of the end was upon us.

The problems began, ostensibly, with the arrival of a 'new' pain. This one was in her left hip. Mum first made mention of it around mid-April of 2016. It began slowly, and quite innocuously, as an irritating ache when walking. At first we thought it was just a slight strain or a pulled muscle, and would pass; and gave it every chance to do so by suggesting more rest, and using over-the-counter painkillers such as paracetamol and pain relief sprays; but it *didn't* pass. Unfortunately, it was a pain that, instead, worsened relatively quickly, and began to limit her mobility much more significantly. Along with the now well-established 'forgetfulness', (and worse), of the Dementia, and the nagging 'atheroma' pain making itself known most days further down that leg, (regardless of the Clopidogrel pills), it was to prove to be one pain/limitation too many for Mum and, despite her determination to just 'keep buggering on', it was soon clear to us that, left untackled, the combination was likely to prove critical, and a threat to her independence; and of course to any last remnants of *ours*, as her main carers.

I think it was at that point, too, that I first dared to introduce her to the idea of having physical 'aids' as *practical* 'help'. For example, it was around this time that I first broached the idea of her having that lightweight wheelchair "just" for longer, out of house, journeys / 'walks'; and perhaps even that 'modern', equally lightweight, commode, for downstairs, so that she didn't have to climb the steep flight up so much; especially during the day.

Well, the offended-cum-insulted looks that spread across her face on just the mention of such *artificial* 'help' spoke volumes; not to mention the disgruntled *verbal* ("I'm not an invalid!"-type), ripostes that accompanied them, with regard to the possibility of being *seen* using either. Even at this late stage, my 90 year old Mum still had enough ingrained nous to know when her self-respect was being challenged, and just didn't like what she was hearing from me. (Or what she might have to face up to, I guess). Like all of us, she still greatly valued her dignity and independence and, despite the Dementia, she was still sufficiently aware of, and just as desperate to preserve, her status as an autonomous, coping, *independent,* person. So, initially it was a firm "No" from Mum and on we 'buggered'.

Alas, and though not *obviously* connected, her deteriorating *physical* mobility also seemed to be coinciding with our latest suspicion of some further deterioration in her *mental* mobility/ agility, as her short-term memory, in particular, appeared to fail her a little more too, and more frequently.

Yet, as I've said, Mum had retained an innate, life-long, and hitherto healthy, determination to preserve her independence and dignity, (especially in her own home), and was keen for it to continue thus. So, even now, that determination remained strong. Accordingly, and despite her difficulties, she was still trying her best to fend off these unwelcome 'boarders'...her own aging, the long-standing atheroma, the latest, and now restrictive left-hip pain, (with the niggling *limp* that it eventually bequeathed), and, of course, the increasing presence of the *forgetfulness,* the critical combination of which, (but especially the frightening 'forgetfulness'), continued to fuel, and now, arguably, increase, her frustrations and to more frequently fire up the accompanying anxiety.

Devoid of the spectre of the Dementia, I'm convinced that she (we) would have managed to carry on coping at home with any *physical* pain that her hip, leg or other part of her body, might bestow; but the Dementia made the critical difference; eventually turning some of her anxiety attacks, as I've said, into those brief, but more intense, 'panic attacks' (which *she* still termed "fear"). It was also, of course, the 'chief suspect' in some noticeable escalation in both the frequency and the intensity of her worst bouts of confusion.

Crucially, though, it was her hip pain that worsened the quickest, and her mobility problems simply increased in proportion; making any *substantial* (especially outdoor) walking effort all the more difficult to bear; so much so that, eventually, we *did* manage to persuade her to at least *look* again at the need for both a 'downstairs' commode and a lightweight wheelchair, ('just for emergencies'); alas, she was *still* resistant, and (like Ethelred) declared herself 'unready' to embrace either...albeit for but a few weeks more, when, in June, and following 'significant developments', the former would finally arrive, free, (with other 'aids'), from the local social services, with the latter, funded privately by ourselves, following barely a month later. (Our hopeful application for a free *wheelchair* from the social services/ NHS failed miserably; their *very* tight criteria requiring the receiver to have need of it more or less *permanently and continuously* both indoors and out, and once aware that Mum was still fairly good at pottering round the house the application was quickly consigned to their 'abject failure' bin. So, in late July I'd logged on, and, for a penny under £100, purchased our very own neat, lightweight, but very serviceable, wheelchair, via the omnipresent Amazon UK...and then, of course, had to spend a not inconsiderable amount of time learning how to 'operate'/'drive' it safely).

The *Medics* & The Hospital.

i. Medicalising Mum - Round 2.

So, on we'd 'buggered'; Dementia, atheroma, and all; but now with Mum's increasing complaints of further *physical* (back) pain, (especially from that left hip); and with *its* accompanying impact on both her level of mobility, and of "embarrassment"; and now with the pressing possibility of both a commode and a wheelchair in her life. Of course, it was all bound to impinge on the *quality* of that life; and it did. So much so that I was finally, if reluctantly, forced to 'bite the bullet' and to suggest to my siblings that we book Mum in for that further 'precautionary' consultation with the GP. This time regarding the *hip* pain...and that was the *third* significant, and equally crucial, 'turning point'. For me, with hindsight, it was the 'leaving home' (on a runaway train) *game-changer*, of a 'turning point'. The (turning) 'point of no return'.

I often think back, even now, with self-flagellating misgivings, to when I made that fateful proposal to seek further medical advice at this *particular* juncture. For it was certainly I who had *initiated* the making of what turned out to be a pivotal, Routine-wrecking, game-changing appointment; even though my willing sister, in her accepted role as 'female health lead' with Mum, had duly booked, and then accompanied her to, her 'appointment with fate'.

What if I'd suggested the need *earlier,* or even let Mum struggle on for another week or two before asking my sister to book the appointment? Might Mum have then seen a *different* doctor at the GP practice? If so, would the diagnosis, and therefore outcome, have been different? (Perhaps avoiding a rushed, panicky, outcome altogether?). If not, might the *A&E* doctor that Mum saw have been different? If so, would he/she have accepted the obvious X-Ray evidence that Mum's hip problem was no more than a common, bone on-bone, worn joint problem, and NOT *admitted* her for those 'further tests'? If so, might she have been returned, same day, from whence she came? That is, back to her own (and of course very familiar) home and Routine. If so, how *then* might things have turned out? Of course, I'll never know the answers to any of these questions for sure; because 'fate' had already 'played its' hand'.

At my suggestion, then, my sister had made the appointment as soon as the surgery opened for a new week, and had taken Mum to keep it just a couple of hours later, on Monday the 6th of June (2016). With hindsight, it was to prove critical, and, in my view, *did* mark the 'beginning of the end', and I remain ever aware that *I* bore responsibility for its instigation!

Mum had not been complaining of the hip pain whilst seated or asleep; but only when she tried to stand, walk or put undue pressure on it. In that circumstance, it seemed pretty obvious that her hip pain was stemming from age-related wear and tear in the joint. So, I was expecting the upshot of the appointment to be just some sort of stronger painkillers, at least in the short term, with perhaps a standard, *non-urgent*, referral to the hospital's outpatient dept. for X-Rays, by way of confirmation ...and perhaps some physiotherapy if we were *really* lucky.

Alas, the GP of the day didn't see it that simply, and came to a totally different, wholly unexpected, and surely fateful conclusion.

On scant alternative evidence, and for whatever reason, the GP came up with the novel suspicion that Mum's (relatively new, and worsening) hip pain might actually be a reaction to a hip *fracture*(!), and that she might have fallen at some time without us knowing. And that despite us visiting her daily, and usually for several hours by then, (though not normally through the night), and despite there being no discernible bruising, cuts, or the like, or any sign of disturbed or broken furniture, and Mum still being able to tell us about such things for the most part.

So the GP had sent her straight home with my sister, with the directive that an ambulance was to be sent there, to take them both the 7 miles to the nearest hospital's A&E Department for an *immediate* examination and X-Ray. (A bit drastic you might think, as I did, but fair enough to err on the side of safety again).

It was at that point that I received a totally unexpected phone call from my concerned sister, and duly arranged to *meet* her, and my brother, at the hospital's A&E Dept., to offer moral support. By the time I arrived on site, though, it was late afternoon.

Despite the A&E X-Ray showing NO obvious fracture, and indeed the young junior doctor on duty actually taking the time to *point out* that it was clearly showing a loss of cartilage in the left hip *joint*, and was therefore suggesting a 'bone-on-bone' *arthritic* situation, (as I'd suspected), and after spending fully 3 hours in A&E, (and once again to 'err on the side of safety'), my 90-year old, Dementia-troubled Mum was actually, and eventually, to make her very first (but not her last) acquaintance with the hospital's MAU (Medical Assessment Unit). To all our surprise, the young doctor was proposing to *admit* Mum "for tests"; advising that Mum's stay there would just be precautionary, and brief; and "probably" for just a "night or two"...but once admitted responsibility for Mum's care immediately transferred to the *MAU* doctors; and nurses. And the A&E guy's suggested 'night or 2' turned into a very slow-moving, very frustrating, night*mare* of a 2 WEEK *confinement* (!) on *medical wards* that were only testing for, and dealing with, *medical* issues relating to the hip pain. Even then, sadly, the 'testing' process, and indeed the experience in general, failed to fill me with confidence, and proved to be the first of a *series* of pretty 'testing' hospital experiences for more than just Mum!

The whole set-up just seemed so hard-pressed, and to grind so very slowly, and, worst of all, inefficiently! Let me cite just a couple of examples.

Firstly, without any *notice* of an intended move, I turned up on the MAU for my 3rd afternoon visit in a row, only to find someone else in Mum's bed; and to be told that the MAU bed had been urgently needed for this other patient, and that Mum had been moved to a more permanent and appropriate bed on Ward 44. (Ominously, signalling that there was no 'brief' stay or early discharge in the offing). Ward 44 turned out to be a ten-minute walk away, and elsewhere on the campus. When I eventually found my way there, Mum again seemed (predictably) confused, disorientated, and unsettled, and I spent the rest of the visit trying desperately to offer simple explanations that I thought she might understand and absorb, and to provide her with much-needed comfort and Reassurance.

Secondly, and perhaps more worrying, and on the very next day, I turned up on her 'new' ward dead on time for the set (2-00pm to 4-00pm) afternoon visiting session, to find Mum had a 'Nil By Mouth' sign hanging on the wall next to her bed. My enquiries to the nursing staff revealed that Mum was awaiting imminent departure "for tests" and that an empty stomach was required for at least one of them; and that, in consequence, Mum had eaten nothing at all so far that day. I accepted the plausible explanation. Once again, though, Mum seemed unaware of where she was; or indeed why. I became concerned that this long, and (to me) needlessly drawn out, stay, in what were clearly 'strange' and quite disorientating surroundings for Mum, might be contributing adversely to a further deterioration in her (tolerated but entirely untreated during the stay) Dementia! Yet, when I raised the matter with the Ward sister on duty, I was supposedly to be reassured with her bland advice that Mum's 'tests' would hopefully be completed "soon".

If I had been reassured on *arrival* by that advice, I most certainly wasn't as the minutes ticked by, and my hungry and bewildered Mum was still abed, and untested, as the, 4pm, 'end of visiting' time approached. I was even more exasperated when at exactly 4pm that same Ward sister arrived bedside to apologise profusely, and to tell me that the proposed 'tests' would *not* now be carried out that day, because Mum had (rightly) been judged insufficiently compos mentis to self-sign a consent form earlier; and the hospital had failed to get it signed by one of her offspring!

No-one seemed too concerned that an extremely vulnerable patient had, in the meantime, been left unfed all day. Nor that one of her offspring had actually been sat beside her, trying to 'hold the line', and to offer reason and reassurance, for nearly 2 hours, by repeatedly telling her that the 'test' was imminent; only to find that it had lately been postponed because of a basic failure of the hospital to get the paperwork sorted!

To 'add insult to injury', I was then advised that the test had been rescheduled for the following day; but only on condition that I went directly over to the relevant office on my way out, to sign the requisite form! It was scant consolation that one of the nurses brought Mum some overdue tea and toast by way of belated recompense for the palpably poor care and nourishment she'd received so far that day; albeit with the promise of a scheduled, more substantial, tea-time meal in the offing. As always, I made my complaints politely, but firmly, with both the busy ward sister and the office bureaucrat, yet the sense of sheer impotence to affect 'the system' continued to hang around me like a bad smell.

Then, just over a week in, and my worst fears were *realised*. My abiding concerns about a further deterioration in Mum's mental health and cognition, whilst an inpatient, were given very scary 'legs' when her overstay on the busy ward caused her confusion to spill over into a brace of quite chilling, never-before-seen, bouts of *delirium*!...both occurring 'before my very eyes', as a well-known magician of another age used to say. (According to the hospital's own leaflet, which I stumbled across quite by chance on the following day, and hiding among a variety of other leaflets in a large rack in 'Reception', "Delirium is a condition which can cause someone to become suddenly confused" and is also called "acute confusional state". Well, that certainly fitted the experience *I'd* been party to). Firstly, then, I'd witnessed my poor Mum getting upset because she'd somehow got it into her head that the woman in the next bed was now my *sister*, who had been admitted because she too had fallen ill. Secondly, and similarly, I was still bedside with her when she somehow got it into her head that an elderly man who had wandered unhindered onto the female ward in his pyjamas and dressing gown was my long-dead father!...both incidents taking all my patience and Reassurance skills to (eventually) placate her. I was truly shaken; but once again, my expressed concerns were respectfully, even sympathetically, heard, but brought no noticeable change. Conclusion - in busy hospitals, where staff and patients change regularly, both delirium and Dementia often go untended. (And once again my research on the subject turned up plenty of *academic* support; one national newspaper having printed a very timely article which cited work that had appeared in the journal JAMA Psychiatry, and which had concluded that, "Noisy hospitals could be accelerating the onset of Dementia in elderly patients", and that, "people with existing Dementia had a three-fold risk of the condition worsening after an episode" [of delirium]. It didn't bode well).

Slowly, slowly, the days dragged by, with Mum's Dementia giving increasing cause for concern for me and my siblings; but still appearing to generate little by way of either concern, or indeed urgency, from amongst the medical ranks; until, eventually, all the X-rays and (medical) 'tests' were deemed to have been completed. The doctor in charge of her case confirmed that they showed *no* fracture of the hip, and that Mum *had* simply developed a severe case of *arthritic* pain in the joint, due to the loss of cartilage and advised that the 'race was on' to identify the best course of (essentially pain- killer) treatment. *Several* were apparently 'trialled', before the doctor identified the 'BuTrans' skin 'patches' as the most appropriate. These 'patches', he advised, came in differing strengths, and contained the active ingredient 'Buprenorphine'; which, he added, was a strong *opioid* painkiller related to morphine; and when attached to a 'clear' area of skin such as the upper arm or shoulder, allows the Buprenorphine to be absorbed steadily into the bloodstream, through the skin, over several days. To tackle the hip pain, he was proposing a '7-day' patch of medium strength in the first instance. (Conceding, when I raised the issue, that it "should" also help 'kill' pain elsewhere; say that being caused by the atheroma). And with that authoritative recommendation, Mum's diagnoses, 'tests' and 'treatment' were finally deemed concluded. The only thing preventing her discharge was now a legally-required assessment by the hospital s*ocial worker* to confirm that a supported *return home* should form the basis of his 'care plan'.

I was finally contacted early on the morning of the 21st of June 2016 by the Ward Sister and told that Mum *had* been seen by the social worker, and, along with another round of prescription medicine, (-1), including now, of course, the innovative morphine-based 'patches', was ready for discharge.

I arranged to collect Mum from the hospital at 11-30am on the same morning, (and for my brother to collect the missing prescription item later)...as I say, 2 long weeks after her supposed 'brief' admittance 'for tests'; and certainly much the worse for wear 'Dementially'. By then, of course, 'the damage was done'; or at least *more* of it was. The intervening fortnight had only served to complicate, confuse and exacerbate, Mum's already 'delicate' situation; especially with regard to her Dementia. The ostensibly compassionate NHS 'system' had repeatedly 'erred on the side of safety' at every level but alas, only seemed to have made matters *worse*! The '*system*', with its well-meaning, but inflexible, so-slow-moving, processes and procedures, had caught her up in *its'* tentacles and (like the Dementia) had reeled her in...this time like a medical 'Venus fly-trap'; *this* 'intruder' simply 'spitting her out' with yet more toxic (this time *morphine*-based) medication to manage and a couple of basic 'disability aids'. (e.g. walking frame).

Try as I might, the regular and reasonable raising of my concerns and misgivings at various points in the processes had been unable to prevent the experience playing out as fully, futilely and, alas, negatively as it undoubtedly appeared to me. Yet there was, hopefully, one crucial consolation - the hope-cum-expectation that she would, at least and at last, have access to some proper pain relief following her ordeal...in the form of the 'Patches' that all those tests had supposedly 'matched' her up with, and lately seen prescribed.

In short, and to cap a critical, probably life-changing, yet arguably pointless and unnecessarily long, not to mention distressing, hospital experience, for both Mum and us, and preposterously ironic after all the professional 'tests', time and ado, the much-vaunted hospital medics had decided (as I'd suspected from the very outset) that Mum was suffering from a severe bone-on-bone arthritic condition in her hip; and that the best option for treating it was...stronger (albeit 'patch-based') pain-killers!

"At least the experience is over", was the consoling thought that my mind kept coming back to as I took Mum home; or was it?

End of Round 2.

It took about 2 weeks of our closest daily supervision, and a couple of early overnight stays, to get Mum back to anything like a settled level of either emotional or practical functioning at home. It was never again going to be *wonderful,* I suppose, but eventually we felt like we were making a modicum of progress. Mum had been returned to the comfort of her own familiar home, environment, and most of all Routine; and at least I felt hopeful again.

That said, the 'patches' were being used as directed but, disconcertingly, without any *greatly* discernible reduction in the hip pain; or the Atheroma for that matter. Mum certainly couldn't *walk* any further after several weeks of using them and of absorbing their (potentially strong and possibly anaesthetising) side effects (including the 'common' ones of headaches, dizziness, nausea and constipation) and, with hindsight, never would.

Then, when her *appetite* started to fail just a few weeks later, and the GP was again consulted, late on the morning of Monday, the 22nd of August, by my worried sister, the same 'safety first' policy saw Mum being whisked off to A&E *once more*; following another advance referral by the GP. And yet again a supposedly cautionary *outpatient* visit turned into another desperate, and even worse, in-patient one. (Talk about 'Groundhog Day'!)

After being seen in A&E, she was *again* admitted, tested and treated (medically) on the MAU ward, but this time for just 3 days in the first instance! During the subsequent observations, she was initially encouraged to eat by using liquid 'Build-up' drinks of various flavours, followed by a slow increase in her intake of more appropriate 'solid' food and meals from the standard hospital menu. Good; but once again the Dementia was largely 'left to its own devices', and received no discernible consideration; and if any potential link between her loss of appetite and the new 'patches' was ever considered, it certainly wasn't raised with us; (see this chapter's postscript); whilst back in a 'strange setting', Mum's cognition seemed to be regressing yet again. Consequently, when I was telephoned unexpectedly by the Ward sister, early on the morning of Thursday the 25th, and advised that Mum was ready for discharge, I was more than a little surprised. Yet, I was ready to take the hospital's word for it, (if only to see Mum freed from her uneasy confinement there), and willingly made haste to collect her from the ward.

Even though she still appeared both tired and weak when I arrived bedside, the hospital advice remained unchanged, and I held on to the hope that she was bound to improve in the familiarity of her own home and Routine.

Perhaps I'd been naive, because her discharge (again) had more than a hint of the farcical about it. I arrived at the agreed time of 11-30am, to find that the promised replenishment of her current prescription medications had yet to be dispensed by the hospital pharmacist and that (once again) a 'missing' element of the prescription wouldn't, apparently, be ready...this time until at least 4-00 pm that afternoon. In that far from perfect circumstance, the hospital's (deadly serious) proposal was for my significantly confused, fully dressed, and bag-packed Mum to just sit it out in the high-backed chair by her bed for another 4+ hours!

As you might imagine, I was less than happy, (for us both), and, (again politely but firmly), said so. Having made what I thought was an understandable fuss, however, the doctor was summoned. *Her* hurried phone call to the pharmacist duly followed, and she herself set off to collect the 'lost' medication. My hopes rose but when she returned some 40 minutes later, she was *still* minus that one item that would have completed the prescription and officially re-activated the 'Care Plan'. The missing item was still, apparently, *en route* from the supplier. A compromise was duly reached.

The hospital would agree to discharge Mum (and the medications that *were* available) into my care, so that I could take her home; but (again) with the 'rider' that I collect the missing medication from the ward later that evening. (In a phone call to my brother, it was agreed that *he* would again take on the task, so that I could concentrate on trying to resettle Mum back at home. Unbeknown to us at the time, alas, the fate of the missing medication wasn't actually going to *matter* too much!).

Once home, Mum managed just a little light soup, by way of lunch, and still seemed ill at ease. She then spent most of the afternoon sleeping. In truth, her poor presentation at discharge had barely improved thus far, but she appeared to rally after her sleep, and after the first of my sister's 2 'flying visits'. So she agreed to go on a short drive with me, and to take my arm as we hobbled round a local mini-market together, in order to stock up again on some grocery essentials; and to get some 'fresh air'. My sister then made a second brief visit, and Mum seemed a little *more* settled during, and then after, her stay. We then watched a little TV together until bedtime.

At around 7-30pm, I saw her off to bed, and, at her prior insistence, (rather reluctantly), saw myself out, once she was 'well away'; having added the usual 'rider' that she ring any one of us if worried in *any* way whatsoever. (With hindsight, it was remiss of me *not* to insist on staying over on that occasion. I can only assume that my own exhaustion had, not for the first time, significantly affected my clarity of thinking).

The very next morning, (Friday, the 26th), my sister visited 'first thing', as agreed, and found Mum up, but still neither fed nor fully dressed; and still rather 'groggy', and a little disorientated. My sister had immediately sought the support of my brother, who lived nearby; and together they decided to telephone the GP for yet further advice. That, once again, and almost predictably by now, was to 'play safe' and recommend that Mum be returned to the hospital; this time offering the (obvious with hindsight) advice that she'd probably been discharged "too early". And with the GP again agreeing to forewarn A&E, my siblings duly returned her there later that day

This time, she would stay a full 3 weeks on a *different* MAU ward...for even further (generally unproductive, and specifically *medical)* 'tests', but alas, beset by the 'perfect storm' of further regressive confusion in unfamiliar surroundings, further 'muscle loss' from prolonged bed-rest and inactivity, and no obvious let up in her *physical* (hip and lower leg) pain, this confinement really would signal the end of an era...and she would never again return to live in her own home!

ii. Medicalising Mum - Round 3.

So, during this critical and longest stay to date, Mum's already limited cognition had, sadly, (and unsurprisingly), regressed yet again; but still remained essentially tolerated rather than actively catered for, on this (alternative) MAU ward, as they continued, ('patches' and all), to search for a *fresh medical* (rather than an *existing*, mental, or, possibly, 'current medicinal') reason for Mum's returning poor appetite and now equally poor physical, as well as psychological, condition.

It wasn't long, then, before she once again started to complain regularly of "fear"; both to *us*, and to the *ward staff* - yes, even in the supposed safety, and permanent populace, of a hospital ward! (So the source of the 'the fear' really *didn't* seem to be specific to her own home as some had insisted was the case, and my long-held suspicion that it was more likely to be a 'fear' of the mental, the isolating *internal*, infarctions that came with the Dementia's increasing presence in her head and, at least in part, transcended her *physical* situation, appeared to have received further legitimacy).

The nursing staff's response to the "fear", (and to my subsequent enquiries of them), *was* to finally refer her elsewhere but the outcome was not as I'd hoped and on one of my afternoon visits in early September (unfortunately, I failed to log the exact date), I was unexpectedly approached bedside by a young female psychologist (?), who was seeking my agreement to 'treat' Mum with yet another toxic pill, this time a "small" dose of an *anti-depressant*, that went under the name of Mirtazapine.

From my (albeit limited) knowledge of anti-depressants in general, I readily recalled that they usually took quite some time to take effect, *and* could carry quite significant side-effects for some patients despite the lack of 'guarantees' that came with their use, anyway. In that light, and given the array of medication that Mum was already 'on', my gut instinct had been to say "No" to putting her through yet more body-sapping, sense-suppressing, medication when, in my opinion, a more personalised, off-ward, type of care, that worked towards getting her home with appropriate support, was the ideal, and more likely to reap the most positive benefits; and I had thought that might be the end of the matter. (My evening internet check suggested that my 'gut' instinct had indeed been correct, as this drug had the potential to impart a whole *raft* of significant side-effects, including headaches, nausea to the point of vomiting, and confusion!).

However, my *sister* had then been approached in my absence, and had been persuaded to sign the consent form anyway, so, on my next visit, the *ward* sister not only advised me that the hospital now *had* their required signature, but also that the Mirtazapine *had* now been added to Mum's burgeoning list of medications, and activated! Of course, I was deeply unhappy about the way I had been circumvented on such an important matter; and there was obvious potential for 'in-house' disagreement all round. My sister subsequently professed to have been unaware of my earlier refusal, and there seemed little to be gained now from looking for a divisive argument after the event; but the hospital, clearly having little else to offer, and nowhere more appropriate to 'house' Mum and her significant 'extra-curricular' mental and emotional needs, had finally found a way to implement their proposed, their only, (*chemical-cosh*), 'alternative recommendation'; and indeed, already had it 'on stream'. The (less than perfect, 'Big- Bother'- like) 'system' had prevailed again.

End of Round 3.

The *Social Services* & The Hospital

Aware that, psychologically, the mind retains a powerful attachment to routine, and to familiar surroundings, and in the face of her still worsening cognition and Dementia, (still barely taken into account), throughout her time as a hospital in-patient, I had campaigned for Mum to be allowed to yet 'see out her days' in her own home, as had been her most abiding and unswerving *compos mentis* wish to me, but with Mum being persuaded to 'purchase' a further package of support from the likes of the local social services. I had lost; not least because the previous social services 'help' had been to merely point us in the direction of the supposedly 'approved' *private* agency that had subsequently failed miserably to deliver; particularly on basic *daytime* consistency (of both time-keeping and personnel); whilst our tentative enquiries about 'night cover', (to both the local social services *and* the private agency), had revealed that no such home-based service was available from either themselves, or from elsewhere in the locality. So I had perhaps been 'clutching at straws', and already *starting* from a pretty weak position. Not too surprisingly, then, (given this abject lack of any quotable success from any *previous* support 'packages'), both the medical opinion and that of my siblings was that the 'risk' factor was currently too high; and that Mum had probably passed the 'point of no return' anyway in terms of ever living independently again in her own home. The final 'nail in the coffin' for my proposal was 'driven in' by the *hospital* social worker, and *his* two penn'orth.

With the post-hospital position less clear, and indeed less than unanimous, on this occasion, and under the Mental Capacity Act of 2005, the hospital social worker had once again been obliged to visit Mum in her hospital bed, both *during* our visits and in our absence, in the course of his legally-required assessment ('of an adult who is considered to lack the mental capacity to make particular decisions for themselves'), and equally-legally-required production of yet another Care Plan, prior to her discharge. As part of that process, he had also accepted my invitation to have a more open discussion, away from Mum's bedside on this occasion; and indeed, away from the prevailing medical aura of the hospital setting. So, on the morning of the 6th of September 2016, my siblings and I met with him at Mum's house, to discuss the more complex aspects, viewpoints and options relating to Mum's predicament this time around. He already had access to Mum's previous medical and social services records, of course, but by the time he left he also had a more in-depth awareness of some notably important differences present in her three offspring's opinions, expectations and perspectives. Alas, given her steady '*in-hospital*' decline and disorientation, Mum had, sadly, been unable to help her own cause too much; because *he* had been unable to get any consistent or coherent answers from *her*. Accordingly, to 'err of the side of safety' yet again, the social worker came to the conclusion that, in the current circumstances, an admission to a Care Home, (at least in the short term, and until and unless her mental capacity could be deemed to have shown pretty substantial improvement), was probably the best 'Care Plan' and option on discharge; although even here there was a significant degree of reinterpretation and confusion afoot, as his subsequent written report dated the 9th of September would assume that such a move had been agreed as 'permanent' from the *start*, when, for me at least, it most certainly had not! (To be fair, and in a strict, safety-first, 'jobsworth' sense, I too would probably have felt obliged to conclude that a Care Home should be the 'first port of call' if *I'd* been the assessing social worker; not least because I would have known that anything else would have been a very 'hard sell' to, and probably blocked as 'too risky' by, line, and higher, social services management).

Ironically, however, the social worker's recommended option, (and therefore Mum's discharge), was immediately, and open-endedly, rendered impossible to execute, because not a single *vacancy* was identifiable, in a single Care Home, in the responsible Local Authority and though Mum was deemed *ready* for discharge, it looked as if she was simply to be left languishing, (in effect living), in her demented confusion, within the confinements of her hospital bed and her bedside high chair, on the self-same (general medical) ward as hitherto, for as long as that lack of Care Home placements remained. (Her only relief to date had been provided by the handful of occasions that I managed to persuade the day's ward sister to take time from her busy shift to go and find, and let me sign, a 'responsibility' form, and thence let me take Mum off the ward, in a 'house' wheelchair, and down two long corridors to the public cafe, for a stimulating change of scenery, and some welcome tea and cake).

Despite the prospect of a lengthy, potentially open-ended, delay, and her virtual 'imprisonment' on the ward, there was still to be no reconsideration of the Care Plan. It seemed that I was *irreversibly* outvoted. The majority view was that, in the absence of a 100% 'safe' alternative, Mum *should* be left languishing so, and should *not* be tried back at home in the short-term/foreseeable future, for fear that she could not currently cope alone there, and would need the sort of 24/7 supervision that was neither viable nor available, in order to be deemed other than 'at risk'. Short of one of us actually *moving in* with her, on a *permanent* basis, (which, as I've said, and for logistical reasons in our own domestic lives, just wasn't really sustainable even on a short-term basis), no-one, it seemed, was prepared to *take* the risk that a still well-supported return to familiar surroundings, and to a familiar routine, might actually *improve* her functioning. Of course, the 'nay-sayers' had a powerful argument in terms of strict *physical* 'risk', and, in the end, the sheer weight of their numbers, and democracy, won out. I was forced to concede defeat. With Mum's consistent compos mentis plea to "never" be put "in a home" ringing in my ears, and consumed by guilt, (for having failed her/ reneged on my promise there), my only condition-cum-insistence, thereafter, was that it would not be *me* that actually *took* her to any such 'home' (put her there) in the first instance. Even so, being forced to *actually* renege on that solemn promise, for all but on a 'technicality', was always going to weigh heavily on me; and so it did. Not least because I knew, from my own work experience, that I too would want to avoid the inherent flaws in all such (institutional) Care Home set ups if at all possible.

In the course of my twenty-odd-year career as a 'frontline', inner-city, Local Authority social worker, I had been required to visit a variety of LA, and indeed, private, 'Care Homes' on a regular basis. In the early days, that included visits to a variety of 'old folks' homes'; and after specialising in child-care for the latter half of that career, to a variety of residential settings catering for a genre that went under the broad title of 'Children & Young people'.

On first reflection, you might think that residential settings catering for such disparate groupings would have little in common, but, 'structurally', you might be surprised.

Sadly, there was not a single residential setting (for either young or old) that did not leave me convinced that living alone in one's own home and community, as an adult, (or with family, if preferred or possible), was *always* a more attractive option than living in any of the supposedly 'specialist' care institutions that crossed my path over nearly 3 decades.

Put simply, for me, and in principle, the main, arguably the only, positive from what amounts to *involuntary* Care Home/ residential living is the *physical* care, safety, health and food provision, etc, that you would expect to be able to 'take as read'. (Though there have been innumerable newspaper and TV investigations highlighting instances where, even here, such basic standards *cannot* be taken for granted!).

On the other hand, however, my social work experience had convinced me that there were/are some very real *mental* and *emotional* disadvantages, indeed 'risks', to such 'institutional' living. *My* view was (and remains) that these essentially revolved around 'limitations', and far outweighed any (potential) positives; 'limitations' that seemed more akin to the sort of strictures one might associate with a move to *any* form of *involuntary* communal living; and might typically include aspects of enforced detention, confinement or imprisonment. Uppermost amongst these I placed the limiting of one's personal independence, freedom of movement and independent decision-making, in general, of basic privacy and personal space in particular, and of access to long-standing personal and familiar routines, surroundings and possessions of choice, of immediacy in terms of access to family and friends, of everyday personal preferences (for say food, home-entertainment, going out and bedtimes), that most people in this country would associate with self-determination and being 'free'.

Moreover, be they for the elderly or for the young, nearly all the care 'institutions' that I came across in the course of my employment, but especially those run privately, had, in the end, to run *economically;* that is, had to compete 'in the market', and remain *financially* viable or 'go to the wall'; ipso facto, ultimately, (and especially when cuts to social budgets are 'policy'), there isn't even certainty of tenure in such residential care. (See later).

Accordingly, in order for such 'businesses' to *remain* financially viable, they usually needed to cater for a minimum number of residents; all of whom were usually required to subscribe to the same, economically-viable, 'all-under-one-roof', in-house 'arrangements'. For example, most 'care' settings usually tried to incorporate 'set meal-times', where forward-planning of 'menus for the many' was usually assumed. Similarly so with set, and invariably *staggered,* bedtimes; where the residents were again expected to go to bed at times determined by the availability of sufficient supervising staff, rather than at times chosen by themselves, as self-determining 'customers'.

And again, in the course of daily living in such 'care' settings, there was usually 'competition' for a limited range of shared facilities. For example, Care Home residents invariably had to accept, and share, *communal* and limited bathroom, toilet, kitchen, seating or TV facilities.

Staffing levels, too, (in terms of both numbers and qualifications), were invariably a problem that limited the ideal functioning of nearly all such 'institutions'. (The status and pay of those employed in 'institutional' community care was generally poor, and the sector was rarely seen as a good career move, so attracting good staff, and more importantly getting them to stay, and to build lasting and meaningful relationships with the usually dependent, and hard to engage, residents, was a more or less permanent problem). Even when fully staffed, the working of long, often demanding, on occasion crisis-centred, 'shifts' inevitably lead, first and foremost, to a get-the-essentials-done pragmatism, and a lack of regular and really personalised 'quality time' with the residents; and a consequent lack of 'ongoing enthusiasm', and therefore of genuinely stimulating interaction; and all taking place within a necessarily 'approved' set-up that had to comply with a whole raft of relevant State legislation and guidance.

As if the 'fall out' from all that wasn't hard enough for most residents to wrestle with, and, at the end of the day, (literally), there was usually a key change of personnel to adapt to, following the exodus of many (if not all) of the day staff to their own families, homes and lives, (and some to their 'days off'); and of course, the early-evening 'handover' to the (invariably fewer and even less interactive) *night* supervision personnel. All of which, I felt, contributed to an inherent sense of powerlessness, uncertainty, isolation and slowly 'shifting sand' for the 'inmates' of such 'institutions'. (As I eventually came, in a mixture of both fondness and cynicism, to think of them).

As well as such *generally* unattractive aspects of 'institutional' living, I also had serious reservations in relation to the elderly, in particular; and even more so when Dementia was likely to be an active ingredient; and this, more than anything, was perhaps where, and why, I came to hold a markedly different, potentially alternative, and more risky, perspective from my two siblings, regarding Mum's care.

My siblings (with the predictable 'safety-first' backing of the hospital, medical and social work establishment) had, understandably, made the strongest argument for putting Mum's *physical* safety first; but my siblings were also convinced that, mentally and emotionally, Mum would be, *deserved* to be, and would *appreciate* being, properly 'looked after' in such an 'approved' setting in her 'latter' years. It was all lovingly meant.

However, when it came to mental and emotional benefits *I* was convinced that they were both looking through 'rose-tinted' glasses, and had an *idealised* notion of how things would progress for Mum in a Care Home setting. They tended (hoped?) to see Mum living out her days, and indeed extended years, in stress-free cosy contentment with other (always) genial 'inmates' of similar generation, memories and age-related interests, abilities and limitations; and doing so under the watchful eye of (ever) consistent/ contented/ committed, and rarely-changing nursing, care and admin staff; all of whom Mum would just 'get along' with, and happily share her life and likes.

To me, if that model was *ever* likely to be sustainable, then it always sounded more likely to be the *lifestyle choice* of someone still significantly compos mentis; and still reasonably rational, active, involved and fundamentally independent and in some sort of 'hotel' or 'retirement', perhaps holiday, or condominium-type, accommodation.

My employment, and others', experiences, therefore, persuaded me that my siblings held an *unrealistic* view of what might be on offer to Mum, and that it was never likely to work out as well as they hoped. Indeed, *my*, more cynical, view was that Care Homes for the (limited self-care) elderly were, at best, 'holding areas'; but, at worst, places where the residents were, effectively, waiting to 'shuffle off their mortal coil'; in concerns run privately, and as I've said, for profit. In fact, and on more than one occasion, I had heard the larger ones referred to, disparagingly, as "granny farms".

I was also of the view that the added presence of Dementia in such settings was likely to preclude such a cosy, contented, 'happy-ever-after', living and outcome; and, by now, I was, most certainly, expecting the vast majority of elderly Care Home residents, like Mum, to be beset by some degree of Dementia; and that most were not, therefore, likely to be in residence by free choice. I was therefore pretty sure that, when combined with physical aging, it was unlikely that most residents, in most Care Homes, would have retained the necessary skills, wit, general health, agility, attention-span, and most of all memory, to interact either 'meaningfully' or 'socially' with each other on a regular 'group' basis; and perhaps not even in a rudimentary way. It also seemed pretty obvious to me that these 'inmates' were themselves bound to *change* from time to time; that is, would inevitably continue to age, and, therefore, lose more of their faculties; and, alas, be more likely to 'pop off' than to return home...and only thus might 'vacancies' ever arise. Otherwise, Mum would *never* be offered a place in one, would she?

My siblings either couldn't or didn't want to accept my pragmatic, and yes pretty downbeat, and I guess, to them, fairly depressing, perspective; preferring to see Residential Care as the *only* feasible option now; even if it be the 'best of a bad bunch' of limited options. It seemed unlikely that both views could prevail. Of course, for all our sakes, but especially for Mum's, I sincerely hoped it *wasn't* going to be mine that prevailed; but my concluding, (perhaps over-dramatic, yet honestly-expressed), 'prediction' was that Mum's Dementia (as it had in the hospital) would certainly worsen further, and probably quite quickly, in the inevitable confusion of yet further strange and unfamiliar surroundings... and that she would be lucky to survive "6 months" in *any* such setting; let alone experience long-lasting contentment into an even riper old age.

Regardless, and with the weight of the medical and social services opinion on their side, I was, as I say, outvoted, and Mum's post-hospital future, (at least in the short term), lay in some sort of Care Home situation.

Postscript

Long after the event, and, indeed, long after Mum's sad passing, (in fact in August 2019), one of the main worries and regrets that I'd harboured at the time, regarding Mum's 'medicalisation', came back to haunt me, when I read the following shocking passage about Buprenorphine – the morphine-based drug permeating the 'patches' that had been visited on my poor Mum by the medics, following their supposed 'tests' to identify the best way to alleviate Mum's hip pain of 2016.

The passage was part of an article written by the 'medical correspondent' of a national newspaper after studying recently released academic research and read, "Doctors...warned that a... study showed an opioid painkiller called buprenorphine, which is taken by 120,000 Dementia patients in the UK, tripled the risk of psychotic and neurological problems – such as personality changes and confusion. They said they believe this drug may also increase the risk of death".

So sorry, Mum for you having to bear the risks and suffer the side-effects of those toxic 'patches'; especially when they didn't even bring you the promised pain relief.

CHAPTER 5

The Dementia Diaries.

What follows in this core and pivotal section is based on the personal memories and experiences of myself and my two siblings, and on a significant array of relevant, alternative and accumulated paperwork, but, in particular, on a series of (5) logbooks (diaries) that we made use of, from the autumn of 2012, to keep track of Mum's deteriorating condition and changing needs in her latter years, as the cruel and merciless Dementia began to reveal itself more markedly, and to exert its slow, creeping, and alas inexorable, stranglehold.

Throughout this key chapter, direct quotes from inputs into the 'diaries' (logbooks), from all 3 of we siblings, will routinely appear, and make up a significant part of the narrative. They are entirely my personal selections, specifically chosen to give either a 'flavour', or the 'essence', of a visit, issue or situation. Most will have been extracted from, and remain attached to, a particular date in one of the 'diaries' (logbooks), and will, (hopefully), be either self-explanatory, or explained in further and adequate detail. To save repetitive notification and acknowledgement, where the quotes have been 'lifted' from my *brother's* input into the diaries, and especially where no further explanation appears needed, the letter '(T)' will appear beside them in brackets. Where they are 'lifted' from my *sister's* input, the letter '(L)' will similarly appear. Unless otherwise stated, all other quotes are attributable to me.

As I've already said, Mum's cognitive functioning had been giving us mild cause for concern for some time; likewise our perceived short-comings of, and therefore increasing frustrations with, the, doubtless overstretched, social and medical services for the masses, in that their availability to us had seemed both hard-won and cursory; whilst any actual advice to us, as Mum's main carers, had hitherto been found to be, at best, imprecise, impersonal, ineffective, impractical, and seemingly ad-hoc, and not therefore of much tangible or sustained support at all; let alone offering a smidgen of hope of actually *improving* many, if any, aspects of Mum's increasingly affected mental (and therefore social) functioning.

It had already taken many months of fitful, seemingly uncoordinated, appointments with the medical services to receive *any* sort of official diagnosis, and even that had been only verbal, essentially focused on *assessment*, and, dishearteningly, unaccompanied by any active 'plan'. So, again as I've said, we'd reluctantly been drawn to the conclusion that we would have to try and navigate our *own* way through the gathering 'fog', rather than to sit around waiting for, or expecting, the so-called 'professionals' to clear a path to any answers.

Accordingly, and following our frequent and extensive discussions during 2012, we had come to the inevitable conclusion that, for Mum's own safety, and for our own peace of mind, *we siblings* would have to find ways to keep that closer eye on her level of cognition; and therefore on her practical, every day, functioning.

To that end, and with a (verbal only) diagnosis of *(vascular)* Dementia having been finally teased from the medics, I'd hit upon the idea of opening that first 'logbook'; and of keeping it on the book- shelf beneath Mum's small telephone table, in the far corner of her small terraced home's 'front room'. In it, (and the others that we should have known would follow), we would henceforth note anything that we individually judged *worthy* of such note from our respective daily visits, phone calls and contacts.

Again as I've said, that very first log-book was opened late in the afternoon of the 14th of August of 2012. Mum would have been half-way through her 86th year. Its main purpose, just to reiterate, was to try and provide a simple yet convenient, DIY, means of logging the latest 'state of play', of providing an accompanying, if journeyman's, often 'best guess', assessment and interpretation of that 'state of play'. That is, of providing a very latest 'update' for the next-visiting sibling of both positive, as well as negative 'developments'. In this way we hoped that any such 'developments' (or otherwise) could be kept in some kind of constructive context, might provide useful information/ evidence for 'action', and might provide 'clout' in any future dealings with both the social and medical services; and might thereby allow both us, and, by dint, them, to have access to some sort of personal yet comparative timeline and to try and make some sort of longer-term sense of what the hell was going on here! So, before I embark on the challenging, indeed emotional, task of documenting and describing the relevant contents and associated analyses of all the 'diaries' in appropriate depth, (particularly the first, as, with due hindsight, 2013 would prove to be yet another unwanted, ensnaring and yet again irreversible, 'turning point' year that would set a new *pattern* of, at best, established but noticeably worsen*ed* symptoms of the Dementia, and at worst of its still ever-so-slowly worsen*ing* trajectory), let me first remind you of the point we had reached, by both re-summarising, and re-setting, the 'baseline' for you, from which the introduction of the very *first* 'diary' was deemed necessary.

As far as we were concerned, Mum was still only in the relatively early stages of Dementia as we entered 2012. Indeed, we were *still* awaiting *official* confirmation that Mum was beset by Dementia at all; let alone what type. For us, the problem was still intermittent rather than routine, and she was still functioning relatively independently, in terms of her self-awareness, and everyday issues such as managing her personal hygiene, food preparation, housekeeping, bedtime/sleeping and overnight needs; albeit with a daily visit of at least a couple of daytime hours (including for her shopping needs), from at least one of us, on a loose rota basis; and backed up by regular telephone check-ups, as necessary. Indeed, she was quite capable of teasing us by going the odd fortnight or so without really exhibiting any *significant* 'forgetfulness' at all; but we still saw the *insignificant* stuff regularly enough to know that it hadn't gone away, and had reached the point where we felt the problem needed further consideration of the available options, by way of better forward planning. To that end we were even minded to re-contact the local social services, for example.

Ironically, we had *previously* made general 'social' enquiries about available services with them in 2011, and their sole 'offering' then had been that (at 85) Mum might benefit from the weekly social contact and stimulation to be gained from attending at their lone day-care centre over in the town. As I've said, in the absence of tangible alternatives, we had then persuaded a reluctant Mum to 'give it a go', and, with our measured encouragement and reassurance, she had forced herself to attend for several months, bless her, on each Monday, during the rest of that year and much of the next. However, she was never entirely keen on going, and was well able to cite instances where other attendees were actually much worse, and more needy, both physically and mentally, in terms of dependency, than she was; and was equally, and repeatedly, well able, in consequence, to tell us that the day, and setting, tended to just make her feel rather patronised and depressed. Accordingly, and unsurprisingly, she eventually started making excuses, and refusing to go when the free mini-bus called for her; her refusal duly leading to a phone call to one of us, from the centre, to tell us so; and that call invariably obliging one of us to attend on her at home as a matter of urgency, to allay her sense of culpability and guilt, and to offer her early comfort and reassurance that she had 'done nothing wrong'. In the end, given her consistent, and quite well reasoned, worries and reluctances, we had to accept that she had 'given it a fair go', as agreed, and should be allowed to follow her expressed wish to 'call it a day' there. (Despite us raising the *option* to return there, on a regular basis, she never asked to, or did, attend again).

By the time we 'opened' that first diary, in that August of 2012, then, Mum was in her 86*th* year, and was still largely, and willingly, living independently in her own home; and once again devoid of all tangible outside, non-family, support or agency input. Moreover, and to her eternal credit, she remained keen to preserve her self-respect, and, therefore, to *retain* prime responsibility for looking after herself. This had included (thus far) taking charge of all her medication in their individual packets, kept neatly together in one corner of one of her kitchen cupboards.

That said, as we saw off autumn our increasing suspicions that she might be taking them out of sequence, perhaps in the wrong combination, or even missing some altogether, on occasion, had found us persuading her to let us pop the right combinations of the *next* day's dosage into an egg-cup for her, in easy view on top of the breadbin, on a daily basis, just to be "on the safe side"; a subtle change that she only accepted after some lengthy, but gentle, reassurance that we were not "bossing" her or "trying to take over". (These 'suspicions' had also been triggered by our realisation that she had occasionally forgotten to tick off the calendar after completing each day's intake, as previously agreed, and might therefore be at risk of taking them more than once; and by the fact that, on a very few occasions, she had simply run out of some tablets early, and had one or two others left over at the end of each 4-week 'batch').

By the turn of the year, the 'egg-cup routine' was pretty well established, and working well; apart from the couple of times when the chemist failed to deliver on their promise, and the automatic renewal of her prescription failed to arrive on time - cue anxiety all round, and our rush to telephone down, and to pick it up ourselves before 'any damage was done'.

Throughout 2012 then, Mum remained pretty well established on a daily intake of 6 prescription drugs - 2 "Carvedilol" 'heart' tablets (1 taken each morning and evening), and 1 "Amlodipine" 'blood-pressure' tablet, taken each morning, (each of these having been imbibed for over *14 years!*), plus 1 "Clopidogrel" 'Atheroma' tablet, taken each morning, (for the past *11 years!*), and 1 each of her "Simvastatin" 'cholesterol', and "Bendrofluazide", 'water' tablets, (taken, we think, for maybe 4 years, though we cannot put a precise date for the inception of the latter 2). Then, for some considerable time prior to the opening of the first 'diary', (perhaps as long as 2 years), she had also been prescribed boxes of "Laxido" sachets, to be dissolved in warm water, and drunk at her convenience, to help with her claimed bouts of increasing constipation. (Whether the latter condition was in any way related to the possible side-effects of any of the other tablets, or combination of, still remained a largely, but niggling, suspicion and conjecture on my part, for now). At various points, the usual 4-weekly prescription renewal went through periods where boxes of paracetamol (for general pain relief), and tubes of Voltarol, to rub on a couple of increasingly arthritic finger joints, (and which she occasionally rubbed, *in*appropriately, elsewhere, to cause severe chafing of her increasingly thin skin!), were added. In addition, her *non*-prescription/over-the-counter *oral* medication of choice included the likes of 'heartburn' tablets, menthol sweets, and liquid 'Milk of Magnesia'; whilst her non-oral buys included small bottles of 'medicinal' olive oil and 'Deep Heat' sprays, for massaging more general muscle aches.

In sum, by the time of the first diary's inception, and medically, our 86 year old Mum, who was suspected of suffering from a slow-burning Dementia, was still effectively able, willing, and encouraged, to self-administer quite a 'cocktail' of oral and non-oral, prescription and non-prescription, medicines. 'Socially', she was agency-free.

And so *to* the 'diaries'.

2012

Aug. 14th: In the continued absence of any truly tangible initiatives from the, yes, almost certainly over-stretched, cash-strapped and certainly rather bureaucratic, for the most part disappointingly ineffective, and particularly snail's-paced, social and medical services for the masses, and to actually try to manage and improve things ourselves, 'off our own bat', so to speak, and on *Tuesday, the 14th of August 2012*, I arrived at Mum's with my standard, lined, refill pad of 80 sheets, bought from our local newsagent.

My first job was to try and tactfully (positively and light-heartedly) explain to Mum the purpose of the logbook, before she raised her own (almost certainly anxious and pessimistic) suspicions that 'something was wrong'. Put simply, and hopefully inclusively, I couched its' arrival thus that, "these days", like *her*, *we too* sometimes forgot to tell each other important things, and may need to leave each other notes "occasionally". Luckily, (and perhaps once again *with* the help of the Dementia), she seemed to accept my explanation readily enough, and raised no particular concerns. So, on we got, with our (soup and ham sandwich) lunch, and out we went on our usual (and another trouble-free) Tuesday afternoon household-shopping expedition.

On our return, with the shopping safely packed away, and over a welcome cuppa in the front room, I casually picked up the logbook again, and, as that keen Star Trek watcher of the time, (sometimes even on *Mum's* TV), and to reinforce that aura of fun and frivolity, and lack of real importance, at least at this outset, I spontaneously wrote on the turquoise-blue frontispiece, in strong black biro, 'Captain's Log, Stardate Aug. 14th 2012'. Next, whilst trying to amuse her with a childish imitation of a pseudo-inter-galactic American accent akin to Cap'n Kirk himself, I read aloud what I'd just written, and duly declared the thing "Open"; Mum smiling, and laughing accommodatingly, as I did so. Then, as she departed for the kitchen to prepare an evening meal of fish fingers and peas, fruitcake and another cup of tea, and left me alone in the front room watching the TV, I took the opportunity to make a discreet first entry, on the first inside sheet. And it was with more than a touch of additional irony that it was being entered during one of Mum's better, indeed good, days/periods, and was therefore entirely uncontroversial, and essentially sat alone there for the rest of the month. It was made with Mum's full knowledge, and simply noted that we'd "Been to Coop. Mum chatted and laughed with CL (a neighbour), & checkout girl; also to Aldi for flowers. Went cemetery put 'em on Dad's grave. So far so good. Fish fingers for tea. Neighbour says he has builders in next Monday for a few days. Could get noisy".

And although there were still occasional moments of what could (and would) easily pass for *everyday* 'forgetfulness', and others that followed when Mum had perhaps seemed a bit quiet, 'down', or "iffy" as I sometimes used to described her, on some of our arrivals, she'd usually responded and rallied so quickly and well to our arrival and presence thereafter that we'd each presumed it was just her understandable reaction to the equally 'iffy' weather, or perhaps just a tad too much associated solitude.

Accordingly, the logbook was effectively left unused, and 'confined to barracks', with my inaugural entry not added to, for the rest of August. Indeed, the next few entries too were uncontroversial in terms of Mum, her functioning and her Dementia, and related to much more *practical*, every day, matters as, for example, with the very *next* entry.

Sept 8th (Sat): Rather than commit to an entry in the new-fangled logbook, my brother had fallen back on the old tried and tested formula for contact, and had chosen to telephone me on the previous evening to report 2 things. Firstly, that he'd noted a thickish coating of ice forming beneath the lower freezer drawer of Mum's fridge-freezer, as he'd taken something out, (it wouldn't shut smoothly), plus some standing water below the salad drawer in the fridge section, on his latest (Friday morning) visit, and had discreetly cleared the problem in both areas. However, in trying to avoid unnecessary worry for Mum with his suspicion that there might be a fault there, he had chosen both to say nothing to her about it, nor enter anything 'official' about it in the logbook in case she might somehow stumble across it, and/ or his 'suspicion' turned out to be wrong; and secondly, that the latest issue of the local "rag" had noted the sad death of 'Billy O', a neighbour who had suffered ill-health for some years, and a man that Mum, (and indeed we offspring), had known for so many more; and because I was due to take the next day's (Sat) 'watch', it was to me, and no doubt with more than a modicum of relief, that he was passing on these issues now.

Luckily, on arrival, on the 8th, I'd found Mum in pretty good spirits, and busying herself with the final preparations of the usual 'Sunday lunch on a Saturday' delight that was a traditional roast beef dinner, (with the 2 veg. creamed mash & gravy as basic, but minus the Yorkshire pudding), plus my favourite home-cooked rice pudding made with full milk, and a couple of chocolate digestives with a cup of tea, to follow. It had been the standard Saturday fare, and a veritable treat that I'd looked forward to each week, for so many years now; very probably since Dad died. Paradoxically, though, and as mentioned elsewhere, this very 'treat' would soon be central, amongst other 'triggers', in persuading me to suspect, detect, and 'benchmark', a crucial and perceptible shift, (escalation), in the Dementia's progress and grip; more of which later.

However, with nothing much to worry about with Mum today, I decided that the time was ripe to gently break the sad news of 'Billy O's' passing, rather than leave her permanently 'in the dark' about it, or have her hear/ read about it elsewhere, and to advise her that my brother had read about it in the latest issue of the local "rag". I did so calmly and 'matter-of-factly' during the tea and biscuits. "Poor Billy, he's suffered enough.", and after a short pause, "Eeee...Another one gone", I heard her mutter, amongst other equally resigned but suitably respectful remarks, as she got up, carefully stacked and lifted some of the used items of crockery, pottered over to the kitchen sink, and began to wash up, with (presumably) her related thoughts, but with what seemed, ostensibly, a quiet acceptance of 'Billy's' fate that bordered on the predictable, inevitable and reconciled.

As she washed and stacked the wet crockery on the drainer, I took the opportunity to put stuff back in the fridge; this providing me with the perfect moment to sneak a peek below both the lower freezer drawer and the salad tray, and yes, the ice and water were, respectively, back in evidence. Clearly, there was a problem here that needed addressing soon, so remaining as calm as I could, and playing the problem right down to just a "spot of ice" under the lower drawer, I neatly distracted her from dwelling too long on the loss of 'Billy O' by casually asking Mum if she still had the receipt for the thing, as it was originally guaranteed for 3 years. She had. She went directly to an old biscuit tin on the shelf in the front room, where she kept her old bills and such stuff, (she never threw anything away), and found it almost immediately. Not only was there still more than a month left on the guarantee, but there was also a description of the fridge-freezer, with make, model number etc. Result!

Hence the next entry into the logbook, made on the 8th Sept., read:

"Mum good all day today. Told her about [Billy O]. Seemed to take it in her stride. Checked fridge. Yes, I think there's a problem.

Found receipt, & called in at DW's (retailer), whilst we were out shopping. DW has rung through details to manufacturer, and will follow up on Monday. Await contact. Have given him my mobile. Salmon sarnies for tea".

Fairly 'run of the mill' stuff, I know, but that's my point. I've laboured a bit over the detail from the 8th because it was just typical of so many mundane entries made during the rest of 2012; nearly all of which tended to avoid over-egging our concern with the Dementia. (Given the limited instances of *significant* 'forgetfulness' of recent weeks, perhaps we'd allowed ourselves to believe that it had 'stabilised' in some way; or might even be in remission). Instead, we'd tended to concentrate on the sort of 'life must go on' issues that were more immediate, pragmatic, household, commonplace, and to all intents 'normal'; in a word, Ordinary. By way of reinforcing the point, here's a few more examples.

15th Sept: "T/c from DW. New fridge arriving Monday between 2 & 3pm. Can either of you be there?"

27th Sept: "Mum worried about taking laxative - in case needs too much toilet in night. Taken @ 5-45pm anyway".

20th Nov: "Measured up front room & hall for new carpet, as discussed" (T). (The sizes were also written in the logbook; for posterity, and in case someone else needed or wanted to be the one to follow this up).

4th Dec: "T away 16/17 Dec. Going Scarborough. L to come up & cover Sunday & put her bin out" (T).

12th Dec: "Everything ok at hospital. Been discharged, back to GP if needed. Still some lung infection on X-Ray – but apparently 'nothing to worry about' – Prescription being del. Weds PM". (L)

However, our relative optimism, (cum-complacency), didn't (indeed couldn't) last.

Come the New Year then, and we were brought back to earth, and to reality, again. The destabilisation of her 'good run', and the 'interruption' of her established routines, by the "to do" (as in 'what a to do') of Christmas, (as Mum had taken to calling the hustle and bustle of such celebratory occasions), and, this time around, a rather more 'fretful' one, (for no more detectable a reason than the inevitable melancholic reflections on, and/or persistence of reminiscences about, loved ones past that I guess penetrate the thoughts of *most* mature adults at this time of year), and despite our continued close attentions throughout, alas continued *beyond* the Yuletide festivities. (Although she'd insisted, for weeks beforehand, that she wanted a "quiet" Christmas, with "no fuss", "at *my* age", we'd still arranged it so that *I* spent the afternoon of Christmas *Eve* with her until her normal, now 7-15pm, bedtime, whilst, as had become the norm, my brother had her round for Christmas dinner and a similar period on Christmas *Day*, and my sister likewise on the *Boxing* Day).

Following 'Sod's Law', then, and just when we thought we'd maybe weathered the Christmas 'storm', and might look forward to better times ahead, came a combination of factors that seemed to embody the *'perfect* storm'.

For starters, her apathy and 'fretfulness' was both compounded and reinforced by the sad and untimely news of two further 'passings', in quick succession; and these with Christmas and the New Year still 'warm'.

The first was that of her 94 year old sister-in-law, who had moved to Scotland many years ago, whilst the second was that of the, "only young", (as Mum saw it), and very local, daughter of a long-gone good friend. This 'young' woman, (at 63, she was just a few months older than my brother), had, sadly, lost her fight with cancer, and had departed this life leaving behind her husband and 2 young teenagers; which particularly upset Mum, and just seemed to make her 'forgetfulness' and low mood the worse. (Although she never said so, my best guess is that it only served as a mid-winter reminder of the mortality of all, and, in that vein, of the relative proximity of her own likely departure). Anyway, coming on and around the time of Mum's own (87th) birthday, these 'losses' did somehow seem to further raise Mum's anxieties, and her propensity to a more depressed frame of mind; and to destabilise things further for her. Alas, and most poignant of all, they appeared to have tipped her *Dementia* into further activity!; and all this flying directly in the face of her relatively good, *pre-Christmas* mood, in the wake of that comforting, anxiety-reducing, 'all clear' regarding her *physical* health, after my sister had taken Mum for that routine, outpatient, follow-up for an old lung infection, on the 12th.

2013

In line with her repeatedly expressed preference for a "quiet" 87th birthday, too, we'd arranged to *overlap* our home visits to Mum, on the day, so that she would have company for the bulk of her waking hours; arriving with useful 'household' presents, new essentials in the clothing department, and cake. Indeed, we'd arrived hopeful that we'd seen the worst of winter, and pointed positively to the lightening nights, and to both the regular flitting of her resident robin, and the first glimpse of snowdrops, in her little backyard garden patch, as reasons to be more cheerful and to be looking forward to the Spring. We'd hoped such 'signs' of 'renewal' might at worst re-stabilise, or at best 'renew', *Mum's* general demeanour and disposition; but instead, and despite her willing efforts, she'd still seemed mired in the more 'iffy', more often, and for longer. So, both on the day, and afterwards, it would probably have remained a bit of a struggle, (both for her and for us), to raise and maintain her morale even *before* the news broke of the demise of that additional pair of long-established contacts from her own *personal* contact 'pot'.

Whilst she'd appeared to take the 'single-shot', September, news of 'Billy O's' demise well enough, this time the '*double-barrelled* blast' appeared to have done some damage, by both worsening her lethargy and further raising her propensity to anxiety, low mood and depression, and this whilst simultaneously seeming to both fuel her 'forgetfulness', and to negatively affect her already less than perfect *concentration*.

It had been *on the very day* of Mum's low-key 87th birthday, then, and with my siblings only recently departed, that I answered a tea-time phone-call that precipitated the following logbook entry.

Jan. 31st. (Thurs): "VH [our cousin] rang. 4-25pm to say Auntie Mary died last Tues. Age 94. Have told Mum. Initially upset of course, and tearful, but not too bad later, after reminiscing. Nothing to be done our end. V & Mary's son, John, attending funeral in Scotland *next* Tues. Mum seemed OK when I left, but just be aware."

Mum had occasionally spoken to Aunt Mary on the phone over the years, and particularly at Christmastime, but she hadn't actually *clapped eyes on her* since she moved to Scotland nearly 20 years ago. (Whether she'd spoken with her over the Christmas period just ended, I really can't recall).

The second death was, both literally and emotionally, more 'close to home', though, (the deceased having been a near and long-standing good neighbour, living only a dozen or so doors, and barely 200 yards, away until her demise), and was recorded in the logbook thus...

Feb. 9th (Sat): "T rang to say Marlene H had died. Told Mum immediately, during lunch, as she'd overheard my chat and picked up on my subdued tone with T, and kept asking 'What's happened'? Was getting worked up. Was upset, and tearful. Said, 'Oh, poor Marlene. It makes you frightened. And those poor kiddies'. Later went shopping at Aldi's. Mum seemed OK on leaving".

Feb 12th (Tues): "Mum & I bumped into Marlene's husband & daughter in Tesco's. Confirmed Marlene died last Weds 6th. To be cremated next Thurs. 14th. Mum offered her condolences. I said she wasn't well enough to attend funeral. L covering for me on Thurs".

As I say, the imparting of the news of these two 'new' deaths seemed to leave its' *own* mark on Mum. It was the first time too (but wouldn't be the last), that I'd heard her dwell on either the *thought* of being 'frightened', in general, or the specific phrase, 'It makes you frightened'. (See quote of the 9th).

Then, and threatening to 'add insult to injury', up cropped another potential problem, this time one that I'd prayed (to the ether) would *not* arise as we became increasingly committed in our support to Mum - a problem with one of we 'carers'.

Feb 25th (Mon): "L not too well. Old gall bladder complaint has returned. I can cover Weds PM if needed; as well as Thurs. Mum aware, and getting anxious. Have told her it's not serious. Try to play it down." (T)

Luckily, at this stage my sister's complaint wouldn't worsen substantially, but would occasionally flare up again. With the help of prescription medication, however, she would recover sufficiently to carry on, for now, with the bulk of her visits and input; but it gave fair warning of 'time out' for a future operation ahead, and rise to yet another 'wing' of Mum's care that we had to cater for.

Anyway, this 'turn of the year' run of unhelpful news certainly seemed to have taken its toll on Mum; leaving her more tired, forgetful, harder to motivate, with poorer concentration, and, in consequence, generally more fragile, and less confident. As well as (involuntarily) incubating any Dementia factors, she now seemed to be regularly hosting many of the classic signs of anxiety and depression, to boot. So, whilst fielding my share of both the everyday 'mundanery' of Mum's needs and predicament, plus those presented by the current downturn, and not for the first time, during my ongoing, but generally unproductive, mostly random, and increasingly despondent, search for likely causes, (let alone 'solutions'), I alighted again on a familiar 'chief suspect', and still a recurrent source of worry for me, that of her prescription medication; and, perhaps more pertinently, any associated 'side-effects', that might yet be influencing her mindset.

Feb 26th (Tues): "Stupidly took Mum to cemetery this afternoon. Far too cold. Came back shivering & felt unwell, until warmed up with tea & toast & hot water bottle. Ok when I left. Just logging in case of any after-effects".

(I included this succinct log as a chastening reminder that, despite my best intentions at all times, and my sporadic, frustration-based, criticisms of others' shortcomings, I often 'got it wrong', myself!).

29th Mar (Fri): "Batteries needed for clock" (T)

2nd Apr (Tues): "Batteries found in cupboard. Just 'cos she *says* she's 'got none' doesn't mean she's 'got none'. Always worth checking these days – be it batteries, sugar, beans, etc."

This was now typical of the sort of the developing and disquieting 'forgetfulness' that we were meeting all too often. When drawing up a shopping list with her, for example, she would now regularly claim *not to have* something 'in stock', when even a cursory inspection of the relevant cupboard, or whatever, would reveal that she did indeed already have the said item(s) in there. It was like she couldn't, (as in didn't know how to), or couldn't be bothered to, check such basic things for herself at present, and opted to just play safe by *presuming* she had none. (It was just so unlike the domestically well-organised Mum we'd known 'down the years'). I discussed the problem with my siblings, of course, and on each occasion could not prevent myself from further raising my concerns about the likely role that her medication might still be playing; and indeed whether she was still even *taking* the correct dosage on *every* occasion, despite the 'egg-cup' approach! We resolved to try and see what information we could 'dig up' but our resolve was further, and quickly, compounded when this happened...

6th Apr (Sat): (I would henceforth deem it 'The Don't Know Where I Am Incident', or, for convenience, just 'The Incident'; also see earlier).

It was early evening, and a pleasant Spring Saturday on the 6th of April 2013. We had only recently returned from our usual supermarket shopping trip, had put our buys away, and had eaten. All without problem; though Mum was tired now. We were just relaxing together in the comfort of her familiar living room. Mum was ensconced in her favourite fireside chair by the window, (with one eye watching the 'world go by' beyond), and I was comfortably couched nearby in the middle of her beige 2-seater sofa. We were both ostensibly watching TV. (*I* was waiting, apprehensively, for the latest Oldham Athletic result to trip through on the BBC's 'Final Score' football printer). Mum had already been quiet for a while, when she slowly seemed to become the more so; that is, more noticeably, and more deeply, so; and then she seemed to become sort of remote and 'vacant', and more than a little disorientated, pre-occupied, and detached from her familiar surroundings and whereabouts. Her faintly gurned facial tics and contortions clearly signalled something more than just day-dreaming, and that she was really struggling to make sense of something. But it wasn't something on television or out in the street. She was still looking at the TV, but now seemed to be looking right through it, and not really *watching* it at all, if you know what I mean. Her eyes were open, but they weren't 'active', and her mind was clearly elsewhere, and more inward looking. She seemed strangely self-absorbed and her 'look' had definitely moved towards troubled. For the moment, she didn't even seem to notice that my own gaze had now shifted firmly in her direction; nor cared, as far as I could discern. Even when I actually spoke up, and quietly asked her if she was "alright", in a bid to try and gently break the focus of her apparently imprisoned mind-set, she seemed not to hear me. Instead, she still seemed abnormally fretful and self-engrossed; yet when I enquired a second time, but at a decibel higher, she did seem to have heard me, and began looking around for recognisable 'signals' that might help her to 're-connect' to the moment, to the present, and to the current reality. She was clearly pretty *confused* still...when she turned slowly towards me and quietly piped up with, "I don't know where I am, Keith"; and began to cry.

As I've noted earlier, the 'incident' itself was short-lived, (probably lasting no more than 5 minutes), but it was still very traumatic, (for us both), and it took all my emotional dexterity, and all my social work skills, to support the situation without 'blinking' myself, and to bring it, and Mum, back to something that resembled 'normality' on the day; thankfully, and for the moment, though, I *had* been able to do so. And on we went.

My sister had already agreed to contact the GP's surgery, and now did so with additional urgency on the very next Monday, (the 8th), regarding both our latest and our continuing worries here; the upshot of which, remarkably, was an almost immediate home visit (exact date surprisingly unlogged, probably the 10th, but definitely before Thurs. the 11th of that month, 'cos see logs of that date, and mine of the 13th), from the surgery's attached 'specialist nurse', and in the presence of my sister. It resulted, to my amazement, (and I assumed with the prior agreement of the GP), in the *immediate, there and then,* cessation of 2 of those prescription drugs, (the Simvastatin and the Bendrofluazide that Mum had been taking for at least 2 years! (The Simvastatin, we understood from the package's leaflet, had been prescribed to help manage a patient's cholesterol levels, but carried the potential side-effects of feeling weak and of dizziness, whilst the respective Bendrofluazide leaflet suggested that it was a diuretic, or 'water' tablet, prescribed for hypertension, and used to clear excess water from the patient, but carrying the, albeit 'mild', potential side-effects of fatigue and pins and needles. Of course, my nagging worry here was that, (certainly to someone struggling with the symptoms and confusions of Dementia, and especially following 'the incident'), even the relatively 'mild' side, or withdrawal, effects of either of these drugs, (and indeed any others), to a clinician, or other compos mentis user, might just as easily be received, experienced and interpreted as 'strange', anxiety-provoking, or worse, by the unsuspecting Dementia sufferer.

My brother's next entry into the logbook, on the *morning* of Thurs. the 11th of April, had followed this up, then, by simply listing her 3 *remaining,* and most long-standing, medications, ready for well-intentioned progression; but then, before adding anything else of relevance, simply logging that he was heading off to buy lunch; thus...

"Captain's log 11.4.13
Carvedilol (heart)
Amlodipine (legs)
Clopidogrel?
Going for fish & chips"

I'd already taken the bait here, and was 'ahead of the game', so to speak, by having looked online to see what more I could find out about them there; and I'd also spent much of my 'down time' having 'a jolly good think' about any further workable ways to improve things for Mum; both medically, and domestically; thus, at some point during my *afternoon* 'shift', on that same day, I logged,

11th Apr. (Thurs): "Dr. Keith advises:-

Clopidogrel – Prevents Blood Clots – reduces risk of thrombosis – thins the blood, helping it flow more easily. That's probably why it's harder to stop bleeding when Mum cuts herself. May account for some of her 'pain' e.g in her legs – the thinner blood flows better but still has to carry her normal bodyweight.

<u>Amlodipine</u> – supposed to stop blood pressure rising too high; but lists headache, confusion, visual disturbance, back pain, increased need to urinate – to name a few – as possible side effects. Enough to make your blood pressure rise!

<u>Carvedilol</u> – a 'beta-blocker' used to treat high blood pressure, heart problems. As you know, I'm still not convinced Mum ever had a heart problem. Side effects include dizziness, unusual tiredness, lack of energy, & nausea! Just these 3 pills taken together, over time & it's no wonder she's not always herself".

Having racked my brain, over several days, to try and come up with *some* way of helping her, in the face of this suspected downturn and deterioration in her functioning, and drawing, as so often, on my years of social work experience, assessments and training, I came up with a 2-pronged 'attack' Firstly, and following from the above, (basic), digging / 'research' into her long-standing prescription pills, I suggested that, medically, we needed to raise our concerns yet again with the GP; this time regarding the continued appropriateness and potential effects of even the 3 remaining, (and most long-standing), items of medication. Secondly, and domestically, I came up with the idea of invoking what I termed "The Three Rs", as a *practical,* but easily remembered, way to try and introduce some additional consistency for Mum, in the face of any 'rooting' uncertainty or confusion, on the home front, and thereby, hopefully, improve things for her. (Also see earlier). Thus, my log of the 11th of April finished with my intentionally 'throw-away' introduction, for others' initial perusal, and for further thought and discussion, of the following postscript.

"Ps When dealing with Mum I recommend:- the '3Rs':-

1. Routine
2. Reassurance
3. Repetition/Reminders

Pps Dr Keith has now left the building."

By the Saturday, (and not just for posterity), I had also (re)-checked online regarding any likely withdrawal effects, and previous side effects, of her recently, (and hastily), revoked Simvastatin and Bendrofluazide in the hope that we wouldn't be taken entirely unawares should Mum display any (further) associated changes. Thus, my next log read,

13th Apr (Sat): "So both the [Simvastatin & Bendrofluazide] have been stopped <u>suddenly</u>! Normally you would expect them to be withdrawn 'one at a time', & slowly; e.g. withdraw Simvastatin, say, every 3rd day, then every 2nd day etc, until its influence has left the body. Then same with Benzo. Poor practice to withdraw <u>both</u> & <u>suddenly</u> in my eyes. Would not be surprised if Mum does not have some 'funny turns' over next couple of weeks, maybe more tired, irritable etc whilst 'adjusting'. That said, she's made a start, so we might as well help her stay off both now we're under way. She may need us to be <u>more</u> sensitive & supportive for a while. Remember the '3Rs' (Routine, Reassurance, Repetition). Mum said she woke up 'confused' this morning; could well be withdrawal effects, adjusting to the 'loss' of the effects of these tablets after being on them for so many years.

Later, up to 2-00pm Mum was 'whingy' & reluctant to go out. My tactic: <u>One step at a time</u>:

1. 'Let's just try getting ready, Mum'.
2. 'Let's just go for a drive where you're just sitting'.
3. Whilst out – 'How do you feel now, Mum'?
4. 'Not too bad', she says.
5. 'OK, let's drive to Aldi's. We don't have to get out if you don't want to'.
6. Arrive Aldi's. Mum says 'I'll try'.
7. Reassurance – 'Good'.
8. She coped perfectly well in-store once her mind was <u>distracted</u>.
9. Came back – she was in a much better mood."

It would have been easy to have accepted Mum's poor mood, and just reinforce it, by languishing indoors watching TV, but, thankfully, I was in the mood for NOT giving in to *her* mood on that occasion, and for looking for something to try and both stimulate and distract her, and we'd both been suitably 'rewarded' for our efforts by Mum's much improved change of mood. So, I'd logged this step-by-step account of what turned out to be quite a successful, mood-changing, afternoon drive out, and culminating in our scoot round Aldi's, to try and show what was possible, and that gentle perseverance, resilience, and not giving up, *could* bring positive rewards; not only as a confidence-building re-read for *me* on future 'downbeat' occasions, (and there would be many), but also in the hope that my *siblings* would note the possibilities, and not take the easy, stay-at-home, do-nothing, option themselves.

16th Apr. (Tues.am): "If Mum's legs ache she stood for 45 mins watching out of window, 2 men sawing a tree down. She was full of chat for over 2 hours". (T).

Mum had been saying that her legs had been aching more in recent days (despite the Clopidogrel). I have included my brother's full but succinct log here not only to illustrate the stark contrast in mood, compared to that of the 13th, but also because it gave fair 'early-warning' that there would be good days, not-so-good days, and distinctly bad days ahead, and that Mum's mood and mindset would become increasingly unpredictable, from here-on in. Hence, on the:

18th Apr. (Thurs): "Not a great day - not helped by weather, and by fact I had dog with me today. Says 'weak', and moaning about 'legs', 'arm'. Managed to coax her out for drive, to newsagent for local rag, and briefly to cemetery. Better than nothing. Put her legs up on a chair for 10 mins when we got back. Seemed to help. She then got up and made beans on toast for tea. Perhaps L is right - we need something to put her legs on. Later, complained of poor vision in right eye (we know she has a floater there). Soon cleared when she settled. OK on leaving"; whilst on the very next day, the:

19th Apr. (Fri): "Mum in good spirits. Very chatty. Eye not mentioned. Seemed good on her legs. (Had a plaster on small cut on her leg)". (T)

Another useful, yet succinct no-trouble, offering from my brother. (Mum even appeared to have dealt appropriately with a cut she had sustained to her leg during our absence).

22nd Apr. (Mon): "Went Post Off. Had toasted t-cake & custard out. Mood ok at the moment. [Cut on] Leg doing ok". (L).

23rd Apr. (Tues.pm): "No major issues – just ups & downs re 'tired'; but managed Tesco OK. *Later* – complaining of 'upset stomach' – went out for Boots Salts – seemed to help a bit. Finally, covered the leg sore with dry lint, for bed. Mum didn't want it but coaxed her to just have it covered".

To reiterate, all three of us were beginning to experience 'mixed' days and reception with Mum; and then, due to my partner's changed (to full day) work requirements on most Thursdays, I was also required to bring our lively 2 yr. old Cocker Spaniel, Molly, with me on those days; rather than leave her alone and unattended for up to 8 hours. That had pros and cons too. Molly provided useful in-house distraction and furry positive *stroking* comfort for Mum, but, in truth, the dog's busy presence and needs would come to add yet more on-visit pressure and responsibility to my Thursday 'shifts', whilst limiting the out-of-house options for us.

25th. Apr. (Thurs): "Mum OK on arrival, but went into 'tired' mode after dinner. We had a sleep, & by 2-30 Mum was better. Given rainy day decided not to exert her further. Walked dog for [local paper]. Mum more lively by time I returned. Had beans on toast for tea. Mum said 'tablets due' and she was right. Checked boxes & all dates to 26th (tomorrow). Rang chemist. They promised to deliver 'remaining 3' tomorrow afternoon. Whoever coming Fri might want to check with chemist; 'cos if they don't arrive Mum will have none left, and the potential for anxiety will be high!! Leg seems to be healing OK. After tea Mum was 'frightened'; wanted doctor to give her 'tablets' to stop 'fear'. Had panic attack and said she couldn't breathe. Got her to sit quietly, and breathe slowly & deeply 2 or 3 times. She improved slowly, but then 'tired' again. Has happened before as my time to go has approached. OK in the end".

27th Apr. (Sat): "Stardate Apr 27th. Please find enclosed copies of stuff on anxiety. Read as your 'homework'. Oh what fun!

Arrived to find Mum weepy. She said she'd been fine until 'an hour ago', but now 'frightened', and 'not able to go shopping'. She had made my dinner though. She went to loo and pronounced her crap 'normal'. Said she was 'thrilled to bits', but 'weak'. Had sleep. Seemed better, & to have forgotten she was frightened. The change was <u>remarkable</u>. She made a cup of tea & when I suggested going to Aldi again, she just got ready and came. Once out she bucks up significantly, again shows the benefit of persevering/ distraction. 'I get frightened' is now a common utterance - seems to be fear of being alone & too quiet. Try it yourself sometime. It can feel weird. Reiterated the <u>good</u> things she did today".

Mum had never been afraid of being alone pre-onset-of-Dementia, and had, for example, revelled in singly looking after our previous dog whilst my wife, daughter and I went on holiday on occasion; for example the 2 weeks, in the autumn of 1996, (yes, later in the year that Dad died), whilst we went on our pre-booked holiday to Disneyland. Whenever she took on similar such roles though, she did it willingly, well and without problem. Consequently, and especially with due hindsight, I'm convinced that it was the onset of the mental 'blocks' caused by the Dementia that came to cause the "fear"; and hence its' appearance later, in other 'safe' settings, such as the care home and the hospital.

"Stay calm when the anxiety attacks happen. <u>Remember</u> - we stay calm & pass calm (Reassurance) to Mum. Not she gets anxious & passes it to us. (NB Read the Boots letter - what the F is that all about. Might complain. Now <u>we've</u> got to remember to order the stuff 7 days before; a recipe for trouble if ever I saw one. Later on, Mum getting upset & 'frightened' because she couldn't remember what tablets to take. Went through it umpteen times. 'One of each taken each morning from the egg-cup, Mum & 1 more [carvedilol] taken after tea. OK?', I repeated. I get the impression she hasn't been taking the evening heart tablet sometimes. We need to be consistent; otherwise she'll <u>never</u> stabilise".

This was one of my longer logs to date. It touched on several, and *varied*, topics as they arose. There would be longer ones; not least because, as Mum's Dementia problems slowly increased in both frequency and complexity, *I* increasingly felt the need to try and offer my *siblings* whatever relevant (social-work-type) advice I could muster, in consequence.

29th Apr. (Mon): "P Office done. Tablets a <u>mess</u>. All over the place – need to talk about this – found 3 heart tablets in egg cup" (L).

My sister was so freaked by the 'mess' she found regarding Mum's tablets that she went straight out and bought something called a 'dosette box' from the nearest chemist, to replace the egg-cup. They come in various sizes, but, as mentioned elsewhere, this one was a thin, rectangular, 6" long, white-plastic, container/organiser, separated into 7 equal sections; and each with a 'light-clip' lid; each with a day of the week (Sun Mon Tues Weds Thurs Fri Sat) printed on it in sharp, contrasting, black. My well-meaning sister had then filled the container with the correct combination of tablets for the rest of the week, and decided to take the rest of them home with her so that Mum couldn't make further such 'messes'. Thus, when I arrived on the next day, I was confronted by the new system... and Mum's *latest* source of confusion!

30th Apr. (Tues): "[Mum] still confused about tablets. Asking 'Where are they?' Also, the container works Sun to Sat; so tablets will have to be put in on a Sat for the Sunday morning. Bring them back, put them upstairs, & I'll fill the container each Sat, for the week. Mum fine around Tesco's. Bumped into relation of CH [old neighbour], and then cousin Sue; daughter of Vera. Mum OK for rest of day; but will need Reassurance about tablet system for a while yet. Apart from that she's been as 'normal' as I've seen her for a while. All good".

1st May. (Weds): "In good mood. Quite alert again & chatty. Went through pills again. Seemed to have grasped it". (T).

2nd May. (Thurs): I arrived (with dog) to find Mum a little 'down'. Mum openly tells me she feels "frightened sometimes", and that her legs are "weak". I immediately went into '3Rs' mode, chatting quietly with her and concentrating on quiet Reassurance; and Mum was soon up and making our soup lunch. Coincidentally, my latest home research (internet) meant that I was also carrying a new, (and hopefully both physically and mentally beneficial) 'trick up my sleeve' today; and after lunch I managed to persuade Mum to join me in the inaugural session of some simple 'breathing and relaxation exercises', gleaned from the on-line, NHS website. These would become our *regular* after-lunch exercises, following which Mum would usually have a short nap of about half-an-hour, and awake the better refreshed and ready to tackle the afternoon fare; usually involving going out somewhere.

On this first occasion all went well, and afterwards, she readily agreed to a short walk round the (local) cemetery with the dog. There she met and chatted nostalgically with a woman who had known her deceased sister, and all was going well, until Mum suddenly decided she didn't feel well, and couldn't see properly. We headed home. There it emerged (can't remember how) that Mum had been out in her *reading* glasses! Once made aware of this her anxiety subsided, and after a long-blown 'raspberry of realisation' a relative confidence returned.

Around tea-time I (magically) produced Mum's evening heart tablet, and of course, my attentive Mum's first question was, "Where's that come from?". (She thought that my sister was still holding them, and we hadn't said otherwise, in case Mum went looking for them upstairs in our absence). I was forced to tell her that I'd brought it with me; only adding to the confusion. (Well, what would *your* response have been?). Mum then sensibly suggested the pills should still be kept at the house, in case the 'bringer' can't come, and she's then got *none* to take. I had no answer to this, beyond saying we need to discuss the matter again with T & L, and we go on to talk about other things, have tea, and watch some TV. Before I leave though, I log roughly as above, but suggest that, in the meantime, we each log daily that we have either put out or given the single, evening, Carvedilol heart tablet just to be sure. It's been a long, but reasonable, day, and Mum is fine when I head for home.

Mum then continued in similar, but relatively settled, mode for the next few days, with the only log worthy of note being my 4th of May recording for my siblings that her tablets were now located "in the bottom-front-right-corner of the upstairs cupboard". Accordingly, I was logging much the same on

6th May (Mon): "Seems to be always in 'tired' and 'can't go out today' mode when I arrive. But with coaxing always does. Lovely day. Too nice to stay IN. Went [WH] Garden Centre. (There was horse-riding going on – but couldn't get Mum to go on one!). Bought Begonias for graves. OK for rest of day. In fact quite lively for her these days".

For whatever reason, I had covered my sister's Bank Holiday Monday 'shift', and she had agreed to cover the morning of the following Tuesday, and had had a very different experience, leading to *this* (perhaps a tad *over*-reactive) log...

7th May. AM Tues): "Worst day of my life. Went [next town]. Big mistake – [Mum] Had a funny turn. Went in cafe – needed toilet – had poo. Went on about it and washed her hands in toilet bowl! Not good at all". (L); which I read when I arrived PM; and responded thus:

"Had to laugh about above. HA HA HA. Would have laughed longer, but I too had difficult early afternoon...weepy, 'frightened', 'can't go out today' pattern. Pretty similar at present. I do think they're anxiety attacks, accompanied (classically) by depression and 'fear' that 'somethings going to happen'. Had sleep. [Mum] woke confused, but had forgotten her 'fear'. She did express her confusion, in knowing she'd been to [next town], thought she'd been to Post Office (she had), but confused that I was here 'on a Monday' (it's Tuesday); shows the importance of Routine; I think today's confusion is based on change to Routine; and anxiety attack appears to have been triggered by anxiety-provoking need to go to public toilet in [next town]. Mum reluctant to go Tesco's. Says 'weak' and me 'forcing' her to go. I said she needed milk, and offered bags of Reassurance, and she slowly got ready. Once in car, distracted by passing sights, she was happy to go round Tesco's, and improved as we went...so much that she then suggested we go round cemetery too! Took her home, and she did seem tired. She made tea. Gave her the evening tablet. No questions asked. Suggestion; May have overdone things today in rush to 'distract'. Perhaps best to limit trips out to 'safe'/ local

91

settings of about 1 to 1 and a half hours max. per day, 'cos not a good day today".

8th May. (Weds): "Called unexpectedly – was fine & having dinner + no tears yet. Very alert. Left tablet". (L); whilst, and in similar positive vein, I opened my log on the following day with:

9th May. (Thurs): "Arrived to find Mum in best mood I've seen for ages! Really surprised me after last few days. Brought her a pouffe for her legs. After lunch and 'exercises', drove for [local paper]; then cemetery. Mum stayed in car 'cos raining; I walked dog to dad's grave. 4-o'clock tablet given. (a bit reluctantly, as she had had such a good day so far; and I didn't want to spoil it). And Eureka! 4-35 Mum complaining of 'dizziness' & 'not well'. Started to say she wouldn't take 4-o-clock tablet anymore. Became very argumentative. L arrived & further discussion. Suggestion (esp T @ Friday) – do NOT put out the 4-o'clock tablet on Friday; and let's see if she copes or still rings someone. I suspect the effects of the 4-o'clock tablet cause anxiety & then she rings someone. 7-o'clock & all's well". (By the time I left, and had fallen back on the '3Rs', Mum had long since returned to calm, and had readied for bed without issue).

10th May (Fri): "Called with Sue. Stayed for dinner. Found her alert & chatty. Did not mention the tablets until we were going. Explained what was going on [with the evening pill tonight]. She seemed to accept it. What will happen tonight? Will I get a call? She has knocked the scab off an old cut. Sue bathed it and put some cream on. [Mum says] has been putting her feet up on the pouffe". (T).

11th May (Sat): "Arrived to find Mum OK, but 'tired'. Had dinner. Seemed chatty. At one point said, 'I think I'm coming back to myself', but then 'tired' again. Filled white thing with tablets for the week. Told her 4-o'clock tablet not necessary at present. Seems OK with that. (I'm not aware of any issues on Fri night). NB Here are some notes on use of the 3 tablets + side effects. Feel free to copy but keep main copy inside this log for ref. – common to all 3 is possibility of fatigue + dizziness, as side effect. (NB. Will need to tell chemist by Fri that pills need renewing). Went Aldi without problem. Walked up High St to chemist. 'Tired' & 'a bit frightened' back at home, but OK after rest. No 4-o'clock tablet given. Mum worried about [grand-daughter's precautionary] trip to eye hospital. 4-55. No obvious reaction to not taking 4- o'clock tablet. Seems OK. 6-o'clock – L rang. 'Some improvement' re [grand-daughter's] eye problem. Mum (& I) much relieved. Mum washed her feet, & I tried to cut her (thick) toenails. May be worth asking GP for chiropodist visit. 7-o'clock and all's well. After-thought/reminder – [my partner] in Turkey for 2 weeks from Mon the 13th – so I'll have dog when I visit. Might make shopping more difficult".

Within the realms of the changed, (to less confident), moods of recent weeks, Mum appeared to be going through a *relatively* 'settled', 'chatty', few days. (Handily, and thankfully, coinciding with the bulk of the 2 weeks that my partner was away on holiday, and whilst I, in consequence, had the dog in 'full' tow). That said, the foregoing still served to remind us of the fairly-well established mixed ('some good, some not so'), mind-sets that, by now, we'd been coming across on a day-by-day basis with Mum; and of the still oft-recurring times where 'tired', 'frightened', 'something might happen', and emptying her bowels regularly, plus the seemingly never-ending 'pills' issues, continued to need our close and careful management. On the other hand, they showed that Mum was still relatively compos mentis, (most of the time), and *aware* of (conscious of) at least *some* of the more 'vacant' moments, and debilitating effects, that the Dementia was continuing to put before her. Indeed, her ongoing attempts to try and resolve things here were (and would remain) behind a large part of her increasingly obvious frustration with her condition.

And, for me, all this still served to further reinforce, and to suggest evidence for, my long-standing suspicions about the effects of the prescription medication. On a wider front, it also highlighted the fact that, regardless, life was still going on elsewhere, (even within our own lives and set-ups), and was bound, occasionally, to impinge on, and sometimes complicate delivery of, our support to Mum; as in having to bring our dog with me on all my visits over the next 2 weeks, whilst my partner took her holiday. (Alas, *Mum's* daily needs and predicament meant that I currently felt distinctly uncomfortable about being 'off the set', so to speak, and taking one myself).

All that notwithstanding, there were still plenty of *practical* domestic problems to keep us busy during the 'lull'; such as a problem with the use of her Post Office card, and the need to renew it for her, a problem with her TV that required my brother's late-night call-out, and some runny-nose symptoms of a cold, that thankfully seemed to respond to the over-the-counter hot-lemon drinks, and didn't progress beyond that.

Once again, though, even this relatively settled period wouldn't (couldn't) last and it wasn't long before we found that *the statutory agencies* were 'back into the frame'.

16th May (Thurs PM): "Already moaning when I arrived with dog. No shopping in – basics like bread and milk needed. Can't take Mum shopping whilst I have dog. Had to leave dog with Mum & go alone. Short trip to cemetery, but Mum not confident & holding on to me all the way. On return Mum very 'frightened' for a long period. 5-00pm wanted me to call Dr. – for tablets [for fear]. Said she felt 'dizzy'. I made the tea today. Worst I've seen her for several days. Maybe a GP home visit might be reassuring. There is a pattern of unpredictability, anxiety/panic on a regular basis, and a consequent reluctance to go out. GP visit might boost confidence again. She asked me to stay several times around tea-time; but by 7 – o'clock wanted me to go - appeared to have forgotten the earlier upset".

17th May (Fri): I rang Mum in the late afternoon, as was my norm on my 'days off', only to find both my siblings still in attendance, having visited, gone home, but been called back by a very anxious, pretty weepy, 'frightened' Mum, who was having one of her worst 'attacks'. They had therefore been present for most of the day, so I agreed to drive over to take on the evening shift and give them both a break. I also wondered if they might be tiring, and starting to show their own anxiety, and if Mum might calm better if just she and (a relatively fresh) I sat quietly together. Not least because my worried sister had already called the local social services for advice, and had been told that someone going under the grandiose title of the "Community Assessor" would apparently deal with the referral; but coming so late in the day and working week, that it would not now be seen/ read by that designated 'grandee' before early Monday. So they had simply been given an 'out-of-hours' number to ring, but only for absolute emergencies.

Before my siblings departed, I was able to tell them that I had, coincidentally, telephoned the GP's surgery and that a Dr. Ahmed (not his real name) was coming for a home visit/meeting @ 12-30 on *Tues.* next; and also that I'd telephoned the chemist for delivery of due prescription on *Thurs.* next. Once alone, I got Mum to sit quietly with me in the front room, as planned, and tried to calm her down: first by gentle and repeated Reassurance, (that 'nothing is going to happen'), and then by attempting just a couple of deep breaths, and sit-down exercises for the hands and feet; and then simply let her nod off naturally for a short nap; and what followed was much more encouraging, and was logged thus:

"5-30pm: Mum made soup for tea, and we shared a toasted tea-cake. She then made brews ok; so I was sure she wouldn't starve; & she seemed better for having actually done something. She then washed up. Then she got frustrated and we argued, (can't recall what about, but was definitely something petty); but again she seemed better for the argument. – Hey, & what about this? – she let out a large fart (yes fart) & when I asked her, [tongue-in-cheek], when she'd bought a new motorbike, she actually saw the funny side and laughed long and loud. It was lovely to see. Later, I found her outside sorting the bin. Seemed more settled at last... almost back to normal. As I left she was 'tired' & 'ready for bed'. 7-30- All's well that ends well. I hope".

At home I rang my siblings to update them; reminding them, as tactfully as I could, to employ the '3Rs' wherever possible, and of the need to try and prevent our own anxieties from showing in Mum's presence. Thankfully, neither had heard anything further from her since I left. We were all agreed that it had been the worst day we'd faced to date; but, of course, we hoped it was a 'one-off', and over. It wasn't; and lead to one of my *brother's* lengthier logs.

18th May (Sat): "Came up at 9-30 [am] after she cried on the phone. Made a phone call to Keith. When I came off the phone she more or less told me what we had been talking about and begged me not to put her in a home. Did a strange thing – kept walking up & down the hall from the front door to the back saying she did not want to go in a home & crying. When I went to her she told me to go away or get out. Sat in the chair. In all the time I was here, until 11-30, she did not sit down for more than 10 mins. STRANGE. Worrying to say the least. Then lo & behold we started to have normal conversations and her mind became more or less as it should be and the conversations started to make sense. Fine as I left. 'WEIRD'.' (T)

My sister had also been summoned for late support by my brother, and had logged this...

"Came while T was here. Not bad. Like T said, didn't want to go in a home – now thinks we want to get rid of her. Making Keith's dinner". (L).

Following T's early morning phone call, I had no idea what to expect, and I arrived for my set afternoon 'shift' with more than a touch of trepidation; yet my logged contribution read:

"Sat. Part 3 - pill boxes refilled for week. L still here. Read logs. L left. I let Mum finish the washing up. Relaxation exercises; then 20 mins nap. Mum woke relaxed. Heard her singing (yes LA LA-ing) as she made my cup of tea. (2-00pm). No opposition to going to Aldi. (Weird is the right word for her current unpredictability, mood swings & sudden changes of mind-set).

Met someone she knew outside Aldi & chatted happily to her for a couple of minutes; and also to me on way round. Less confident crossing road to £1 shop. I could feel her grip really tighten on my arm. Returned home & left her to put shopping away while I popped out for about 25 mins. Shopping all away when I returned; but now 'tired' & 'weary' & 'eye playing up'. But she stayed fairly alert. Confidence waned a little after tea but coaxed her along and she held it together well. All very 'weird' today, but 'phew'. 7-o'clock & all's well!"

Mum was clearly going through a particularly bad 'patch', (with the Dementia particularly 'active'), and it had been the second very stressful day in a row; with all three of us involved and drained by another of Mum's currently very hard to read mood swings and states of mind. She had obviously been upset enough whilst on her own to ring my brother early in the day; but then got even more upset when she overheard his mid-morning telephone conversation with me; which had involved the very first mention of whether she could still cope 'home alone', and whether a 'Care Home' might soon have a part to play. The oddest thing for me though, was that whilst she was clearly struggling with some further Dementia-related difficulties, they were not permanently-debilitating ones, in that she was still able to listen in to, and interpret, (accurately), what was being discussed there, and its relevance to *her* situation and not just in isolation!

19th May. (Sun): "Arrived after cutting grass. Got ear-bashing because grass all over kitchen floor. She was alert & chatty. She remembered the woman's name from outside Aldi. The conversation died down for a few minutes and you could see her mind thinking. Then the dreaded statement came. '[T], I don't want to go in a home'. I reassured her that we did not want to put her in a home. She did not mention it again. She went to the toilet twice. All in all a good morning". (T).

Something must have 'stuck', because she had clearly *remembered* both my brother discussing the option of a 'home' with me, on the telephone, on the previous day, (and, indeed, still seemed to be harbouring some worries about the possibility), *and* meeting that old acquaintance outside Aldi's. My brother's Reassurance that we were *not* looking for a 'home' for her seemed to 'do the trick' (at least in the short term), and there followed another couple of *relatively* unproblematic days; certainly ones much lower on the 'trauma' scale for us! On the other hand, my sister's Friday call to the social services had brought a response and this log:

20th May (Mon): "Mum seems happy & well. Went P.Off. Told her next door neighbour had visitors. Never seen her move so fast! Social Services coming Thurs @ 11-30, feel a fraud now!" (L).

What with the booked visit from Dr. Ahmed also due on the morrow, (the Tues), it suddenly seemed like the 'march of the agencies' was in full swing.

21st May (Tues): Following 'House Meeting' with Dr. Ahmed: For this I had provided a printed A4 sheet, (see Appendix 1) with the main bullet points set out, in the hope of both focusing everyone's attention, and reminding *myself* of the matters I wanted to raise. The meeting lasted less than an hour, and the log that I subsequently wrote read:

"Outcome:-

1. OK to knock the night-time Carvedilol 'on the head'. Permanently.
2. Dr. Ahmed to refer Mum for Psychiatric input.
3. Not possible for [the surgery] to offer preventative home visit on a monthly or other basis.
4. Will refer my complaint re Boots to practice manager.

2-00pm [After others left] I made us hot-soup lunch + choc roll & tea (yum yum). Mum already positive that Dr. Ahmed had said there was 'nothing wrong' [with her], and saying 'I'll have to pull myself together now'. After lunch: Relaxation exercises; then she slept for 45 mins. Awoke 3-35. Too late to go out, and Mum had had a busy day. Awoke OK; and seemed quite alert. Actually said again, 'I'm glad I'm OK', after asking what Dr. said once more; and [again seeking] my Reassurance that all was well. 4-15 - She made pastie & chips for tea. Briefly 'scared' when eye played up, but coped ok making tea. [I] was able to use the Dr's 'all-'clear' to continue Reassurance. 5-30 Walked dog. Away 20 mins. No issues on my return. 6-00pm: She asked again what Dr. said. I said 1. Refer to psychologist to see how memory working, 2. Dr. said 'Everything OK for 87'. From lunch onward, generally another good day. 7-o'clock & all's well".

23rd May. (Thurs): Following, (and with specific regard to), the actual, hour-long, meeting with the Social Worker, I had simply logged:

"Met S.W. Gave him copy of my sheet for GP meeting. Discussed all options. Mum will be assessed & an amount of Personal Budget identified for her 'care needs'". (At least in part, the brevity was because, unchangingly, and disappointingly, 'Day Care' appeared to be the main/sole option on offer from the social services, for those Dementia sufferers still living in their own homes).

However, Mum had been present throughout, and it had soon become obvious that she was getting upset, nervous, and fidgety at times, and indeed disturbed to the point of tears on one occasion, by the conversation *about* her going on *around* her without fully including her; not least because her Dementia was preventing her from *fully understanding* what was being discussed anyway. All that notwithstanding, she had clearly picked up sufficient snippets, including mention of the word 'care', to set her on edge, and a-worrying that *something*, some potential change/consequence, was being 'planned' for her. Consequently, with everyone departed, my *post*-meeting logs reflected my efforts to deal with the 'fall-out' here.

As with the GP meeting, then, once everyone else had left, I was required to re-visit the point of the *social worker's* summit in more, oft-repeated, (hopefully) easier-to-understand, detail with Mum; initially over our increasingly routine (Big) soup lunch. "What's he come for?", she had asked repeatedly; both over lunch and beyond.

For some time afterwards, she clearly retained the recollection that someone had been, and had internalised enough to know that the meeting had been about *her;* and her 'care'. More than once, I was required to explain that the social worker had just been here to look at what help *might* be on offer for her from social services; and that 'day care' had indeed been mentioned. (As I say, 'Day Care' appeared to be their main/sole offering for those still living in their own homes). My next brief log that day then read thus:

"Relaxation exercises followed by 35 mins sleep. Woke OK, but not confidently; & not keen to go out. Cuppa later, and she was willing to [come on] drive for local paper". Whilst out, and as if by chance (!), I drove past, (briefly slowing to a stop), 3 of the different Care Homes named by the social worker as also offering 'day-care'; and later logged accordingly:

"1. Ashwood Ho. 'Quiet'. 'Drab' [Mum's words]. Church across; some cars going to nearby [primary] school; but no activity around the house. Rainy.
2. The Moorlands. Only seen from Daisy Lane, but 'No, No, I don't want to go there'.
3. Hillside Care. – worried about distance from home to road; & when we got there, she saw an old guy sat (left) outside in a wheelchair; and said she didn't like it, & was 'too big'. (It was). Back home walked dog while Mum made beans on toast for tea. No problems on return; but kept saying, 'I'll have to pull myself together'; again seems better for having been out. 7-o'clock & all's well."

So we had held 2 home-based 'agency' meetings within 3 days, and despite the conspicuous lack of real 'productivity' from either, both had passed off relatively smoothly, in that Mum's predictable anxieties before each had not spilled over into *prolonged* upset. That said, as I say, her repeated queries, afterwards, suggested that she had taken in just enough from each to tax her mind still, and to leave her, still, with some degree of unresolved worry. It may also have taken something out of her physically, as the next day's succinct log from my brother suggested Mum had quickly slipped back into her (now almost normal), 'tired' mind-set.

24th May. (Fri): "Sue [T's partner] had started to make dinner – [Mum] broke down again. 'Tired' & 'scared' again. Not her best day". (T).

25th May. (Sat am): "Tablets done – seems good but has a cold. Spoke to Matron at Hillside Care – do take day care but patients [have] quite bad Dementia; so maybe not good choice". (L). Whilst following my later 'shift', I was a bit more positive.

"Usual low-key 'tired' stuff when I arrived, but OK; even better after 'relaxation' & nap. Nice & sunny so went Aldi's – no probs. Then to cemetery – no probs. 'Tired' again at home, but OK. She made tea; up & about after that until 6-00pm. Rest. Best I've seen her for some time! Shows what's still possible. Hope springs eternal! Not much else to record. 7-00 o'clock & all's well."

To try and sum up so far - The 'normal', fully compos mentis, fully-coping, independent 'Mum at her best' was becoming a rare sight, and quite hard to track down, let alone tease out and stabilise; yet it still cropped up in various guises, and on enough occasions, and for varying lengths of time, to preserve our ever-fainter hopes that things might *not* get worse. That said, the creeping Dementia appeared to be slowly taking its toll, though, and to have moved her subtly, probably irreversibly, to another level of deterioration; yet certainly not to a level sufficient to prevent her from regularly, and often quite forcibly, making it known that she did not want to leave her own home. Even so, her moods and states of mind were now much more unpredictable, often shifting at short notice, and more frequently underpinned by anxiety ("fear"), and therefore more emotional; and we had felt obliged to at least *seek* further contact, advice, and potentially support 'services' from both the medical and social agencies, in the hope that, in their absence, they might somehow have identified, or come up with, improved options and offers. The recent home meetings, then, represented the renewed, and latest, points of contact. Alas, in reality, neither had brought anything new to put before us by way of support in the community; not least because, as I say, Mum still retained both a sufficient and a significant degree of cognition, in both the general, and in the particular, to know that 'something was going on', and to repeatedly express her wish to 'remain in her own home'. In this regard, though, she knew, for example, that the matter of her 'care' had now been raised both between we siblings, and separately at the 2 recent 'agency' meetings held *in* her home.

Where would we go from here? Well, essentially, it was a case of 'Keep calm and carry on'. However, the pressures were beginning to build.

27th May (Mon): Called. Was crying & scared, having toilet problems. I made toast. Feels sick. Confused. Wouldn't go out for walk. Found half-open sachets of [prescribed laxative]". (L).

28th May (Tues): "8-30am. She phoned at 8-15 feeling frightened. Susan stayed until Keith came. I feel another summit meeting is required and a decision will have to be made". (T).

I arrived for my usual Tuesday afternoon 'shift', to find Mum in her usual 'tired', and downbeat mood, and, having read the above, morning input, had picked up on my *brother's* clearly increasing anxieties; yet, in the light of the distinct lack of new offers from the recent agency meetings, I had soon, and rather frustratedly, even brusquely, logged, in capital letters, thus:

"WHAT ARE THE OPTIONS? THERE'S NO EASY ANSWERS. WE HAVE TO LEARN TO LIVE WITH UNCERTAINTY & NOT BE AFRAID OF IT"!

Luckily, I too had been feeling the pressure, and in my 'clutching at straws' search for something positive to try, had spent some of my 'down time' working on a set of simple but positive MANTRAS that I thought Mum and I might initially repeat together, (and, in time, she whilst alone), from which she (and we) might take heart in times of anxiety. Printed 'landscape', and in capitals, on a white A4 sheet, and in various 'rainbow' colours to attract her attention, they read:

BE POSITIVE
KEEP TRYING
STAY CALM AND RELAX
LAUGH ABOUT IT

I immediately showed these to a rather anxious, fearful, depressed-looking Mum, and then read them out loud to her, before blue-tacking them about 6 ft up in the middle of her least obstructed kitchen wall, where they would be in full view from anywhere in the kitchen. I then persuaded her to work *with* me to make a simple soup lunch, with bread, followed by a fruit scone and cuppa, and logged what followed thus:

"All the while I was offering supportive chat around the 'Be Positive' list on the wall, with the repeated Reminder that every time the panic comes, she works through it, AND NOTHING HAPPENS. Mum already much better – already distracted. 1-20 Relaxation exercises + 35 mins sleep. Woke slowly & still a bit 'frightened'. Suggested we go out. Mum not keen & got worse (!) when I said we needed to go out (for money & basics). She said I was 'forcing' her. Continued to coax, cajole & reassure. BIG MOMENT! – to press on or give in to her renewed anxiety?

My thinking: - Is there any pain? Answer 'No'. What's the alternative? Return to depression of earlier & sit in. Answer 'No way'.

Decision: Press on a step at a time. Helped her get coat on. She was weepy and uncertain. Helped her put her shoes on. Still weepy. Assured her I would 'not leave her'. Shuffled to door & out to car. Immediately a bit better – like overcoming a big 1st hurdle. Drove to P. Office & by time I parked she was ready to come with me. (She had been saying I would have to go in alone). Went to P. Office – drew out [money] together. Back to car ok. Suggested a [drive] to Ashwood Ho. Did so. All quiet. Rainy again. She started to say she wanted to 'stay in her own home' again & would have to 'pull myself together'. On the way to Tesco, decided to review The Moorlands. This time found the entrance. Parked right outside. Could see the day room – no-one in it. However, didn't say she wouldn't go – so perhaps a possibility? Looks nice. Drove to Tesco. Mum Ok by now; but holding on to me until met V&R (my cousin & partner) when she let go of my arm. Shopped OK. No probs. Drove Mum home [& popped out]. Came home. All groceries put away & Mum almost 'normal' again, pottering about. I put it to her that she had tackled the anxiety 'brilliantly' (reward for desired behaviour), and asked her to compare with how she felt this morning – surprisingly (even to me) she could hardly remember *being* upset this morning; again an almost magical change of mood – I'm glad I didn't give in to the Big Moment earlier – because the reward in her changed mood/ behaviour was well worth the (undoubted) risk. She cooked tea OK, and held it together well. Over tea was again saying 'I don't want to leave my house'. 5-30pm minor panic when Mum couldn't find P.Off card; turned out to be in other purse compartment – panic over – shows how easily the anxiety is triggered though &how easily I/you can get sucked in. I had my shoes on ready to go P.O. A tough, but rewarding, day. 7- o'clock & all's well."

29th May. (Weds): "Well what a difference a day makes. Mum more than chatty. When I arrived she was ready for her hair appointments. She said she lay in bed Tues night and thought 'I am not ready for a home and am not going in a home. All they want (the home) is my money and they are not having it'. (Made me laugh). L arrived so I read your saga. Could make a best-selling novel with all that's happening, but all 3 of us would be entitled to any royalties. As I am writing this she is in the kitchen brewing up and singing". (T).

30th May. (Thurs): "9-30am - Came up for flying visit. As soon as I came through the door she was looking for an argument. Told me to get out etc. Never 2 days the same. Would like to know why. Guess what, she wanted to go in a home. L came. She got call at 9-00am. Mum wanted Lemsip & aspirin. Guess what – she [L] took an ear-bashing as well. Your turn next". (T).

For the first time ever, my brother had logged that Mum had now said that she *did* want to go in a home! Was this just to get attention, or a definite change of attitude?

"Arrived to 'Have a cold'. Seems like she might have sniffles. She made [Big] soup lunch OK. 1-00pm Relaxation + Sleep (1hr). Still sniffling – so decided not to take her out. Walked [my dog]. Gone 35 mins. No probs on return – that said, she has been indoors all day, and may be susceptible to more depressive options tomorrow. 7-o'clock & all's well".

And on we went like this, with little change in sight. Sometimes she was in (relatively) good order, sometimes she wasn't. As I've said, her mood was also more susceptible to shifting *during* our visits, these days, too.

For me, however, my necessarily long, usually 7-hour+, stints, (due to living much further away than my siblings), plus my social work background, had actually enabled me to *work on things* with Mum; and a pattern was slowly emerging.

This pattern, of my lunchtime arrival, followed by a Reassuring chat over a simple shared lunch, (invariably Heinz Big Soup these days, though she was still capable of surprising me with something more complicated), continued Reassurance as necessary, my regular referral to, and Repetition of, the 'Be Positive' mantras on the kitchen wall, and the now habitual post-lunch relaxation exercises recommended by the NHS website, followed by Mum having a nap, invariably resulted in a much better waking outlook than when I arrived.

It usually meant that Mum was then in a calmer, more Reassured and better frame of mind; the better to accompany me on, and to further benefit from, the sensory changes and distractions built-in to some sort of social *outing*. (Shopping, walk round nearby cemetery, park, etc).

All in all, putting in a lot of time and 'legwork' *at one go* (compared to the shorter, more frequent, more 'pop-in', versions available to my locally-based siblings), was tending to bring me greater rewards, in the form of a more settled Mum as my 'shift' progressed.

In short, I'd stumbled across a generally serviceable *Routine* that worked pretty well, (both for me and for Mum), during my long (nearly always) afternoon/ evening 'shifts'.

What *was* beginning to emerge now, alas, was a worrying pattern of Mum struggling the more, psychologically, with being on her own for too long; especially overnight, and when faced with any Dementia-lead moments. With her 'independence' worries also taking root, (following the 2 recent, home-based, 'agency' meetings, and her lingering suspicion that we might be 'in league' with them over potential changes to her home/'care' status), and along with the ongoing responsibility for managing her (newly-Carvedilol-reduced) dosette-box medication, (and any side-effects), each morning, I guess being 'home alone', (even *without* any increasingly scary moments of Dementia-lead anxiety), was always going to 'test her mental mettle' anew.

As mentioned, too, (and perhaps not surprising given the foregoing), she had actually said to my brother, on one fleeting and worked-up occasion, that she *did* now want to go in a home. All this tended to *confirm* for me that being 'home alone' for long periods *was* now a significant issue for Mum, (and therefore us); a combination of factors probably preying on her (already mixed-up) mind, and draining her of valuable energy and confidence; and probably contributing significantly to her regular claims of feeling 'tired' and in 'fear', when we arrived or to when she felt upset enough to call one of us. So it was *no* surprise to note that she improved in prolonged, consistent company, and with ready Reassurance, relaxation, distraction, etc, and, therefore, as our day progressed. What to do to help and/or improve things further here, though?

Moving in with her might have seemed one obvious solution, but would have been both logistically impractical, as we each had commitments to service in our own lives, and profoundly unfair, (and potentially damaging), to whoever actually agreed to take on that challenge. Accordingly, and for our own self-preservation, and recuperation, we still tended to agree that the most appropriate maxim to work to was, 'A trouble shared is a trouble halved', if we were to offer Mum our *optimum* support. Moreover, we were equally agreed that a compos mentis Mum would have been *horrified* at the thought of one of her offspring effectively giving up their life to permanently service hers, anyway. And indeed, we were *already* being drained ourselves, by doing everything else *but* move in. The only other option, of course, *was* for her to become 'looked after' in some sort of 'care home'; an option that she was still essentially hostile to, and (with that one fleeting exception), regularly making it known that she did *not* want to take up. Then, just for a moment, and apparently in the 'nick of time', it looked like 'the cavalry' might be 'riding over the hill' to our rescue.

4th June (Tues): "When I arrived [am] she had the settee out and hoovering. Alert & chatty. <u>A message from L</u>. The Mental Health people (1 person) are coming at 10-30 on Thursday. They want to see her on her own and are insistent that none of us are there. L will come up to let them in. Then she will go home and await a phone call from them. Then come back up. L knows the person who is coming. They want to see her at her worst to assess the situation. Its odds on she will have a good day. She does not know they are coming yet". (T).

At the end of that same day's afternoon shift, I had taken up the cudgels here, and logged:

"She was in quite a good mood, & over our soup lunch advised her that the 'specialist social worker' [I was trying to avoid the use of the word 'psychiatric'] was coming on Thurs. (6th). Initially saying she did not want to see him/her; cos didn't want to go in a home. Reassured her that it was only to assess memory & <u>advise</u> us of options. Generally came round to the idea...and possibly will see the 'specialist social worker'".

I had jumped in, and tried to prepare the way with regard to the CPN (Community Psychiatric Nurse) visit, but we should've known better!

5th June (Weds): "Rang as usual. Mum not in good mood. Put phone down on me. L took her out but [Mum] became frightened and her legs went. Got call at 1-00pm from L. Felt obliged to come up and give her support. L went to work. Mum went to sleep, woke at 3-15. All the time she was saying she was frightened in the house on her own. Asked why CPN was coming on Thursday. I explained that she may give us some more answers to what her problem was. Reassured her that she was not going in a home. Phone call from L. CP Nurse is NOT coming on Thurs. She has a meeting. Someone will phone L on Friday to arrange another time & day. [Mum had] rallied round and insisted that I went". (T).

The 'cavalry' had beaten a hasty retreat!...and on we went, still battling alone, and 'under our own steam'.

6th June (Thurs): A M: "Arrived she was on one again. Calmed down once she was told that no-one was coming today" (T).

It seemed clear that the impending involvement of the CPN really had been playing on Mum's mind, and the cancellation of the visit certainly seemed to make for an easier afternoon visit for me.

"Arrived expecting the worst, but Mum not bad; apart from usual moans of 'tired' & 'Oh, mi legs'. Having moaned, she then said, 'I don't moan' – I just laughed helplessly out loud and so did she! Relaxation session + 25 mins sleep. Drove for [local paper]; then walk round cemetery with [my dog]. Met someone she knew. Chatted. Generally 'tired', ('oh, mi legs', 'Oh mi back'), but OK through tea/evening. 7-o'clock & all's well".

7th June (Fri): "Called out @ 7-00pm. She said she was frightened. I came up. She was crying. I made her a cup of tea and stayed with her until L came at 8-45. She made some hot milk and gave her some paracetamol. [We] stayed until [Mum] went to bed and was asleep". (T).

8th June (Sat): "Sat Morn – update on last night. We stayed until 11-00pm. Decided not to stay the night as when we checked she was well away. She says she has had no tablets for Sat morn but I am sure she has taken them and forgotten. She had no recollection of what went on on Fri night". (T).

"Sat brainstorm - wonder if Mum might have taken Sat pills last night? Hence the 'kick-off'. She insists she hasn't taken any pills this morning yet can't explain why Sat slot [in dosette box] is empty. T said she'd had soup for lunch, but she put herself some of mine in a bowl, and had more. Relaxation + 30 mins nap; [then] willing to 'try' going out. (For info, SW's no and email is [xxxxxx];. best to have them involved. If you act privately they'll just assume you don't need social services).

Usual shopping @ Aldi without problem! Also walked to Dad's & gran's graves @ cemetery OK. 4-00pm. Still saying she's had no tablets today. And if I'm right, it has major implications (L) for suggesting tranquilisers!! & their side effects! 4-15 & she's saying she doesn't want to go in a home; well there's a surprise. She made tea ok & seems generally ok just now. (I suggested we get full-size cardboard cut-outs of the 3 of us, with attached interactive voicebox, to sit with her when we're not there. She laughed, but could make my fortune). Bye for now".

The matter of her medication had never gone away, but appeared to be raising its ugly head anew. My sister had been coming to the view that a course of tranquilisers might help, but if Mum was now starting to misuse the dosette box too, we *already* had yet another major medication problem to manage. That said, they say that 'laughter is the best and cheapest medicine', (it was also on the 'Be Positive' list), and, Mum had always had a good sense of humour, so it was always worth trying to lighten the mood by cracking a (here the cardboard cut-out) joke with Mum; and if she laughed, I'd log it for my siblings use and amusement!

10th June (Mon): "Called out by Mum at 9-00am. You know the rest. (He had telephoned to update me). She insisted we all went so she could have a sleep and she would be alright. I stayed with her, with L, until 9-00 pm. She went to bed at 7-30pm". (T).

The "rest", referred to above in my brother's brief log included a full, and draining day for my siblings. The fact that so little was logged reflected the hectic nature of events. Mum had been complaining of both high anxiety, and of not feeling well, from 'the off', and had barely improved despite the close attentions of my siblings. My brother had eventually called my sister for support, (both lived just a couple of miles from Mum), and together they had spent *all day* dealing with Mum's claimed state of ill-health. This had included an upset stomach, and attendant toileting issues, in which her 'water' had emerged a deep brown colour. My worried sister had then called the surgery for advice, and had ended up with a home visit from the GP. They then had to be present to deal with that too. The GP had simply prescribed something to calm her stomach, and arranged a precautionary follow-up outpatient/ check-up appointment at the hospital. On the following day my brother was back, and logged thus:

11th June (Tues): "Arrived at 9-30am. You would not think there was a problem. Can't bloody well believe it. Been chatty, alert, doing jobs (including your dinner). Happy to be going to the doctor tomorrow about her bowels etc. L phoned The Mental Health People. Said we would contact them when we needed them. L been for her money & paid papers until July. Fine as I left". (T).

Similarly from my afternoon shift:

"Arrived to quite a good mood today. Over lunch chatted with Mum about yesterday. She had little accurate recollection; for instance, when I suggested her 'water' had been brown, she thought I meant the water coming from the tap and blamed the Water Board! When I asked about the doctor coming, she remembered little, and had no recollection of him seeing her in her bedroom. I'm not going to 'look a gift horse in the mouth'; at present she's talking about a list for Tesco's. I also think we should seek [the CPN's] input as soon as Mum's medical visit & consequences are known; not least because SW will probably be seeking their input for *his* assessment. Relaxation session + 35 mins nap. Drove to Tesco & shopped without problem; in decent mood until I left. Are you sure yesterday (& last Fri) happened, or are you 2 conspiring to drive me to loony bin & claim my fortune. 7-o'clock as all's well".

12th June (Wed Morn): "Received phone call at 8-30am. Guess what. She was on one. Did not go up until 10-00am. She was on one. Eventually calmed down. Just sat and let her calm down by talking etc. Don't know what happens. I just write what I find." (T).

(Afternoon): "Hospital done. A bit afraid and weepy. Mind everywhere – but considering she had a finger up her [bum] twice this week - not bad. Results – scan at [W] hospital within 2 weeks. Not sure what for". (L).

13th June (Thurs): "Thurs. Thinking: Once again Mum seems to improve as the day goes on. Why?

1. Could be mornings are coping with new input of medication which has done its worst by late afternoon.
2. Could be that company (when otherwise too quiet) relaxes her.
3. Could be that stimulus/distraction on the days she goes out changes her mind-set.
4. Could be that it dawns on her 'nothing has happened' after morning anxieties.
5. Could be some other reason (or combination of), who knows?

(Let's organise a raffle in the village, with prize for who gets it right!).

That said, it doesn't take much to 'destabilise' her. Anyway, she made beans on toast for tea, with appropriate 'afters', and caused me no further bother. (Hey, suggestion – cameras in house, kitchen & bedroom?). 7-o'clock and all's well".

Of course, (and probably because I could more easily empathise with 1-5 above), I had completely forgotten to list her Dementia amongst the most obvious reasons for her changes in mood.

14th June (Fr): "Mum thought she was going hospital – didn't know T was away. Fish for dinner. Angela from Mental Health coming Tue 25th June @ 12-30. On hols at the moment. Got emergency numbers if needed". (L).

T was away, and I was covering his Fri afternoon shift but sometimes it's just not your day!

"Well, what a strange day! One where you think you should have stayed in bed!...and not even my normal [visiting]day.

9-00am Rang Mum [to remind her *I* was coming]. Ready for hospital! Not today. Mum upset. Started off with a 'damping' for me and [my dog] about 9-30am near home. Then got proper soaking (enough to hold inaugural meeting of the local Drowned Rat's Society), after further short [dog]walk round [Mum's most local] reservoir.

1-30pm barely dry before L & B [L's husband] left me in the lurch and with news she's going out tomorrow! Mum not in best mood & told me to make my own cuppa. I did, (cuppa & scone), & sat at [kitchen] table to consume. Mum went in house & I thought she'd nodded off, so stayed in kitchen reading the logs, handouts and [Council] bumf.

c.2-30pm (lost track of time) Mum came back & laid in to me, claiming I was not speaking to her, was selfish, always had been, and had 'better go!'. She started to cry, and when I stayed unmoved she rang L & asked her to return. Now you'd think with L not long gone, she'd have gone shopping or something, & with T on his Jollies, Trooping his Colours or something, the chances of Mum finding someone to collude with her [attention-seeking?] looked slim but this was not my day, & yes, L *was* home & came up and on we went. Anyway, L went to work, and to break the negative mind-set, I suggested we go for a drive. Got Mum ready. Got dog ready. Got me ready. Outside front door we bumped into 2 neighbours [for distracting chat]. Where to go? 'Birds'. [This was a small car park near a trail, where people put food out for the birds, which in turn provided distraction at no cost]. Got round there & bugger me the clouds closed in & the heavens opened, with an almighty downpour / thunderstorm. Drove back home. Rain pelting down; thunder and lightning still rumbling away in the distance. Dog unwalked but Mum in a better mood! Once indoors, she made cuppa and then soup & sandwich, and the clouds parted and the sun came out (see what I mean about not being my day). But Mum's mood settled OK, if understandably 'tired' after all that shouting & crying. 7-o'clock & all's well".

The next day, my 'normal' Saturday, was relatively uncontroversial, and the following day, the Sunday, similarly so; but, just to show it was still possible to keep a sense of humour despite the difficulties and drainings of the previous, or other, days, I had gone for a pseudo-biblical, tongue-in-cheek, tone for my next logging.

"Peace be with you. And Lo, it came to pass that Keithus of [my local town] didst journey over to [Mum's village] for a 4th day in a row. And when he came upon Mum he found her sorely moaning & in need of Reassurance. So he set her down upon a chair, and shared chat, relaxation & a 30 mins sleep. And when they awoke, they partaketh of tea & biscuits & lo, the world didst appear better... enough to go forth even into the edge of the land of [the town] & to [local] Garden Centerus where Mum didst exchange coinage for foliage in pots (x 2). And Mum sayeth (without forcing, L), she wouldst have us visit the cemetery and thus we went forth there & paid due homage. And lo, a strange light shone down from the sky, and warmeth all around - aaah. Distracted thus & uplifted thrice we didst return home in good spirits & Mum didst prepare chicken & chips (yummy!), and continued to 'flower'; and peace descended upon this place thereafter. And Keithus returned from whence he came. Thanks be to??? The Dog? 7-o'clock & all's well".

17th June (Mon): T was back from his mini-break, to log:

"Arrived at 9-30am. She must wait for me. She was crying & depressed. [Saying] 'This is not me'. Did calm down after talking etc. [but was] looking for an argument. But I am learning. I kept her talking. What is the answer? I don't know. We will have to see what the experienced people say". (T)

To which I had, at some point, added, both succinctly and cynically, "Wouldn't hold your breath if I were you!!" Thereafter, we enjoyed a few days that, these days, constituted one of our increasingly rare (and relative) 'settled' spells. The next significant interruptions *were* 'agency-induced'.

25th June (Tues): "[Following the CPNs mention of possible medication, expressed my view that I was] not keen on a mental medication-based input; except as very last resort; but Mum nowhere near that bad at present; indeed on a good run. Expressed my view that CPNs read this log from about April to get a progressive view of we 3 siblings' [differing] perspectives. [Argued] that if (theoretically) I moved in with Mum, she would NOT need ANY new medication so use of medication now would be because WE can't be there and not any innate need for it.

CPNs left – back 9-30am on Friday for cuppa & read log. T & L left. Relaxation session + 30 mins sleep. Mum woke 'tired' but persuaded her to go Tesco's. Went OK. No probs. Back late (due to CPNs meeting) for pastie & chips tea. No probs thereafter. 7 o'clock & all's well".

This time the home visit/meeting by the 'agency' workers did not seem to 'throw' Mum, though. She presented no real problems on the Weds; nor for the next day's (Thurs.) logs.

27th June (Thurs): "Arrived 9-30am. Everything ok. Remembered someone coming tomorrow. Remembered the 2 people who came on Tues. Asked what for. She had cut her leg somehow. Got her to clean it up & put a plaster on. L rang. Has left numerous messages for Dr. A' s [named hospital medic] secretary. I also have left a message. At the moment there has been no contact. [Might] see what [GP] surgery can do". (T).

"Arrived to OK Mum. Def on a more positive run. Letter from [hospital] Dr – summarising her trip with L &Sue – mentions Dementia 3x. Lunched ok. For info: have put some stuff on likely (SSRI) medication recommendations from CPNs in back of log – very last resort for me. I think Mum might respond to psychological/behaviour techniques from someone independent, like CPN. Relaxation + sleep. Raining PM; but persuaded Mum to go for drive; *she* suggested brief walk round cemetery – reluctantly agreed, as I had to balance dog-on-lead on left arm, 87 year old on right arm, brolly in middle - now that's magic! Worth the effort, as Mum even better thro distraction. No real problems today, though. Would not like to damage her current good run by further medication. More than willing to try anything non-internal/

non-invasive. As it's more easily reversed if not working. 7-o'clock & all's well".

The letter referred to above was from the Dr at the *Memory Clinic*, at the local hospital, who had conducted the initial hospital-based appointment, and subsequently brought about the CPNs' limited home involvement and assessment. SSRIs (Selective Serotonin Reuptake Inhibitors) are effectively one type of commonly-prescribed antidepressant, but, like all prescribed medication, are not free of side-effects; including ones similar to those she already had to contend with via her *existing* medication; such as the possibility of upset stomach, blurred vision, pain in joints and muscles, and agitation. Nor do they carry any guarantee of success. Not surprisingly, then, I was once again anxious to avoid Mum having to take further such questionable, 'wing-and-a-prayer', medication; especially in the face of any Dementia. For me it was just an easy 'out' for the public 'agencies'; especially when the cost, bureaucratic processes, and limited availability of the likes of interactive, (and therefore more labour-intensive) CBT (Cognitive Behaviour Therapy), had meant that it was not offered first; and, even then, not always without accompanying SSRIs. The very next day's logs tended to point to more (generally inefficient) bureaucracy, and to rather confirm my suspicions and concerns.

28th June (Fri): "Angela [CPN] here – seems ok. Going to get together with [social worker] + GP – coming back Mon morning for another chat". (L).

"L left message with [local hospital] Dr's secretary, because she has spoken to [W] hospital, and they have no record of any appointment for Mum; also [they] do not do that type of scan. [L] is awaiting reply from [local hospital Dr's] secretary, as to what is going on. Mum was ok with Angela. She is coming again on Monday". (T). And again on the:

8th July (Mon): "Nothing entered – L not well. [CPN] was here says Mum. [Other one] coming Fri. says Mum. L phoned about the scan. Mum is on [long] waiting list. She will have to wait her turn. A letter will be sent. She has to have it done at [W] hospital. They have a scanner at [local] hospital but no one is trained to use it. A good morning. Mum ok apart from eye playing up & going to toilet [a lot]". (T).

Luckily, whilst all these 'agencies' appeared to be 'singing from different hymn sheets', and generally faffing about, (with the CPNs appearing to drop in on Mum ad hoc, and reporting little back to us, and the various medics and their respective hospitals and departments apparently unable to sort things out between themselves), Mum was still enjoying her (relatively) good run. On Thurs. the 5th of July, for example, I had actually signed off with, "7-00pm, Isn't it nice to see Mum 'almost normal' again"; whilst on the 13th I was still able to positively log, "Can't believe how much better she's been functioning over the last 2 weeks...relax & prepare for next 'change' while you can", and, (almost the 'norm' in recent days), had abridged many of my other logs to, "usual routine – lunch, relaxation, nap, Aldi, tea, OK".

Yes, and most welcomingly, our respective sibling routines were experiencing a relatively settled spell, with regular 'trips out', (for both grocery and clothing shopping, for lunch, to the Post Office, to the cemetery, garden centre, and local parks, for her hair done), and a few ongoing in-house 'specials', (such as having her carpets steam cleaned, refreshing the jaded emulsion on her living room walls, maintaining and fixing anything that needed it, and planting out fresh plants in both her small back-garden strip, and in the pots she kept indoors on the window sills, etc.). Indeed, anything that we thought might help to maintain and promote Mum's good run and mind-set.

The only minor interruptions during this relatively smooth operational period were our continuing concerns about whether Mum had taken her medication properly, L reporting that she had received notification of a scan booked for Mum for Monday the 5th of August, and, on one occasion, a phone call from an organisation called 'Care-link'. The latter turned out to be a supposed 'support in the community' service linked, (by a button that could trigger a telephone call to the client if the latter pressed it), to a central unit somewhere out in there in the community; which, in turn, would trigger a call to the appropriate 'carers', (i.e. one of us!), if necessary; all of course at a cost to the 'client'. On the latter, my brother had advised that we were still awaiting the completion of relevant medical and CPN involvements and inputs before considering such community services, and had declined the Care-link service at that time.

At least we now had a date for the long-awaited scan; yet we *still* awaited anything *definitive* from either of the 2 CPNs, the social worker, or even GP; indeed, even when the CPN belatedly made contact with me by phone, her latest thoughts (logged below), were hardly encouraging.

23rd July (Tues): "Mum good on arrival. T/C from Angela [CPN] yesterday for update. She told me she tried to assess Mum's memory, but didn't complete it because Mum got anxious whenever she couldn't give answers! So NO memory info! [CPN] again mentioned [SSRI] 'medication' but I was firm in rejecting this esp. as Mum doing so well. [CBT] unlikely as would mean involvement for too long. Only realistic offering – regular visit from a 'carer'; or perhaps a 'sitter' (befriender). Also Day-care. Asked Angela to put her thoughts in writing & leave copies at Mums; and then to arrange a meeting to discuss/ finalise decisions. Told you not to expect miracles!

Have raised above with Mum today, but she's not particularly keen on anything. That's OK while Mum's good, but a 'sitter' might be useful as a friend and to fill in when we're on holiday etc. Feel free to discuss with Mum. Relaxation + nap. Mum woke with problem focusing with eyes – some anxiety. Got her to rest a further 5 mins & focus returned. Shows how easily she can be de-stabilised. Went Tesco. Generally OK. 7-00pm all OK".

24th July (Weds): "Called am – Mum eating breakfast. Worried about her mind forgetting [things]. Reassured her". (L).

"Read the Keith saga. Agree that a sitter or carer should come [on some] afternoons when we are not available. Tried to explain to Mum but she could not, or would not, grasp it. I think the top & bottom of it is that Mum does not want anybody, [but us]. I feel we should stand our ground". (T).

These 2 minimal Wednesday logs put our predicament 'in a nutshell'. Firstly, my sister's succinct *morning* log reminded us that

Mum actually *knew* that she was forgetting some things on occasion. In many ways, this presented the 'worst of all worlds' for her, leaving her sufficiently compos mentis to have her views taken seriously, yet not sufficiently so as to be able to manage the moments when the Dementia triggered vital 'missing links', and threatened to prevent her from having either the ability or the confidence to live as independently as she once did, and would still like to.

Secondly, my brother had already met with some predictable resistance as he'd tried to explain just what might be available, and had identified the key fact that Mum did not really want 'anybody' to interrupt the ideal of her continued independence; with only 'comfort zone' support being provided by the 3 of *us.*

Thankfully, it was late July now, and Mum was still in her good run, ("another smooth operation", "a good morning", and "all's well", typical of our parting inputs into the log-book), so there was no immediate urgency for a sitter/carer; and we siblings continued to take her out, as described, with the minimum of ado. Nevertheless, there were still sufficient "tired", "get a bit frightened", and "want to stay in my own home" moments, to hint that the 'good run' might not (could not) last.

And then, suddenly, there was some 'agency' activity. Or was there?

1st Aug. (Thurs): "Do I take it that scan is at [the local] hospital after all? What are they playing at? Lunch Ok. Relaxation & nap Ok. Chatted about idea of 'sitter' [again]. Mum saying she's 'got us'. [I] said sitter might be useful 'friend' when we're not around & when dark early. Saying she wants to stay in own home, sleeps well, and will 'just have to put up with' dark nights/winter. Mum unable to remember anything specific from Weds visit of Angela & a.n.other. Tea for 2. TTFN".

5th Aug. (Mon): "Hospital done – barium meal, injection in arm, then CT Scanner – she didn't like it. Was trying to get off! – results from GP when they're ready. P.O. done". (L).

9th Aug. (Fri): "Angela came @ 2-30 pm. Stayed 20 mins. A get- together is arranged for Tues. the 20th Aug at 12 noon to assess the options open to us. [CPNs] have made all their visits.

They and [social worker] will have to arrange everything after 20ᵗʰ August". (T).

There were 'hints' of movement, but nothing definite yet; though one worrying thing that definitely occurred anew was:

10ᵗʰ Aug. (Sat): "Tablets done. [Found] <u>shit</u> on floor; cleaned up and [Mum] seems OK. (L).

My sister had simply noted this, (and cleaned it up, of course), but had not expanded on how much, or where it had come from, so that was my first logged query when I arrived later that day for my usual Saturday afternoon 'shift'.

"Shit on floor – where from? Mum 'tired' but OK. Made good dinner. Wasn't aware of 20ᵗʰ meeting. She's not keen on anything. I think the 'sitter', carefully chosen, is still worth 'trialling'; esp thro winter. It doesn't look like CPNs are going to offer CBT for her OCD; otherwise they wouldn't be ending their involvement. (They've been largely a waste of time in my view).

Still need to decide on Care-link option & if included in the £26.50. Mum definitely not keen on Day-Care, but today said it's 'OK if someone wanted to pop in'. Usual routine. No probs. Salmon butties for tea - oooh! All Ok".

I can't recall exactly where the £26.50 figure had come to us from, (probably in the form of a letter), but it represented the weekly allowance that the social services assessment had finally come up with for Mum. She could spend this on the (pretty limited) options available *through* the social services, or any approved *private* possibilities, that might be identified. More worrying to me, though, by far, was my sister's, rather matter-of-fact, referral to "shit on the floor" and an update / possible explanation arrived in her (equally brief, and matter-of-fact,) Monday log:

12ᵗʰ Aug. (Mon):

"P. Office done. [Mum] legs aching and is bored. I think what happened on Sat is – she was weeing in [a bowl in the kitchen]; rather than climb the stairs – but pooed as well. Nice!" (L).

13ᵗʰ Aug. (Tues): AM. "Mum been toilet twice. Very weak after. What are results of scan? Angela coming Weds aft. Said [CPNs] would not be coming many more times. Apparently [social worker] phoned on Sat morn and Mum put phone down on him. Mum had good cry this morning thinking we are putting her in a home because of the meeting next Tues. The honeymoon period could be over". (T).

The clues seemed to be there. Mum had been going to the toilet more frequently. There appeared to be no obvious medical reason for this. She had not complained of any specific pain or discomfort, nor of being particularly constipated, (a not infrequent occurrence in her life in recent months, that I suspected might be a side-effect of her current medication), and we came to the (not unreasonable) conclusion that she had probably been getting over-anxious about the proposed meeting on the 20th, having jumped to the assumption that this was going to result in her going in a home. We presumed that her raised anxiety, and her subsequent increased need for the loo, had somehow, persuaded her to 'save' her legs, minimise the frequency of her climbs upstairs for the purpose, and opt, instead, to relieve herself in an old plastic washing-up bowl, and flush it down the old, (but still operable) outside toilet; the "shit on floor" incident being a 'missed-target accident', and hopefully a 'one- off', once she felt Reassured again! So, rather than confront, (and probably upset) Mum about this 'shitty' (and as I say, hopefully one-off) accident, and whilst she still appeared to be continuing her 'good run', (it was unlikely that she would remember the incident anyway, several days later), we opted to just monitor the situation until after the meeting when, hopefully, she would realise that she was *not* going in a home, and her anxiety and increased loo needs might abate, but it was a worrying new dimension to her (and therefore our), predicament. Then *came* that long-awaited meeting, where I logged:

20th Aug. (Tues): "No SW. Only Angela. No report. No further service from CPNs. (Told you!) Mum getting upset by the conversation; presume she couldn't follow it; [maybe she] thought plans were being hatched behind her back. Suggest future meetings (where discussion is King) are held elsewhere - & a smaller meeting is then held with Mum (say SW + 1 of us) to 'sell' her the 'decisions' of the [original] planning meeting. Soup, relaxation

+ 25 mins nap; then Tesco + cemetery walk (nice day). Mum 'back to normal' by now. Fish finger tea. No further problems today".

The long-awaited planning meeting had been a severe disappointment, with neither the social worker nor the other CPN involved deeming it worthy of their attendance, and with not a jot of written prose for us to take away and peruse, let alone guide us. To be honest, and despite Angela coming to 'face the music', I felt it smacked of more than a hint of 'too much trouble', and of tacit disrespect, and only served to confirm my cynicism about the lack of genuinely useful help coming from the public 'agencies'. We were no nearer to seeing a clear way forward.

Moreover, and sadly, the formality of the meeting *did* tend to serve as/coincide with a 'turning point' in Mum's 'good run'. For, although, on the day, she seemed to have recovered well enough later on, (with the upset that it had clearly caused her at the time; and probably prior), there were renewed signs of a subsequent, and, alas, more persistent, downturn in her mood and general demeanour, and in her ability to concentrate, and an apparent *internalisation* of her worries about going in a home, in the days that followed - and, perhaps as an emotional reaction, an even *more* worrying recurrence of some toileting issues.

21st Aug. (Weds): "Trip to [town]. Mum 'tired', and been to toilet again" (L).

25th Aug (Sun): "Mum not having a good morning – depressed. Came round a bit as we went on. Been to toilet twice. Soiled sheet in the night. Would not settle this morning. Always on the go. Got the same old story of going in home" (T).

26th Aug. (Mon): "Called to find her on all 4s weeding [in the backyard setts]. She said the same to me about a home! Seems ok. Having a sandwich. Forgets very quickly now" (L).

27th Aug. (Tues): AM - "Found her depressed again. The carpet in the hall had been soiled. I scrubbed it clean. Remembers Sue coming Sun afternoon; after she phoned down after I left at 12-30. Sue stayed until 4-00pm. When she phoned down she'd said she was 'frightened & depressed'" (T).

PM – "Mum getting upset about a missing table mat. Getting frustrated @ not knowing what's happened to it – so OTT &

OCD about a table mat. Agreed to buy new ones in Tesco. Definitely 'down' & depressed today. Bit of a worry that she's slipping back towards depression & 'frightened'. Why was the hall carpet soiled? Anyway, stay calm & carry on – The 3Rs (Routine, Reassurance, Repetition). It may not be coincidence that this 'destabilisation' has followed small changes in Routine. Remind her to Be Positive etc. Usual Routine for me: soup lunch, relaxation, 30 mins nap. Mum bucked up a bit. Went Tesco + cemetery. Mum much better. Bought placemats. NB I'll give [social worker] 'til next Monday & then drop him an email. (I'll cc you in); but don't expect soc serv. to produce 'solutions'. It's largely up to us. What SSD give is a bonus if they give owt! Able to show Mum that this morning's mood was just that; since she's been to Tesco + cemetery AND NOTHING HAPPENED. Fish Finger tea. OK generally again. (But as winter draws on she'll need good support to offset depressive moods). Anyway, 7 – o'clock & all's well".

Nevertheless, we had to presume that her 'good run' *was* now over, and to expect a return to her previous concerns. We weren't disappointed.

28th Aug. (Wed): "Been Coop – came back – legs hurting. She seems better as both [neighbours] are at home today+ are outside. Going to phone GP to see if they have results of scan" (L).

29th Aug. (Thurs): "When I arrived she was cleaning windows outside. Definitely better with someone around. Quite chatty today. I feel someone calling in is a must on days to be decided. Had funny turn about 11-o'clock. Said she could not see. There are times when I feel she should not be on her own". (T).

31st Aug. (Sat): "Sat Morn 8-45am – Mum phoned said there was something wrong with the gas. When I arrived I could not find anything wrong. Mum obviously worked up about it. I took an ear-bashing. Keeps opening & closing door of oven so flames go up & down. Legs hurting & feeling frightened". (T).

A number of old problems, underpinned by an increase in her general confusion, and in her almost obsessive return to highly physical activities based around cleaning, appeared to have returned in recent days, and seemed to be taking hold. In particular, there were her more regular complaints of (worse)pains in her legs (probably true but exaggerated by anxiety, by her actual physical activity, or in the hope of garnering further visits and attention), and, similarly, there was the return of the 'fear', (especially when alone), and a subsequent increase in panicky phone calls (especially to my brother, who was both the eldest and the nearest), to claim things in her house were broken or not working properly, or (as in the case of the gas oven), might 'blow her up', that I suspected were a reflection of the Dementia-lead OCD. And yet she still insisted that she wanted to 'stay in mi own home'. So there again, and starkly, was our most pressing and difficult dilemma; and, at that time, one that seemed to be pretty intractable.

For me at least, getting her out and about and keeping her in our established (and of course distracting) Routine (of lunch, relaxation, nap, outing, etc) did seem to help 'in the present', as it were, but once I left again, *she* was left again to deal with being alone with her thoughts and her worries and, of course, with her Dementia.

To some degree, I suppose, it was the sheer lack of predictability, and therefore opportunity to forward-plan with any certainty, (for both Mum and us), that caused much of the stress and strain that was becoming inherent in the situation; not least because we felt we were battling it all on our own, in large part in ignorance of what we were encountering, and feeling totally unsupported in any useful and meaningful way by any other (particularly public agency) inputs, sources and contributions

The start of the new month (of September), looked as though it was going to continue in similar vein, but might there still be the slightest glimmer of 'light at the end of the tunnel', from which the agency 'cavalry' might be re-riding - by way of another meeting?

2nd Sept (Mon): "Not good. Crying + confused. [Mum complained of] pain in legs but mind all over the place. Jenny [other CPN] here. Thought there was an 11-o'clock meeting. [SW had] not told her. [It had been moved to 1-30pm @ Weds, 11th of Sept, at my *brother's* house]" (L).

3rd Sept (Tues): "Arrived 9-30am. Mum Ok until 11-00am. Had panic attack and became confused. When I arrived, she was polishing, but could not remember [doing] it after the attack. Had problem with her eye. Tried to get her to have a nap but she would not" (T).

That said, all hope was not completely lost, and we each still encountered that odd 'better' day.

PM – "Despite T's earlier note of panic attack Mum was actually quite positive when I arrived. Lunch / Relaxation/ 30 mins nap /Routine. Tesco. Met L + Aunt Vera. Went cemetery. Talked about Dad being 94 tomorrow. Fish finger tea + egg-custard – yumeee. 'Tired' later, but generally ok".

4th Sept (Wed): "Am still in shock. Had good day. Been [next town], M&S + Bhs. Bought clothes. No problems. Had toastie + chips in Bhs for dinner. [Mum] just tired. It can't last". (L).

5th Sept (Thurs): "Had a good morning; [but] she went to toilet this morning. Had trouble, so she has taken a [laxative] sachet". (T).

And so on we continued, (logging as we went), with our individual inputs, 'shifts' and 'routines'; and often therefore with Mum's differing reactions to each of us, in consequence; and yet each, by turns, continuing to encounter a mixture of good days and bad days; and indeed a mixture of good bits and bad bits *within* any one 'shift' or day; both she and we still being callously teased with (false) hope, as the Dementia relented regularly enough to give Mum the chance to touch base with 'normality' more than not, and then getting stressed by the bad bits, when it didn't and, of course, when the problems remained.

7th Sept (Sat): "Mum a bit 'down' at 1st, but improved. Dosette done. Lunch/Relaxation/25 mins nap Routine. Evidence of small amount of poo stain on bathroom carpet. Cleaned it up. Evidence of urine by side of bed – may have tipped [chamber pot, whilst emptying]. Cleaned it as best without Mum knowing. May be damp. Went Aldi ok. Left Mum to unpack. No probs. Hope you are preparing 'top' questions for SW/CPN & reading all your 'homework'. G'day".

10th Sept (Tues):

AM – "Has been to toilet twice. Feels very weak. Made cup of tea & biscuits. I feel all the bran & sachets is too much. Tried to talk to her about this [potential] 'sitter' coming in. We may have a problem. She got better as the morning went on" (T).

PM – "Mum ok on arrival. [Usual routine]. [Small] Argument pre-tea when she sought sympathy for being 'depressed'; refuse to be drawn. Went through 'Be Positive' stuff & she came round".

12th Sept (Thurs): "This is my memory of yesterday [11th Sept meeting]: -

1. CPN offered nothing. Waste of time. [Just being] nice not enough.
2. S.W. only offered 'private agency' carer.
3. We agreed to SW offer @ 2 x weekly for half an hour @ 3-30pm to 4pm (£6 per time?).
4. Soc serv. nothing else new to offer either; [except checking on vague *possibility* of Mum + one of us attending Alzheimer's support group once a week].
5. Await further contact from SW.

Am I right??

And so to Mum. OK on arrival. So, over soup lunch raised & chatted about meeting for 'Carers'. [Said] that it was a meeting for ME; but [that] I'd like her to come with me 'for company' – and after some anxiety she said she *would*! (I've got a 'foot in the door' - next time I raise it, I'll say she promised). As for 'sitter' - briefly mentioned it, but felt she had heard enough on the subject, so left it. Talked about Grandma [her Mum] & about things Mum has never done – never been abroad (unless you count North Wales), can't swim, or ride a bike. Never flown. Relaxation exercises & 30 mins nap. [Went shop] for local paper & cards + cemetery walk [with my dog]. Beans on toast for tea. All OK".

The latest addition to our tasks, 'plans', and indeed hopes, then, was to just try and *introduce* Mum to the *idea* of both a 'carer' (as befriender) calling in on her twice a week for half an hour, and (by well-intended deception), of her attending an Alzheimer's support group (with one of we 'carers') over in the town; to see how *that* went.

14th Sept (Sat): "Mum ok on arrival. Dosette box done. (enough left for 2 weeks). Nice dinner. Chat about 'carer' [coming in]. [With gentle persuasion] she agreed in principle to 2 x weekly@ home. Also reminded her of promise to accompany me to MY 'carers' meeting. I'll wait & see! Usual Relaxation & 30 mins nap Routine. Aldi – no probs. Tea Ok. TTFN". (Ta Ta For Now).

As September cooled and winter beckoned, another area of domestic contention began to crop up again, and needed to be re-added to our never-ending list of things to bear in mind.

16th Sept (Mon): "Been P O + Tesco. Bit wobbly on legs. Otherwise not bad. Cold in house. Put heating on" (L).

The decent Spring and Summer, weatherwise, of 2013, had been most welcome, and had meant that the need for the (central) heating to be on in Mum's house had hardly weighed heavy amongst our most immediate concerns for quite some while, but the unanticipated, mid-September, downturn in temperature had provided us with a timely reminder that it had previously been a significant 'bone of contention' with Mum. Coming from a poor, and therefore financially-careful, background, Mum had always budgeted very thriftily, and central heating was a relatively new luxury in her life. Throughout her life, she had become used to just adding extra layers of clothing, and putting up with the cold, so, since the central heating had been installed, (probably 10 or 12 years previously, and definitely post-Dad), she had only used it sparingly. However, her decisions back then were fully compos mentis ones, but her mental decline and forgetfulness in recent months meant that it was now another significant issue for *us* to monitor. My sister had noted that Mum's house was cold, and raised the issue anew. It would quickly resume its status as that 'bone of contention'.

Meanwhile, we continued, (more or less 'on call'), with the general management of the bulk of her life, and current level of Dementia; including, of course, her regular forgetfulness, and accompanying bouts of 'fear', and loss of confidence, the likes of her medication, her recurring, often chronic, leg 'aches and pains', her recently increased need for the toilet, with its newly-suspected 'make-shifts' and 'spills', and most of her needs in sheer practical, household terms, domestically; whilst, in particular, and at present, trying to prepare Mum for having a 'sitter' in the house on occasion; not that we had heard anything further from the social worker yet - to my brother's frustration.

17th Sept (Tues): "Not a bad morning. Mentioned the sitter again. [Mum] still rebels against [the idea]; but hey we still have not had any contact from Keith's buddy [social worker]. Is this going to be another long job" (T).

18th Sept (Weds): "Been out for dinner @ Garden Centre- ate all dinner. Cold in house again" (L).

19th Sept (Thurs): "Arrived to Mum on toilet again. No heating on again" (T).

21st Sept (Sat): AM. "Called in just to see if [hospital] letter had come. It has. [Appointment] not til Nov. Can't be that bad then". (L).

PM – "Mum OK. Seen letter. Agree with L – can't be much if appt isn't til 15th Nov. Dosette done. Good lunch. Relaxation, 25 mins nap Routine. Argument about out-of-date eggs whilst compiling [shopping] list. [Mum said] 'T & L never tell me what to do. Piss off, Keith'! Then Aldi. Still 'tired' but OK. Salmon sarnie tea; then telly. All quiet of the western front".

25th Sept (Weds): "6pm. Mum phoned down. She had had power cut. Nothing working. Came up. Sat for 2 hrs, [until] the power came back on. Mum handled it well. Did not panic. When I got back home *we* had a power cut! I did not panic. I handled it well. Ha Ha" (T).

27th Sept. (Fri): "5pm. Mum phoned. She had made a mess of telly. I came up and put it right" (T).

28th Sept (Sat): "Worst for a while on arrival. Upset, crying, 'frightened'. Doesn't know why. Saying, 'go in a home', 'mi time's comin', 'you think I'm puttin' it on' stuff. Anyway, she'd made lunch, & we chatted round it, and she slowly came round. Dosette filled, [for week], but supplies all gone now! Need Boots visit before next Sat. Lunch/Relaxation/nap Routine. Then Aldi + cemetery. Mum bucked up. Sandwich tea. Not Mum's best day. Just 'tired' all day".

1ˢᵗ Oct (Tues): AM - "Mum on form talking about homes & death. Calmed down after a while. Then R [her brother] came. He asked her if she was ok. She started to cry, saying she was 'frightened' and depressed. Had a cup of tea with R. [and chatted]. Been to toilet twice this morning. Told R about sitters. Mum told R that we were making her have them. Mum feeling 'weak' and 'tired' after going to toilet. Cried again" (T).

PM - "All present for 'constipation corner'. 'Eureka' – all is relieved. Mum better afterwards. Quite amazing how quick recovery can occur. 2-30pm – went Tesco's. OK (You wouldn't have known there'd been a problem)."

4ᵗʰ Oct. (Thurs.): "Nothing from A-care when I left".

"A-care" (not their real name), was the name of the private agency that had finally been forwarded to us via a social services e-mail, with regard to the supply of the 'sitter'. The e-mail had advised that Mum's referral had been forwarded to the agency 'on our behalf', and that we would be contacted directly by the company. We awaited their 'approach' with a strange mixture of both hope and trepidation. Yet another new 'twist in our tale' beckoned.

Then, even 'before a ball was bowled' *there*, came another, a different, 'agency update' so - two potentially fresh 'fish to batter' together (to mix metaphors).

6ᵗʰ Oct (Sat):

"Scan letter from Hosp! (It's behind the gas bill on shelf, so Mum can't read it). Talks of post-infective changes of lung + benign ovarian cyst. (Not sure it's serious – or appt would have been sooner). Mum ok on arrival. Had made Sat. lunch + rice pud ok! Done Dosette. [Usual Routine] + walk round cemetery. Nice autumn day. Mum 'tired' thereafter, but still kept 'on the go'. Salmon tea + telly. 7-o'clock & all's well".

9ᵗʰ Oct (Tues): AM - "Arrived to Mum on toilet. Thought it was going to be like last Tuesday. (I've only just recovered). Not much happening with your mate [social worker] & the sitters. Convinced no-one wants the job. Not enough hours. Whoever covers next Sunday needs to put Mums brown bin out". (T).

PM – "Mum fragile on arrival & easily could be upset. Soup lunch + chat improved her. [Looks like] I'll have to find some

Sunday time. (I didn't want to go out for my Sunday lunch anyway). Re Sitters – will email [social worker] tomorrow re A-care. Checked dosette box – Wednesday's open & pills have gone! Mum can't remember taking 2 lots; but I think she has. Thought about leaving her without for Weds, but guessed she'd just open [next] Thursday's; so decided to refill Weds; but we might be short towards the end of this prescription. I think that's why she's fragile just now. Effects start to wear off soon. Relaxation + nap Routine. Tesco OK. Brief walk round cemetery. Mum much improved. (Shows the effects of the medication on morning mood though?). All OK now. Fish finger tea + telly. All quiet on the Western front".

10th Oct. (Weds): "Been to Mill Yard. Nice shops. I think she gets breathless too much, and this is the lung problem. I can phone A-care if you want. I don't think we should underestimate the problem with her lungs; don't overdo the walking". (L).

Mum certainly seemed in quite a fragile state through October. Almost anything slightly out of the ordinary, and out of her current comfort zone and routine, seemed to 'throw her' and make her rather tense and edgy. For example, just going for her one-off flu jab, or for her eyes checked and glasses mended might now constitute a trigger. Additionally, the colder weather had re-raised the increasingly sticky issue of keeping her central heating on; for it was another rather OCD, rather irrational, and, to us, unnecessary source of potential argument for Mum. We would now regularly arrive to find Mum had switched off all the radiators, (supposedly to save money), and we would explain, (admittedly in our rather 'we know better' tone), that it was cold, mildly 'tick her off', and simply put them back on again. Mum would almost certainly be turning them off again, once we had departed, (and that was a winter worry in itself), but there were times when she had craftily turned some off again whilst we were still *there*, but out of the relevant room. The manoeuvrings, and potential for 'words' on this unnecessarily- tricky subject (yet another), was now set to continue right throughout the winter. Meanwhile, the management of the rest of her life, (still in her own home), and all of her other personal issues (Dementia, medication, hygiene and toilet needs, pains in legs, food-intake and finance monitoring, household maintenance jobs, both essential and non-essential shopping, prominent among them), continued relatively unabated and still devoid of any tangible outside help, but:

16th Oct. (Tues): "Mum best she's been for 3 or 4 visits when I arrived. T/c to L. She's booked optician for 23rd. Advised her that I have today spoken to Alan McD @ A-care & forwarded all the recent e-mails. He's ringing me back tomorrow. I will try to set up a meeting @ noon next Tues @ T's. Check your inboxes. Went for Mum's coat & bag, & noticed some pee by bed. & mat hung over bath. Mum agreed she 'missed' [whilst] trying to pee in [chamber pot]. Thoroughly cleaned it then hoovered all round. We need to check things like this all the time now. There was loads of dust in the corner too. Mum can't get hoover upstairs [as easily]; so we might need to 'offer' to do it every couple of weeks. Need to keep one step ahead; [also] need to keep check as weather gets colder. [Usual Routine]. 5-40pm [OCD incident]. Mum went to put something in bin – and saw I'd emptied Hoover straight in. I looked out of kitchen window & she had the bin upside down! - with all the stuff on the floor. Put the bin upright, but Mum insisted on brushing up all the [debris]. Bit of an argument, but you can't stop the obsessiveness – it's a bit scary. Glad for relax with telly; it's been draining - the obsessive behaviour just drives you nuts! – and will eventually do for her, I think. Anyway, going home for rest".

After a promising arrival, it had turned out to be quite a busy and unexpectedly tiring day for *me*; giving me just an inkling of what it might be like for *her* these days. What with remembering things like re-filling her Dosette box for the week, with Mum clearly having again 'missed the mark'(at least once), whilst trying to pee in the chamber pot in her bedroom last night, (requiring my urgent attention to remedial hygiene tasks), with the 'usual routine', out and about in the community, and with the late OCD/ obsessive behaviour 'bin incident' that threatened to force an unnecessary argument, and to 'destabilise' her near the end of the day, (such behaviour, and petty arguments, had definitely become worse in recent weeks, with her increasing propensity to 'make mountains' out of things of relatively insignificant importance to most of us, and to getting worked up if she didn't have things 'just so'), I had been 'kept on my toes' quite a bit, and was heading home feeling both mentally and physically exhausted - with hindsight, it was perhaps amongst the most typical examples of how the situation now had the potential to inflict 'wear and tear' on we *carers* too, if we didn't find time to stay rested and refreshed.

I guess the root of such 'wear and tear' lay in the steady *accumulation* of worry over, and sheer uncertainty and unpredictability inherent in, Mum's plight these days in respect of how she was coping, and what to expect, and, given all that, how best to proceed. Thus:

17th Oct. (Weds): "Wot all the fuss about! Been [next town], charity shops & hotpot dinner. All Ok – for now!" (L).

18th Oct. (Thurs): AM – "When I arrived she was all ready to go to visit [a friend's] new flat. When I told her [that visit] was on Sunday she got upset and cried. Settled down after a while. She has been to toilet twice this morning. Says she is struggling. Talked about sitters. Says she does not want them, but told her it would be a good thing. Since she has been to the toilet she has felt weak & tired. In fact she spent most of the 2 hrs on the toilet". (T).

PM – "Mum OK on arrival; but has had all 3 of us for company. Soup & cake for lunch. L only gone 5 mins when she went outside & tipped bin upside down again! She said something was in bin but not in a bag! For God's sake! Relaxation + 20 mins nap. Mum woke 'tired' & I stupidly said, 'You shouldn't be tipping bins upside down then, should you?' & got sucked into another argument. Took a while to calm her again, but went for [local paper] + walk round cemetery with dog - nice mild afternoon. Mum Ok by return & forgotten argument – Mem. Loss can be used positively! Also, sometimes an argument relieves her tension. Beans for tea, then telly. Once again, not my best effort, but hey...All quiet on the Western Front".

We were coming to the end of the (80-sheet) founding log book. I had opened it (only back in early August) with my inaugural entry, and as fate would have it, the final contribution would also fall to me. We had logged much, (both good and not so), in barely 3 months, and there had been significant and noticeable changes, (sadly, mostly for the worse, for Mum), along that short way. However, like the first, the final contribution was both relatively positive, and relatively uncontroversial.

19th Oct (Sat):

"Mum OK on arrival. [Usual Routine]. Aldi. Dosette done. 'Tired' & [a bit of] the usual negativity - ('don't want a,b,c,'), but generally a better day for me than the last 2. NB see you @ T's on Tues.

Here endeth my Vol. 1 contributions".

Accordingly, on the very next day my brother, (even hinting at a touch of childlike excitement), opened Vol. 2., equally uncontroversially, with:

20th Oct. (Sun): "I am the first to write in the new book". He then went on to cover the usual matters, noting that the arranged visit to the friend's flat had gone OK, but adding little new or, thankfully, of concern.

My earliest contribution was a basic log and record of the belated, (arranged at relatively short notice), and inaugural meeting with JulieB., the first person (apparently a supervisor), that we actually *met* from A-care! We had arranged to hold it at my brother's house on the *morning* of the 22nd, in order to avoid any potential upset or destabilisation for Mum, (who, these days, found any such meetings a bit overwhelming, and hard to follow); and I had continued on (a little later than usual) to my 'shift' with Mum. Thus, by the end of that day's shift, my contribution read:

22nd Oct. (Tues): "P.M. Arrived 1-00pm (after meeting) – visits to start Sunday 3rd Nov. – JulieB + Carer Deborah to visit 3-30. L to be in attendance – after that let them 'crack on'. Payments to be invoiced fortnightly in my name; but to Mum's address – any of the 3 of us can open /pay in turn. Soup lunch. Mum a bit anxious because of my 'lateness'. Also started to say she wouldn't wear the new [crimson red winter] coat [I'd bought her]. It fitted well & she came round slowly. Argument about collar [being up]; told her it was a 'winter collar'. Went Tesco – in new coat! She likes it!! Fish finger tea + Egg custard (It doesn't get any better!). Don't forget the 3Rs - Routine, Reassurance, Repetition.

Ps I met someone recently who said his father made him walk the plank - they couldn't afford a dog. HA HA HA - thought I'd never stop. Goodbye Ruby Tuesday".

Vol. 2. was under way. Thankfully, though there were doubtless challenges old and new up ahead (not least the unknown effects of the sitters in the *more imminent* of the 'new' category), there was still room for a little light relief and a chuckle - including at the latest 'new coat saga' snippet at the end of this next log.

23rd Oct (Weds): "Opticians done – no changes. New readers may be ready Fri. Not too bad today, but could have gone either way. She won't wear her new coat unless its weekend". (L). So the new ("best") coat was still a typical and current source of her out-of-comfort-zone OCD.

24th Oct. (Thurs): "T still here. Mum having a 'bit of a turn'. Soon got her up & doing. T went. Soup lunch. Boots medication needs collecting at some point. L might; otherwise I'll try. Relaxation & nap. Mum woke OK; but we argued about putting on the new [winter] coat. I said firmly that I couldn't take her out otherwise. She cried, called me selfish & asked me to go. I declined. I did say I'd walk [dog] alone & leave Mum at home. She changed her mind, put on new coat & out we went. [Whilst out] I re-iterated that her new coat was for *everyday* in winter, not just w/ends. I think she's got the message. Beans on toast for tea. Late scare – Mum took scab off right-leg sore. [It] took time to stem flow. Then lint + plaster".

26th Oct (Sat): "Oh dear. Upset & crying – confused about [new] glasses. Had brought down another pair from upstairs for some reason; which added to her confusion. Sorted them. Took 'old' pair back upstairs. Done dosette pills. Soup for dinner. She had made a rice pudding ok though. Clocks back tonight!! It'll be dark by 5-30 from Sunday – curtains closed early – so expect Mum to be 'down' more. [Usual Routine] Aldi – in new coat! Mum [put] all shopping away; and much better in herself. Salmon sarnies for tea. All clocks back 1 hr. (NB beware storm/wind Sunday into Monday). TTFN".

And, from time to time, the support system developed glitches, and didn't run quite as smoothly as its operatives might hope and *improvisation* was not uncommon, which of course often had its' impact on Mum's comfort zone, Dementia and OCD behaviour.

28th Oct (Mon): "Oh dear. No car. Got taxi up to Mums, then went on 11.00 bus – Yes bus! – to Post Office – then taxi back. Mum's nerves + confusion are getting worse [as is] the pain in her legs. I think we need to increase dose of that tablet. I hope she isn't throwing them away! Anyway, she did well on the bus. Walking, yes walking, home now!". (L).

29th Oct (Tues): "Mum best she's been for ages on arrival. Hurrah. Did mention pain in legs but I get that every time now. I think the blood-thinning tablet [could] be responsible for the leg pain – it's an everyday pain. The blood is thinner but carrying the same body weight. Chat about 'sitter' over lunch. Says she'll give it a go. Hoovered upstairs. [Usual Routine]. Fish Finger tea. 5.00pm 'Tired', but clocks went back so body-clock thinks it's still 6.00?

I'd put some oven chips in with fish fingers & whilst I was having a pee, Mum took them out & put them under grill! No idea why. I turned off grill & put them back in oven &Mum had a paddy!! 'Go Go Go. You don't care. No sympathy for nobody. I'm 80 years old. I've cooked chips for years; You're bossing me'. '[They're] *oven* chips Mum', [I said]. Anyway, managed her 'down' again, & by end of tea she was apologetic. It may be letting out tension is useful. By 6.00pm she was OK again, even forgotten the argument, but she complained of increased pain in her legs - suggests tension is at its root. Watched telly. All back quiet on the Western Front".

2nd Nov (Sat): "Mum in pretty good mood on arrival. Sat dinner OK too. L called in to check arrangements for first 'sit' tomorrow. [Usual Routine]".

But what when the day of that first 'sit', (at the scheduled 3.30pm 'slot'), actually neared and then dawned?

3rd Nov. (Sun): "Called to find her crying + tense. Changed clothes. Lots of pain in legs + moaning. 'You think I'm putting this on' she says. 3-45 Still not here". (L).

As ever, Carers working for commercial organisations were, even then, under severe time and number pressures, and it was not exactly surprising to any of us that Deborah did not arrive *exactly* on time, though it was still disappointing; whilst Julie B's promise to be in attendance on this first occasion *completely* failed to materialise. There is no specific log of what time Deborah did finally arrive, as my sister had her hands full preparing Mum for the visit, and acting as go-between, and didn't actually log anything on the day, but around 4pm is a best guess, as Deborah was still there, and actually answered Mum's phone, when I rang with my daily support call just before 4-30pm. Dementia or not, Mum was still sufficiently careful not to give much away over the phone, and in Deborah's presence, but an arrival around the time the half-hour slot was supposed to be *ending* wasn't exactly what we'd hoped for by way of an ideal induction; especially for a 'client' who is already prone to anxiety in general, is suffering from Dementia in particular, and, in that context, is even more anxious about meeting someone new. In theory, we were off to a less than perfect start and it would certainly 'set the scene' for *future* occasions! Yet, despite the carer's lateness, Julie B's complete 'no-show', Mum's previously expressed reluctance about having a Carer come in at all, and our own consequent reservations, the inaugural visit appeared to have passed off without obvious issue, and to have left no noticeable trace of any long-lasting negativity.

4th Nov. (Mon): "[Mum] doesn't remember much about yesterday's visitor but seems happy with her for now. She's bringing scones on Weds! Very tired today. Yawning a lot". (L).

5th Nov. (Tues): "Some complaint of 'legs' & 'arm' pain (from Flu jab?). Mum happy with Deborah. Good start. I'm not happy with lateness - need to keep an eye on this; though we won't know what time she arrives now will we? Also, what happened to Julie? No notice that she wasn't coming! Anyway, let's see how it goes. Big Soup for lunch + scone. Relaxation + 20 mins nap; then out. Tesco. Dropped Mum at home then [popped out]. Back home Mum had put shopping away. Fish finger tea. [Mum] generally tired, but OK".

6th Nov. (Thurs): AM - "Mum OK on arrival. A lot different from yesterday, when she put the phone down on me. Mum happy with sitter. (Well there's a result. We have done something right). Mum broke down about 11-15. Her eye was playing up and her arm was hurting. Also, 'I'd be better in a home'. (T).

PM – "Mum ready to feel sorry for herself, but OK once attention deflected onto other things. On her mood yesterday, I think she was showing some raised anxiety because Deborah was coming PM – may be so again on Sunday but I think she'll get better as she gets used to Deborah. I suspect the raised anxiety was to do with seeing Deborah alone. Usual Routine. Anyway, Mum's 'train' seems back on 'track' (for now)".

Despite the (lateness and lack of supervisor) 'hiccups' at the inaugural 'gig', the Carer's involvement actually seemed to be going OK. Mum liked Deborah. However, as mentioned in my log of the 5th, with no actual presence there on the days and slots in question, (Sunday and Wednesdays between 3-30 and 4pm), we now found ourselves in the bizarre situation of purchasing a 'Carer' service, but with only *Mum's* (unreliable) feedback, (and the promise of regular but as yet unarranged 'progress meetings'), to guide us as to how each day's visit was actually working out in terms of *both* time and content.

I also remained concerned about the number of instances and times when Mum seemed to have some sort of mini- breakdown at around *11pm*, during my siblings 'shifts'; either with general anxiety, or more specific issues around leg pains or eyes 'playing up'. I was still convinced that the taking, or perhaps wearing - off, of her morning medication might be a factor here. I was rarely there myself until around lunchtime, and suspected that it was more than just good fortune and my social work perspective that helped me to avoid some of those 'upsets for elevenses'. (Though Mum could still surprise me with something *approaching* a Saturday roast dinner, and suitable afters, on occasion, a lunch of Big Soup was fast-becoming the norm for the vast majority of my arrivals. They were easily affordable, widely available, generally nutritious, providing both good content and variety, and, perhaps most valuable of all, were still well within Mum's ambit to make, both for my visit, and in my absence. They were a 'safe bet', so we would invariably stock up on them whilst out shopping together).

8th Nov. (Sat): "Rang as normal from 9-30 to 9-45. All I was getting was engaged. Took the decision to come up. Found receiver on the upstairs [handset] was on the floor". (T).

This was a typical example of the many and varied, but essentially small-beer, every day, one-off, issues and worries that we met with, accumulated, responded to and managed. Others were more chronic - such as her medication, and, as winter drew on, her tendency to turn off the radiators.

9th Nov. (Sun): "Mum happily watching [Remembrance] service & singing! Bin already out. Noted tablets not taken, so opened 'Sunday' and threw them away – think it will be less stressful. Sandwiches for dinner". (L).

10th Nov. (Mon): "Tablets not taken again. Told her and she took them no problem, but we need to keep an eye on it. Post Off done. Doing OK". (L).

Then back to the 'one-offs'. Mum had spoken of someone phoning her, but didn't know who.

11th Nov. (Tues): AM – "Arrived. Mum taken tablets OK. Did 1471 on phone, but still don't know who phoned. Feel it could be a different carer 2morrow. L agrees. All in all a good morning". (T).

PM. "Mum good on arrival. Appetite quite good today too. Relaxation exercises + 20mins nap. Whilst Mum was napping I sent text to Julie B. Her reply confirmed someone rang about Care Plans. Text back asking her to go via 'one of sibs' [as previously agreed!] – so still expecting Deborah tomorrow as per plan. Further text from Julie – 'it was the office that called' – it won't happen again [Oh, yes it would!!] – so mystery phone call sorted. Tesco for general shopping. (Wasn't he in command at Dunkirk?!) Are you aware Mum's hospital appt is this Friday?".

14th Nov. (Thurs): "Reluctant to say it, but all going quite well at the moment. Mum confirmed Debbie came as planned Weds PM; and when I rang Mum @ 4-20pm yesterday she was quite chirpy. [Usual Routine]" and there was another snippet of (relative) good news.

15th Nov. (Fri): "Good day at hospital. Good results + laugh with [niece] at hospital. Mum Reassured now – will get letter from GP about lung problem. Thought it best not to do another colonoscopy. You know the rest". (L).

17th Nov. (Sun): "Mum OK on arrival. Cleaning up before Debbie comes. (Have we had a bill yet?) Baz can't come out [of hospital] today. Maybe Mon. If [so] Sue will come up in place of L. L is trying to get extra hours because Baz can't work for a while. All this got Mum tensed up and she started to panic. Reminded her Debbie was coming. She said she only stays 20 mins. Do we believe her, as we pay for 30". (T).

My sister's husband, Baz. had been admitted to hospital following knee problems. When he was finally discharged, he would still be unfit for work. This meant that my sister's visits to Mum might be jeopardised by my sister having to seek extra work hours herself, to stop her own household finances coming under pressure - yet another potential pressure on the set-up and Routine with Mum that we might have to juggle. (Luckily, neither my brother nor myself had yet experienced any serious interruptions in our support roles to Mum).

20th Nov. (Weds): "Been [town]. Papers paid. No heating on. V.cold! Had dinner out. Carer coming later. Will check if prescription due". (L).

21st Nov. (Thurs): "[Usual Routine]. Slight upset when small scab on back of lower left leg came off with her tights and trickle of blood wouldn't stop; partly 'cos she kept ON her legs. Eventually ceased & I put plaster on – just shows how easily Mum's 'stability' can become' instability'".

23rd Nov. (Sat): "Mum OK on arrival. Dosette done. Lunch OK. Read A-Care invoice – for 3 x half-hour – exactly £20. I will post off. (I will copy invoice for records & put in back of log). Then I'll get Mum to reimburse me somehow. OK? [Told Mum] it was a small amount out of her Attendance Allowance. [Usual Routine]. Aldi. Mum unpacked. Salmon Sarnies then TV to 7-00".

24th Nov. (Sun): Mum still complaining about her arm & eye playing up. Reminded her Debbie was coming today. Been to toilet twice whilst I was here. Went to pieces about 11-00am because she could not go to the toilet. No heating on again. Can't get through to her about putting it on when she gets up. Not a bad morning". (T).

25th Nov. (Mon): "Not as bad as I expected today. I think Debbie is having a good effect. Arm bad today. Won't see Doc. Pie for dinner. Bloody cold in here. Just put rads on". (L).

26th Nov. (Tues): "No heating on again. Like a fridge. I said I would get [valves swapped]. She said it was her house and they were not being changed. We can't win. Her arm is sore again, but she won't go to docs. Says it's the weather. OK in general, but her mind is thinking all the time". (T).

3rd Dec. (Tues): AM – "No heating on when I arrived. [Her brother] here. Been to toilet twice. Mum been up the ladders cleaning the windows inside. Been complaining of her arm hurting [again]. Not a bad morning". (T).

PM – "Mum quite good on arrival. Complaining of arm pain. I think it's a strain that she aggravates; noted T's reference to being up ladder – that's the most likely source of arm pain; especially as she says she doesn't have it in bed. [Usual Routine]. Tesco. Fish fingers for tea. [All] as well as could be".

We were into December now, with the winter season, and its predictably lower temperatures, poorer weather, loss of colour and greenery, and long dark nights, holding sway, and tending to set the agenda. Depressing at the best of times for many folk, it was certainly not the easiest season or circumstance for supporting Mum, and her Dementia-infiltrated life; and therefore for keeping up her increasingly flagging morale and the difficult management of a string of personal issues that had effectively become 'normalised' to the point of 'everyday mundane' - including (still) with her heating, medication, food-intake, toileting, and of course, Dementia-induced, (and upsetting for all), propensity to forgetfulness, depression, crying, and anxiety. Physically too (and despite, or perhaps because of, her prescribed medication), she was complaining regularly of chronic pain in her lower left leg, and more recently to her upper left arm, (some of it probably anxiety induced), and was inevitably affected by the perceived limitations and worry inherent there.

Additionally, we had now introduced Debbie the Carer into the equation. So far, thank goodness, the Carer thing actually seemed to be working OK; though it was far from clear that there were *definitive* benefits, and we'd still had no formal progress meeting, and, therefore, no formal feedback beyond Debbie's standard, dated, and hurriedly scribbled "all OK", on an official A-care worksheet kept near the phone. Beyond that we had only *Mum's* unreliable perspective (and the bills, and our best guess) to guide us on how or whether the sessions were working for her - or even taking place properly at all!

On the other, more positive, hand, there were still plenty of good, compos mentis, moments, and indeed days, to appreciate, (for me built round the 'Usual Routine' and the '3Rs'), and so on we pressed with that management structure, and with the good days and not so, and just praying that we three (and our own domestic situations) would continue in good health, order and fortune for the foreseeable future. The pattern was pretty well set. What else could we do? So, typically:

7th Dec. (Sat): "Mum saying she's 'depressed', & crying. Spoke of arm pain. Said she must go to doctor if she wants it looking at. She confirmed that arm does not hurt in bed – strain? Psychological? I was firm in tone & added that she'd been indoors for 2 days [so probably] feeling down. She was also [irrationally] upset by letters (EON bill + A-care bill) and, unfortunately, delivery of wrong Sat. paper. Reassured her that WE have it all under control. Not a good entry, but onward. She'd made dinner OK though – but no heating on. Relaxation + 20 mins nap. Then dosette done for week. Took wrong paper back to shop, went to Post Office [and then] went cemetery & put wreaths on Dad's & Gran's graves. Went Aldi for standard shopping [and] walked up [High St]. Home for tea – salmon sarnies + cake. Mum had bucked up a lot compared to my arrival. Strange day – hard work at the outset; but more settled by the day's end. Anyway, I'm going to apply for a job making mirrors – I could see myself doing that!"

Her often poor mind-set on arrival, (perhaps affected by earlier imbibing of her medication), and accompanying (real or psychosomatic) pain was now common; probably exacerbated by a night and early morning on her own in the winter gloom. As often though, (certainly via *my* shift's regular concentration on 'Routine'), things tended to improve steadily with company; and for me through the Relaxation Exercises, the short nap, and my invoking of the Reassurance element, (in particular), of the '3Rs'. She was usually then in the mood to go out somewhere, including for shopping, and thus, both stimulated and distracted from her 'problems'. More often than not, she would return more settled, and ready to occupy herself making tea for us both. In and around all that, I would discreetly try and fit in any 'jobs' that specifically needed doing by someone other than Mum; such as filling the dosette box, dealing with any relevant paperwork/post, mending and fixing stuff, and cleaning hither and thither as seemed necessary.

Using the old adage that 'laughter is the cheapest and best medicine', I would also try to regularly introduce the odd (sometimes very odd) spot of humour - both directly to Mum (who was still well capable of accessing her lovely sense of humour, and so well capable of enjoying a good laugh in the right circumstance), and hopefully for my siblings' light-relief when they came to read the log. And then we found Christmas was approaching once more - with all *its* emotional entanglements and memories - yet still with the same ongoing problems for Mum.

8th Dec. (Sun): Having spent time with Mum already that morning, and tried to talk to her about keeping warm, this later log appeared from my brother.

"5-30pm Mum phoned. Said she had no telly. Came up. [Again]. Nothing wrong with telly. All radiators off. House cold. What is going on?" (T).

Even at this point, we were still relative, free-standing, (i.e. unsupported), novices in understanding and dealing with the intricacies of Mum's Dementia. With hindsight, such episodes were probably reflecting further 'incident'-like disturbances for Mum; especially those occurring when we weren't there. That is, times when she was actually experiencing the most active, ('mind all over the place'), legacy of her Dementia, (maybe as more mental 'blank spots', and an accompanying sense of scary isolation and confusion, for example), and was just anxiously seeking our attention and support with these situations and issues, by taking an instinctive action that she hoped would bring it - say, by turning off the radiators, *dwelling* on a mild ache, or forcing an argument, when we *were* there; or, similarly, by jumping on the phone to one of us, about non-existent or suddenly-confusing everyday problems (say with the telly), in order to get us round there, and to mitigate her anxiety and isolation, when we *weren't*. And then, 8 casually-scribbled, almost 'throw-away', words, that I could so easily have missed in the middle of an otherwise pretty ordinary log from my sister, had raised the spectre of yet another potentially serious management problem to add to our woes and worries.

9th Dec. (Mon): "I have smelt gas on 2 separate visits!"

Clearly a potentially dangerous occurrence, this was not something I had noted myself, but just the mention of it obviously set off 'alarm bells'! Thankfully, no-one logged any immediate repeat incidents, but it went without saying that we would need to keep the closest watch for any; not that we knew what our response or solution would or should be. Our best hope was that the problem was either an 'olfactory' error on my sister's part, or a two-off malfunction and mistake on Mum's; but we'd be watching. Otherwise, it was 'business as usual'.

11th Dec. (Weds): Dog in tow, and for whatever reason, I was filling in for L, who usually visited Mum in the *morning* on her Wednesday 'shift'; and re-invoking a slightly biblical, yet seemingly slightly-irked, and slightly inconvenienced, tone myself, (such instances were infrequent, but certainly not non-existent), I recorded our opening exchanges and progress thus:

"Peace be with you. Welcome to this (hopefully) one-off 'Wednesday Special'. We are gathered here today to sort out mother again. When I arrived @ 10-45 am she was in another depressed & self-pitying mood- 'Oh, mi arm', 'Oh, I should be in a home', 'Oh, I am in a mess' - drives you nuts after a while; but recourse to Plan A – Distraction.

'A don't think a can go out today, Keith' – cry, cry - Mum.

'Yes, you can Mum. You must, to change your mood' – Keith.

'You're forcing me; L & T don't force me' – Mum.

'No they don't, Mum & you stay depressed, so let's go out, OK'. – Keith.

Got Mum dressed in winter coat (she doesn't argue with me about the coat now). 'Made' her put hat on. Drove to 'Birds'. Bernard (a fellow elderly depressive, but worse than Mum) was there sat in his car. Mum had a good chat & established that he had now moved [house, but] was unhappy [cos] drains blocked. But – I was able to point to someone more depressed than Mum. She bucked up no end! Walked Mum and [my dog] on trail for ½ an hour. Mum said she enjoyed it! Back home for Soup! Mum in much better mood & she's singing to herself - won't last. Anyway, left 2pm, & full of hope. Mum to have sleep before putting on her 'face' for Debbie. Peace be with you".

For once, I had the opportunity to experience her morning mood myself, and once again it was not great as the 'witching hour' of 11-00am hove into being. It all tended to add supplementary 'fuel' to the 'fire' of my suspicion that 11am was the time that Mum experienced the waning of the strongest effects of her morning medication, and thus presented so many apparent issues to my siblings, as they worked through their mostly *morning* 'shifts'. Moreover, my regular reliance (sometimes risky insistence) on *distraction* as a means of helping her (and me) to deal with in such 'destabilisations' also seemed to have worked equally well at this *earlier* time. Persevering with getting her out and about had once again reaped rewards for me; not least, on this occasion, because she (we) had been lucky enough to bump into a fellow depressive, and to be reminded that there were both other sufferers out there and some worse that her!

Meanwhile, and whilst still struggling with a husband with a significant knee injury, my sister, as lead 'health minister', had also managed to get Mum to a doctor's appointment to have her now chronic 'arm' pain looked at.

12th Dec. (Thurs): "Came up for 1 hr before I was thrown out. Mum still getting dressed. Had not taken her tablets. Stressed about going to Doc's. Thought it better not to mention them and took them out of the case. Will be up tomorrow and will check that she has taken Friday's. No heating on again. Arm hurting still. L came. Baz has fallen and his knee has opened up & bleeding. They are going back to hospital this afternoon. Don't mention to Mum". (T).

"Examined by GP. Frozen Shoulder. See leaflets – referring for physiotherapy. Recommended painkillers & gel. Takes a while. Nothing to do with 'flu jab. Simple exercises". (L).

"L here [on arrival]. Read leaflet. Guess what? 'The cause is not clear'. [I still think] the flu jab has triggered some sort of effect on the shoulder muscles. It's too much of a coincidence that the 'frozen shoulder' pain started almost immediately after the flu jab. L left. Mum immediately asking where the prescription was. I presume there isn't one & she has to buy her own paracetamol & gel? Mum made soup. We chatted about the frozen shoulder [diagnosis]. Mum banging on about when to take the paracetamol, [which we already had in], & getting worked up. Told her to just take it if the pain's too much. Anyway, always useful to have a GP visit (psychologically), to say the Dr. couldn't find anything wrong apart from the [frozen] shoulder. (i.e. 'You're in good health – Dr said so'). Relaxation Exercises + 30 mins nap. For [local paper] with dog. Didn't take Mum out. Rainy day & she'd been to Dr's. Beans on toast for tea. (NB No complaints of 'arm' pain for over 4 hours!). Gone to recharge my batteries".

The frozen shoulder, along with other relatively minor issues, continued to 'bug' Mum, and to loom overly large in her oft-distorted, and increasingly OCD-bound, perspectives; for instance:

13th Dec. (Fri): "OK on arrival. Pills taken. Talked about frozen shoulder. She has rubbed it [with olive oil]. Lots of times she seems to forget about the arm. Quite alert. Talked about smaller kettle, one that holds [less]. The one she has is too big, as she fills it to the top, and can't hold it with her sore arm.". (L).

14th Dec. (Sat): "Mum weepy on arrival. Standard stuff these days – 'arm', legs', 'can't remember', and some junk mail about broken gas boilers had got her down + latest A-care bill (will take this and pay). Mum had made chicken dinner + rice pud – yummeee. Done dosette for week. None left now – need new prescription by FRIDAY, (see if they'll put the Ibuprofen in). Relaxation + 20 mins nap. Mum bucked up, so 1. Aldi. 2. Various shops looking for Ibuprofen Gel. (She drove me nuts with her Obsessive need for this; why didn't we get it on prescription – but we couldn't find any. Told her to use warm olive oil). Mum unpacked. No problems on return. Not a bad day, after poor start, so I score it 6/10. And so to bed, ssss".

17th Dec. (Tues): AM – "What is happening, Chris. Day AFT. regarding Debbie. Also what cover is there for Boxing Day?" (T).

PM – "Arrived to meet T on way out, so got *verbal* update. Then got T/C from [admin], re physio @ [local health centre]. Earliest offer 1-30pm @ Tues. 7th Jan 2014 – agreed to this as I can do it; confirmatory letter to follow. Soup lunch. If you, L, do Boxing day as you normally would (although it's a Thursday), I will come up with dog on the Friday + then go back to my Saturday as normal. Regarding Debbie + Xmas Day I will email A-care tomorrow [for clarity]. What about Weds 1st Jan. re Debbie – do we need her? [Usual Routine]. I don't know if Mum was all moaned out, but she hardly complained at all whilst out! (She usually goes, 'I didn't know I was coming to Tesco today'; even though we go EVERY Tues, and 'I don't know if I've got enough money, Keith'; even though we [always] check her purse together, before we leave – but none of that today – she was quite good company – so I've no more idea than anyone else what to expect!!

But then 5-20pm. I could see Mum's mood change. She went very quiet & 'frightened'. It was triggered by a change in the quality of her sight in her right eye. She said she couldn't see because of the 'floater'. She became upset for a while, and it took quite a while to Reassure her that 'Nothing's going to happen'. It must be scary when this happens and you're alone. Hence the T/cs we get. She described it as 'like a film going over' [her eye]. Causes acute anxiety. A re-referral to an eye specialist might be Reassuring to both she & we in the New Year. Mum calmed & eye better by 6-15. So, I still score it 6/10 as I head home a little wiser".

So, from regular, often minor, OCD issues, such as the kettle or the Ibuprofen Gel, to *ir*regular, but scary, 'mental' ones like the 'floater', and the anxiety attacks, (and of course all the other ongoing effects of the Dementia; especially when alone/at night), and now the annual, and rather tricky 'administration and cover' arrangements for the emotional quagmire that is Christmas in these circumstances, there were always tasks and issues of one sort or another to attend to, and never much time to relax, and to properly gauge how we were doing. So, to try and better *benchmark/ monitor* how things were going, (at least for myself), my latest quirky idea was to try and employ a basic *scoring system* for my visits. On the first couple of occasions I had scored my (slightly better than average) visits 6/10, and would try to measure my future visits accordingly.

18th Dec. (Weds): "Had to come up 3-00pm. Had a panic attack. Frightened. The usual. Does not want Debbie – says she'll take her away! Doesn't want to stay alone at night". (L).

19th Dec. (Thurs.): "[Usual Routine]. Mum woke 'frightened'; struggle to get her to go out at all. Helped her get dressed. She said I was 'forcing' her. Told her I would 'make sure nothing happened'. Eventually got her (& dog) to car; but she was banging on about going in a home, 'cos she's frightened at night. Went cemetery for brief walk; but cold. Mum still talking about 'homes' [that] will 'look after you'. Decided to head for Ashwood Ho. & then The Moorlands. Mum 'coming round'; but not sure if she did want such a home now. I suggested going to one for day-care in the New Year. Back at home she talked about her 'nice little house'; and said she'd carry on here. Raining hard but Mum in better mood. P S. No mention of arm whilst we were out. Beans on toast for tea. Not a great day from my point of view - weather shit, Mum 'all over the shop', but better end than I thought. Gone to 'recovery'. 5/10".

Mum's recurring 'fear' was once again causing HER to actually raise the thought of going in a home, to be 'looked after', (a far cry from her oft-stated 'over my dead body' views of such a move from her more compos mentis days), yet when the likely possibilities and 'realities' were actually put before her, via a simple drive-by to view the potential possibilities from the outside, she recoiled to wanting to retain the safety and familiarity of her 'nice little house'. Nevertheless, we had a real dilemma here. If Mum was becoming afraid of being alone in her own home, (a home that she had been happy in for over 60 years), that was a major change, so *should* we begin to persuade Mum to take the 'leap', and actually leave her own home? On the other hand, would such a move be even more confusing and stressful for her? I certainly felt so, for in the course of my social work career, I had had need to work with Care Homes for both children & young people, and the elderly, and I had been decidedly less than impressed with what I found for either group. So, for me, such a move was an absolutely last resort; especially as it would be 'going against the grain' of what Mum had so expressly opposed when fully compos mentis. (Not to mention the extortionate costs involved). Yet, supporting her in-house needs was already absorbing so much of our own personal lives, and was already getting more and more stressful for *us*, too – making it difficult, (short of moving in full time - an option that we'd already agreed would be both logistically impractical for all, and, potentially, exhausting for the sibling 'in residence'), to see how we might further manage, and try to mitigate, her 'fears', going forward. Hence the dilemma. For, if she *was* now (albeit inconsistently) raising the matter of being 'looked after' herself, this was going to be yet *another* key area of her life that we would have to keep under ever closer review. With Christmas upon us, it was certainly the sort of 'present' we could have done *without*!

Still, life had to go on, and one easily-achievable option to try was more *signage*.

21st Dec. (Sat): "Not at her best on arrival. Could have been worse. Hadn't made chicken dinner, but HAD made rice pudding. 'Arm' hurting, 2 x A-care letters + Physio letter all causing her anxiety. Have taken A-care bills. Physio one on shelf. Radiators OFF in both kitchen and front room. Told her off (lightly) & put them on. Have made Reminder sign for the kitchen wall – 'HEATING AND EATING'. Dosette done. [Usual Routine]; then Aldi for general shopping. (I think he should do his own!). No mention of arm while out. Salmon sarnies for tea. Mum quite good at this point (4-25pm) & its been a good day. Would have scored it 7/10; but 5-40pm - anxiety attack - 'legs', 'arm', 'dizzy'. 6-30pm the crisis was past. Mum saying she felt better. Mum OK when I left @ 7-30. Shame about the anxiety attack otherwise been a good day, but that late attack means I score 6/10".

22nd Dec. (Sun): "Not good on arrival. Crying & frightened. Gave me a bad time, but hey ho I've had them before. She calmed down after a while. I have told Mum I will start ringing her at 6 to break the night up for her. She said that was OK. Mum would not settle. All the time I was here she kept walking in and out of the kitchen. I watched her go upstairs to the toilet. Have seen her handle it better. Has been to the toilet 3 times. Says she can't go properly. Had a few words over [overfilling] the kettle, and then saying she couldn't lift it. Tried to tell her not to fill it to the top, but she went off on one and said she will do what she wants. Worst morning I have had for a long time". (T).

24th Dec (Tues. – Christmas Eve): AM - "Arrived 9-30. Mum upset & crying but soon calmed down. Reminded her I will come for her at 11-30 [tomorrow – Christmas Day] and bring her back when she wants. I will try and keep her as long as possible. Reminded her she is going to L's on Boxing Day. Seems OK with arrangements at the moment. Had a card from John & Jennifer [ex-neighbours]. Upset her a bit because they [had] remembered her & sent a photo of their (now 2) children. Wants to send a New Year card to them". (T).

PM – "Mum moping in chair. Worked to get her up & about. Made soup. She wouldn't let me wash up. Relaxation + 20 mins nap. Woke OK; said 'Where we goin', Keith?'. 'Tesco, Mum' & off we went. She did quite well; not holding onto trolley much & not in bad mood either. Back home she was anxious again. Wanted to write note to remind her its Christmas Day tomorrow & that she's going to T's. Fish for Christmas Eve tea + trifle! Gave Mum 2 of her presents – the white hyacinth and the new kitchen mat. There's some smaller presents to open on Christmas day.

[Home] thoughts:-

1. If Mum went in a home:-
    a. Would she be less anxious?

b. Would she like a small room & single bed + communal room?

c. Other residents, likely to be just as bad. Sooner or later some would pop off – how would she cope with that? What if home closed?

d. As visitors could/would we spend the same amount of time with her. What if she got fed up there?

e. Would she get out as much or just 'slip away' sat in a chair - what I call die dying rather than die living!

2. If Mum didn't go in a home:-
   a. What extra support could WE provide?
   b. What extra support could someone else / another agency provide?
   c. Can we get her to cooperate with a psychiatric report/ update? What will it produce?
   d. Would she consider day-care. (No).

Either way, we're looking for things to HELP; but there won't be SOLUTIONS @ 88. Let's get Christmas out of the way & see what's what. I'll keep my mobile with me in case u want to discuss anything over Xmas

6-15 Watching Carols from Kings – Mum seems to be enjoying it - singing quietly to some. Lovely to see/hear. Stay calm. Happy Christmas 7/10".

Christmas Day: "As discussed over the phone. Mum stuck it out until 6-40pm. Once we got in Mum became tense as I was going, but the best day for months". (T).

Christmas was over. The 'Plan' had gone pretty well. Much better than any of us anticipated, with all the emotional guff that's attached to the occasion. My brother had popped in on the morning of Christmas Eve, and I had spent a generally enjoyable Christmas Eve afternoon, until bedtime, with her, and had managed to incorporate not only the 'usual relaxation and nap Routine', and a colourful Christmassy trip to Tesco, without undue issue, but had also found time to think about and log the pros and cons of Mum living in a 'Home', so we'd got off to a good start. Then, we had each telephoned Mum nice and early on Christmas morning, and T had collected her later that morning, (as promised), and taken her to his house/family celebrations for Xmas dinner etc. Distracted by the festivities there she seemed to have coped well, and had been taken home, and seen off to bed, without significant problem by 7pm. On the Boxing day, Mum had then been collected by my sister, and spent the afternoon there, but things had not gone quite so smoothly. Although no written log was made for Boxing Day, my sister's verbal feedback had told of an afternoon managing Mum's reversion to her usual moans and groans; but just in a different setting; though nothing untoward. (It may have been that the previous day's relatively late celebrations had taken a lot out of Mum and that she was still tired).

Regardless, we all breathed a giant sigh of relief that Mum had coped OK, that our Christmas plans and celebrations had suffered no *undue* complications or interruptions, and that we had rather 'got away with it'. Phew!

However, it was certainly 'business as usual' by Friday. Which certainly 'took the shine off' MY smug sense of relief.

27th Dec. (Fri): "I rang Mum @ 9-30am – someone had done a good job, 'cos Mum sounded ok and WAS expecting me today. [Even tho' Friday was not one of my normal visiting days]. Drove over and walked [dog]. Mum not bad on arrival, but easily confused by having to warm soup/cook chicken for Sat/ & get [my dog] food. So 'one job at a time' instigated. [Together we] put chicken in oven/ fed dog/warmed soup – in that order. Mum OK again, but now 'arm' hurting. Asked Mum to talk to me like an adult; and not in a child's tone. After brief, 'I won't let you in' rubbish, she did talk 'properly'. Chat about putting less water in kettle – I emptied out all the water & invited Mum to pick up the 'light' (empty) kettle. Suggested she fill up a teacup twice & pour that in. Less weight to lift. She agreed but just 5 minutes later she filled the bloody thing right up again!, saying, 'Nobody tells me what to do'. Ah, well, keep trying. Relaxation Routine + 25mins nap. Walked [dog]; but too windy for Mum. At this stage 6/10 score. All going reasonably well UNTIL she went to the toilet

149

about 4pm! Got very upset 'cos she couldn't 'go'. 'Call Dr. Keith'. Then <u>Major Shit Scene</u>: She sat & stood straining in toilet several times, & shat a little; but then had minor 'shits' in kitchen. Cried. Back to toilet. Shit 'spots' on toilet mat. Then she stood, legs astride, in kitchen, put a washing-up bowl between her legs and SHAT/bombed 4 or 5 large solid 'logs' into the bowl, from about 2 ft up!; plus splats onto kitchen lino. She was very relieved, very weepy & very weak. Major use of Cillit-Bang in kitchen & bathroom; [I] took bowl of turds to toilet & was nearly sick myself, whilst retching!!

5-30pm – I made beans on toast for tea & yoghurt & cake – doesn't get better. One thing's for sure, I will NOT be applying for any jobs in Old Folks Homes!

6-30pm – Mum sleepy now; TV. [Dog had been] up & down the stairs behind us & licking at the shit spots [before I'd been able to clean them up]. What a few hours that was!!

Lessons: -

1. We need to look @ Mum's diet. (Have suggested less cheese - it bungs you up).
2. Only one [laxative sachet] available – need more now it's been used.
3. Is another GP consultation needed, 'cos she must have been holding this 'load of shit' for while? (May have affected her Boxing Day mood, L).

By 6-30pm Mum could hardly remember the 'kerfuffle'. She knew she was tired & 'had been', but couldn't remember the straining, crying & mess. Hopefully, the fact that she's 'empty' will help. As I leave, Mum ain't bad again. Needs sleep. As do I! Score 4/10".

28th Dec. (Sat): "Mum not bad on arrival. Soup. 'Arm' hurting. Maybe from straining yesterday. Improved over lunch & chat, with Reassurance. Discussed 'Constipation' over lunch! I repeated [advice] from the website:-

1. Sit on loo every day @ same time, (best after breakfast, suggested 9am) – whether u want to go or not – Routine.

2. Drink plenty of water.
3. Take laxative as needed.
4. Eat more fruit & veg. (try prunes).
5. Eat Fibre (Bran) as at present.

Please can u Repeat/Remind Mum on these points - it's worth a try. Relaxation + 20 mins nap. Woke slowly but OK & ready for Aldi. [Mum put all] stuff away on return. Salmon sarnie tea. L called round 5ish. Brought laxative. Mum OK. 1st night I've had no 'incident' for a while. Fingers crossed & home for M o D. 7/10".

The toileting issues had taken on a sort of 'constipated' importance as the year drew to a close. It was bad enough when Mum struggled to 'go' *in* the toilet, but it certainly wasn't easy to see Mum descend from the heights of impeccable cleanliness and hygiene in her heyday, (she cleaned for money in her later working life!), to the point of dealing with her obvious constipation in such desperate ways as openly, and awkwardly, using an old washing-up bowl in the kitchen! Clearly, the Dementia was a factor here, for there was no way that Mum would have embarrassed herself before her offspring otherwise! We were in 'unchartered waters' now on this issue. What could we expect next?

31st Dec. (Tues – New Year's Eve): AM – "Mum OK on arrival. Told her about Eric M [a fellow villager and friend who had died]. Took it quite well. If she tells you once she tells you a dozen times that Eric played in a band. L rang. Won't be up until dinner tomorrow as she is going out 2nite. She said the death of Eric was sudden. The funeral is next Tues at [the] Crem. Reassured Mum that she was fit compared to Eric. What will 2014 bring? We don't know. Happy New Year". (T).

PM – "Mum OK on arrival. In fact quite good. Soup lunch & cake & shortbread. Brief chat about Eric M, but she didn't dwell on it. Relaxation Exercises + 25 mins nap. Woke unsteady, but rose and made cuppa & slowly got better; so out we went. Tesco really busy. Me to cemetery; Mum put shopping away. Fish for tea. After tea, I cut Mum's toenails, but they're tough & thick – may be worth asking for chiropodist to have a go. Otherwise quite a good day & end to old year. 7/10. Happy New Year".

The old year had drawn to a close. In many ways, and with hindsight, 2013 would prove to be something of a 'turning point' year. For, during it, the Dementia had slowly, but definitely, tightened its' grip, and Mum had changed significantly from a still fairly compos mentis, still fairly confident, 'happy-in-mi-own home', coping, sort of Mum at the beginning of the year, to a much less confident, more dependent one, with yet more new 'issues' to be managed, (including, 'arm', toileting, 'fear', heating, 'gas'?, and an actual 'carer'), as it ended.

2014

We were off to a decent start.

My sister had the dubious privilege of kicking off the 2014 log, but thankfully, with nothing 'untoward'.

1st Jan. (Weds): "Bit weepy, but just arm pain + mixed up with days. Very cold – no heating on. I got here 11.00 so hasn't been on all morning. Doesn't help with pain. Had a nice New Year dinner - fish finger butties + warm scones – mmm. Not a bad day really". (L).

2nd Jan. (Thurs): "Mum Ok on arrival. Then Kate [my adult daughter] arrived. Soup & beans for dinner. Mum perked up @ distractions [Kate + dog]. Brief relaxation & short nap. Then short trip to cemetery with Mum, [dog] & Kate. Hard work but worthwhile. Back for cuppa, before Kate left @ 3.00pm. Quiet sit for 35 mins & chat. Beans on toast for tea + cake. No major issues. Mum's had a decent day. 7/10. That's the way to do it, 2014"; but it couldn't last and now another potential 'management' issue (almost literally), 'fell' into the 'mix', and threatened to need adding to the ever-growing list.

4th Jan. (Sat): "Mum upset on arrival. Says she missed the bottom step of stairs & fell into the kitchen door earlier. Obviously she was shocked & may have further strained her arm, but improved once she'd told me. [After checking], I Reassured her 'nothing broken'. Long chat. Seems she was trying to put her cardigan on whilst coming downstairs – and missed the step by not concentrating. Let her know Repeatedly that coming down stairs needs her FULL ATTENTION. Also, kitchen radiator was off. Anyway, soup & chicken for lunch + rice pudding. L arrived. Dosette done. Relaxation Exercises + 20 mins nap. Then Aldi. Not bad round Aldi, but poor confidence back at home - hit by this morning's 'trip' in stairs? Yet still tried to carry shoes + coat + toilet rolls upstairs at one go; then wondered why 'tired'. Then insisted on making tea. 5pm After tea – major panic attack-'Frightened', 'arm', 'eye', 'feel sick', 'weak'. Asking me to stay, [agreed if necessary], to 'get doctor'. 'Go in a home'. Lasted about 40 mins. 6pm Calm [now], but 'tired'. Talking reasonably ok now. 7pm - had completely forgotten the 'attack'. [Still] 'tired', but not now sure why. [No longer asking me to stay]. Not a great day 5/10".

Mum had *never* had a fall, and was still relatively sure-footed, but the *potential* (at 88) was perhaps our greatest unspoken worry for the times, (especially through the night), when none of us (or any other 'carer'), were in attendance. In my 'down time', it was an ever-present worry that I carried on a permanent basis. It *never* went away. ('Was she OK, safe, coping, etc.). It was also at the front of my mind whenever I was due to be *first* to arrive on any particular day. ('What would I find? Might she be dead even crossed my mind!). Thus far, our worries had never come to fruition, but like the 'dual' incident of 'the smell of gas' noted not too long ago by my sister, (thankfully there had been no recorded repetition), the *'fall'* had now shown *its* potential 'hand'. Of course, any regular suggestion of either the presence of 'gas' or of the likelihood of a 'fall' had obvious and serious implications for Mum's safety, and, by implication, for her remaining alone in her own home. Next-up challenge for me, though, was to take her to the local [clinic] to keep her 'arm' appointment with the physiotherapist. It had finally arrived.

7th Jan. (Tues):

"Mum OK on arrival. Had to *remind* her about [clinic]; but ok with it. Brief Relaxation + 10 mins nap, but broken because Mum now had [clinic] on her mind. Anyway, we got ready & went. Arrived on time to see Tim – nice enough guy, but only confused the issue. Tim said it could be *either* a frozen shoulder OR a strain OR a touch of Arthritis! (Honestly, I could have come up with that!) He got Mum partially undressed & got her to move her arms in various directions – but still couldn't say exactly what it was. Upshot – he showed us some exercises to try with a (walking) stick twice daily and then said we had to find our own stick! He gave us a sheet with the exercises printed on (in the back of this pad with the frozen shoulder info). He also said putting gentle heat on it might help. (Well, I would never have thought of that!). Finally, he said to practice the above and come back in 2 weeks; have booked for Mon the 20th. (But I ask you – GP don't know; physio don't know; I'd have a guess as good as them for their salaries!). On to Tesco. Fish for tea. Anyway, get her to try the exercises – go on I dare you & bet you £1. Mum said, 'I do enough bloody exercises as it is. He can go to hell'. 6pm – T/Cs form T & L. Updates given. Quite a good day. 7/10".

9th Jan (Thurs): AM - "OK on arrival. Having breakfast. Asked her to do some exercises with the stick, but she said they were a waste of time. Has not mentioned the arm this morning. I asked about Debbie, but can't seem to get a reasonable answer from her. Been to toilet twice. No heating on. I watched her put clothes on [old]rack and pull it up with no complaint regarding her arm. Strange". (T).

PM – "Mum not bad on arrival. Soup for dinner. Mum is adamant that Debbie didn't come on Weds. I will e-mail Julie B. [Usual Routine]. At 2-30 the rains briefly ceased. Talked Mum into coming for [drive] to fill time. Rains started again. Enough to make anyone depressed. 4pm - Mum is up and down like a fiddler's elbow. Faffing. Beans on toast for tea. It's 5-20. I've been sat down since 4-30. Mum sat down for her tea but is again up & about. [OCD?]. Nevertheless, & given the rain Mum's done well. Decent day 7/10".

11th Jan. (Sat): "Mum OK on arrival; though kitchen radiator off. Put it on. Mum had made Chicken Dinner for 1st time in 3 weeks; plus [home-made] rice pudding. T rang. A-care been in contact. Apologetic about Weds. [Appears Debbie really didn't come, but no-one had informed us, despite their agreement to do so]. [Usual Routine]. 5-30 pm – L came, but broke bulb in lamp; and then left – leaving Mum disturbed. She said the lamp wasn't the same brightness [with new bulb]; then blamed L 'cos she'd got wrong telly channel; then when I told her to try & get right channel herself, she started crying & threw the remote at the fireplace, in temper. I picked it up & threw it on the carpet, saying '2 can do that, Mum'. Luckily, it still worked. Anyway, due to that [late] 'interruption', an 8/10 has to be downgraded to only 7/10".

12ᵗʰ Jan (Sun): "OK on arrival. Doing housework. Suggested a walk. The answer was NO. Went toilet twice. Asked if she'd done exercises with stick. She said they were a waste of time. No heating on. No bed made. Mum got worked up about 11 o'clock [again] for no reason, but it passed with a bit of distraction. Reminded her Debbie was coming & things were back to normal. Not a bad morning". (T).

5pm – called out. Sink blocked. Full of peas, carrots etc. Mum [still] not happy with light in corner. Nothing wrong with light. Just looking for problems". (T).

14th Jan (Tues): "Mum not bad on arrival, but faffing about phone bill. PRESCRIPTION DUE! Relaxation + 25 mins nap. Then OK 'til I asked her to wear a hat in the cold. Said 'No', cried & started shouting at me. 'Go, Go, I'll ring T, you're all for yourself, always have been, you're not bossing me'. All that sort of [stuff] – not quite so Relaxing! Asked her to walk [outside] to see how cold it was - lead to repeat of the above! She finally 'came round' & off we went. P.Off – paid BT bill; Tesco. Fine round Tesco. OK on return. Mum now 'tired' of course, but doesn't remember why, 'cos she's forgotten the row. And so to tea - fish in Butter Sauce + Egg Custard. Still, shouting match apart, not a bad day. 6/10".

15ᵗʰ Jan (Weds): "Trip to [town]. All very good. Walk up street to Methodist church for dinner – soup & choc cake – homemade, very nice. With the 'old folk'. She remembered the row you had Tues. Will get prescription this week. Suggested sleep before Debbie comes. 10/10! So there!" (L).

16ᵗʰ Jan. (Thurs): AM – "Not good on arrival. Crying & shouting at me because she'd lost her cross & chain. Found it down side of her chair. Soon calmed down, but no heat in either room. Mum told me about your falling out (not all that daft). You are further down the will. Started to get upset about 10-30. Kept tapping her forehead & shaking her head. I suggested a walk in the backyard. Her eye was playing up. Could be because of the tension". (T).

PM – "L here on arrival. (Brought prescription). [Usual Routine]. Went for local paper/ cemetery 'run/ & brief visits to 'birds'. Useful break from house = 'distraction' - let it rain, let it rain. Whilst I read paper Mum was rarely off her feet, checking, wiping, etc. Beans on toast for tea. 5-15 – I washed up, but Mum insisted on drying & then cleaning everywhere I'd done. Would drive you nuts 24/7. 5-45 – Mum came to sit down, saying 'I'm not well'; 'I'm frightened'; 'Something's going to happen'. Predictable given she's been on her feet for hours. Advised her to rest, to recover. She calmed down & we watched telly. OK by 7. 6/10".

The dynamics of recent days had been interesting, if pretty stressful. It was clear that her perception of a row with me had stayed in her memory, at least to some degree, and had been regurgitated to T & L in their turn, on the following couple of days. Clearly, her memory of particularly worrying 'interactions' worked well enough on occasion, but not necessarily either accurately or indefinitely. It was also likely that such tension-inducing 'interactions', as Mum perceived them, were having a knock-on effect on her behaviour and moods. However, it was also interesting to read my brother's log where he noted her 'tapping her forehead, and shaking her head', as if she was trying to 'break through' some sort of mental barrier being erected at that time, by the Dementia. There were lessons to learn here. Not least that keeping calm with Mum at all times offered the best chance of her keeping *her* calm and coping. It may also have helped that I had arrived on the Thursday thus, (the first time I'd visited since the 'row'), and shown her that things were absolutely fine between us, and 'carrying on as normal'.

18th Jan. (Sat): "Mum actually good on arrival. [Usual Routine]. No problems. Found Mum's chain on hall carpet – but no cross – but Mum's reaction was very good. She'd normally make a crisis, but didn't. We found another cross in her purse & put that on. Well done, Mum. (For L, don't forget Mum due @

physio on Mon – appt card in wooden bowl on kitchen shelf}).
Been a decent day really, so, for the first time, I'm scoring 8/10".

19th Jan. (Sun): "Mum OK on arrival. Having breakfast.
Keith rang. Debbie not coming. Has phoned in sick. Reminded
[Mum] about [physio clinic] on Monday. Reminder I am away
31st Jan to 2nd Feb. Mum went to toilet at 11-00am. Has flushed
toilet 3 times. It is now 11-25. She has just come back. As I left she
was having some dinner & a sleep". (T).

20th Jan. (Mon): "Did well at [physio clinic]. Some
improvement since last visit. [Further] visit booked for Feb. For
steroid injection if needed. If things carry on improving we can
phone & [cancel]. All in all a good day, though mind all over the
place. Tablets for Tues. are not in box!? Has she taken them?
Doesn't seem to have affected her". (L).

21st Jan. (Tues): "Arrived 9-30am. Mum crying & in vile
mood. Tablets + box all on the work surface near kettle. Phoned
L. She came up. Mum kept telling us to get out as she did not want
any of us. Mum said doctor came last week and knocked 3 off. We
explained that was months ago, but this got Mum more agitated.
She eventually calmed down & said she was sorry. Mum keeps
opening and closing the dosette box to see if the tablets are still
there". (T).

23rd Jan. (Thurs): Arrived to find T still there from his
morning 'shift'. He had had another difficult time, with Mum's
mood generally 'down' and uncooperative. Reluctant to depart
with Mum's poor mood unresolved, he had felt the need to stay
with Mum until I arrived for my afternoon 'shift'; and he had
wanted to share his concerns directly with me, anyway. (Not
actually seeing each other for days at a time, and relying on the
logs for communication, could often leave us feeling like we were
'ships passing in the night', and could leave *we carers* feeling quite
isolated whilst supporting Mum, so the occasional face-to- face
chat also allowed us to share and get rid of some of our *own*
built-up anxieties). With the handover complete, and my brother
on his way, it was time to start again with *my* 'shift'.

"I started to make soup. Mum went and sat in her chair in the
front room & refused to come in [the kitchen]. Need a plan! Ah, I

also need a pee, so I'll use that. 'Mum, could you watch the soup on the oven please, while I go to the toilet'? Went upstairs. Had pee & shouted again for her to check pan and waited (the tension builds!) and I hear her shuffle into kitchen. I count to 10 then creep down stairs & she's supervising the soup. Game on. 'Oh, thanks, Mum'. Sat her down at table as she looked unsteady, and I made the soup, scone + tea. Mum saying she wasn't hungry – 'Mum if you don't eat you will get ill'. Buttered some bread & gave it to her. She ate it all. Result. Reassuring chat over lunch, telling her 'nothing's going to happen 'etc. I then washed up; though Mum then got up & wiped & dried everything I'd done. Hailstone shower – useful distraction; then quiet sit, Relaxation Exercises + 30 mins nap. Woke calmer. 2-15 – Mum up making cuppa, more or less back to 'normal'. Cuppa was late, so went to look; she had the spinner out for 'smalls'. I made the cuppa. Mum much better by now but still vaguely remembered 'arguing' – Reassured her that it was just discussion – seemed to accept it. [Suggested] paying papers. She agreed & off we went. [Then] drive to cemetery. Busy dog on left arm, doddery old codger on right arm. Brolly up. Beans on toast for tea. 5-15 – Mum faffing again – washing up, washing dog's towel, cleaning floor. She thinks keeping busy 'stops her being frightened'; but more likely to bring it on if already tired. 6-00 [Mum said] 'I go to bed @ 7 o'clock & I'm happy. I like going to bed with mi wireless on'. All-in-all a draining for all. 6/10".

25th Jan. (Sat): "Mum not bad on arrival. [Usual Routine]. Mum woke up during nap, saying arm hurt. Started argument along the same old stuff – 'don't care', 'go in a home'. Decent argument as I asked her to talk like an adult, not a child. She cried & told me to go. Eventually tired. I let her sleep. Most people of her age would sit & watch TV, listen to radio, knit, do jigsaw, read, etc. But she won't do any of these – just 'keeps going' til knackered, then sits & moans about being tired etc. - but no idea that she's made it [so]. Mum woke & at first seemed calm, but 'went off' again, saying 'No body cares', 'Go in a home - 'Go Go Go' – unfortunately, I 'took the bait', and said I was 'going & not coming back'. Mum got very upset & rang L. [Afterwards] I asked

Mum to either 'come shopping or let me go home'. She chose shopping. Took a while getting her ready. Drove round a bit, to distract her & let her settle down, then Aldi. She was already in better mood & coped admirably round Aldi & up to Poundstretcher.

4.00pm. Back home. Mum about 'normal' again now. She put stuff away, but 'tired'. Thought: I think Mum's anxiety does build up while we're away, and it's almost like she needs to argue to get it out of her system. Although she rarely appears to remember the argument for too long, it does drain her (& me). Thought for me: I really do need to work harder at NOT taking the bait. I should know better. In theory I do, but in practice I'm definitely getting 'slack'. Salmon sarnies for tea. 5pm - Minor obsession with tiny 'gap' in front [window] blind. Chat with Mum about her anxieties, but the key one [at present] is 'something's going to happen' fear. No easy solution beyond Reassurance. Mum ready for bed/sleep. A day that started quite well beset by anxiety; even so, no real problems 6/10".

Mum still appeared to forget most arguments soon after their occurrence and completion, but occasionally that was NOT so. In such instances, Mum would rarely remember them too accurately nowadays, but the perceived upset might still have 'lodged' somewhere in her dementing brain, and might mean that she 'carried' some *warped* version of that upset, internally, so I needed to revisit the theory, and then find again, in practice, the ability to *resist* her 'bait', and not 'swallow' it. More than ever, it was becoming apparent that Mum's personality and behaviour was changing - from the pleasant, affable, organised, inoffensive, Mum that we knew, to one where the confusion from the Dementia was causing her all sorts of anxiety and fretfulness; and a degree of accompanying, well-out-of-character, behaviour that we barely recognised. Accordingly, we needed to train ourselves to be less surprised by it; or irked by her more frequent argumentative outbursts, as she tried to make sense of what was happening to both her mind *and* body, and to make yet further *allowances* for them. Though that be easier said than done, we owed it to her to keep trying. If she was becoming less and less in control of her faculties, we should hardly be surprised that it showed in increased anxiety and 'fear', etc. After all, in the circumstances, (of the Dementia,) it wasn't really her fault anyway. Like those employed in the emergency services, we too needed to stay both as objective as we could, and calm under ALL 'fire'. We could but try. The point was poignantly made for me in my sister's next log.

27th Jan. (Mon): "Post Off OK. Walk round Coop. Started crying. Came home. Cried again. Told me she had been up all night crying about the Sat row with Keith. I read out [Keith's log] of what happened + how sorry he was. She asked me to phone Keith. I did. He wasn't in. Hopefully, we can put it behind us now. I am with T. Don't fill her head with too much info – it doesn't register anymore". (L).

My brother had also chipped in with his '2 pennorth' of parapsychologist's advice for me, logging that when he had started his job as a hospital porter at a hospital that catered mostly for the elderly, and many with Dementia, he had been advised to "Go with the easy option", and not look for trouble. I could see some *short-term* benefits, and resolved to try it occasionally, but I couldn't see, longer-term, how that approach would resolve any fundamental issues that might be troubling the 'patient,' in this case Mum.

Anyway, all advice logged, I was back to my calmer, more relaxed, more stoical, self when I next visited Mum on the following Tuesday, (the 28th), and, with my usual patience, usual, and on this occasion even more, affectionate hug for Mum, and the 'Usual Routine' and Reassurance, I was able to set Mum's mind at rest that, despite occasional 'differences of opinion', she was, and would remain, much- loved by me, (and indeed by us all), and that all was, and always would remain fundamentally OK between us. Accordingly, we had a good day together; including reciting nursery rhymes together over our fish-finger tea, (triggered by us spotting a black cat crossing Mum's backyard, following which I just spontaneously recited 'Pussy cat pussy cat where have you been'; and leading on to other rhymes in which Mum merrily joined in), and I scored it 8/10.

30th Jan. (Thurs): "Good on arrival. Soup for lunch. Mum [fed dog &] opened 'cards' (from T & Me). Relaxation exercises

+ 30 mins nap. Mum not keen to put hat on (in an icy wind) & she seemed ready to argue. SO! – took the 'easy option' & didn't take Mum out. (No argument – just told her was icy cold). Walked [my dog] to paper shop. Mum OK on my return. ('Easy option' worked? If I always took the easy option she'd never go out!). Beans on toast for tea. (Note to L – Alzheimer's Society meets first Weds in month @ Central Methodist Church). Brief anxiety attack during and just after tea. I think its over-tiredness (@88) & reluctance to rest/sit quietly. She spoke of 'fear of something happening' – even though I'm sat here! In truth, her basic 'fear' is hard to find a solution to, because its TRUE – if something [actually] happens when we're not here what will she do. My answer [to her] was WE ring or come round several times PER DAY; and if we got no answer we'd come round – best answer I can think of. Anyway, she was Ok again [later]. 7/10".

31st Jan. (Fri: Happy 88th birthday, Mum): "L there already on arrival. Mum 'dressed up' to go for Birthday Lunch. Drove to {Garden Centre]. Really packed. Chucking it down outside. Mum ordered Soup & Toastie & ate the lot. We then ordered 2 apple& pear crumbles + custard between the 3 of us & Mum ate quite a bit of that too. Cuppa back at home. L left. Mum cooked tomorrow's chicken. Relaxation session + 30 mins nap + quiet sit & chat. Moved to kitchen for 'light' tea of ham & tomato sarnies + trifle. Phew, I'm full! 5-30 – Mum trying to stack dishes on top shelf, despite my efforts to get her to put them [lower]. Predictably, 1 dish fell & broke on kitchen floor. Crying started, but Reassurance helped. But her obsessiveness won't respond to even firm advice – every dish has to be in its place! That said, a nice birthday lunch & not a bad afternoon. No real problems. Happy Birthday, Mum. 8/10".

January, and 2014, had set off well enough, had presented downside problems old and new in the middle, and then finished back on a relatively positive note, with Mum's 88th birthday. I was back on duty on the following day, too, Saturday, the 1st of February, and Mum's good birthday mood had extended into the new month; and, sticking largely to the 'Usual Routine', I was able to log another nice day, and score the second 8/10 in a row, but we were soon back to normal - for Mum was soon back to the 'fear' and anxiety stuff, and there were the ever-present issues around keeping her heating on in the cold weather, and whether she was regularly taking her medication, and the like; but in particular, her propensity to display the *OCD* behaviour seemed to come to the fore in early February. For example my brother found her outside cleaning the bin and out of breath, whilst my sister logged that "Debbie caught her in the garden doing her pots", and "with no coat on"; and, on more than one occasion, I had watched her 'keeping busy' by cleaning and re-cleaning the kitchen floor, or redoing areas that I had already done for her, and had had to answer her repeated questions about mundane things that might have nothing at all to do with Mum's life, (such as the barrage of OCD-like questions that followed a knock on her door, by an unknown man asking if we knew the whereabouts of one of our neighbours! We didn't)). We were still of the view that this OCD stuff was, at least in part, an OTT attempt to offset her 'fear', and to cope with the steadily deteriorating quality of her cognition these days; but, frustratingly, we still had no obvious solutions for her...and as for the 'easy option' so much quoted at me by my siblings:

8th Feb. (Sat): "Called 10-30. Mum brushing her hair. When she saw me she had a mini strop! So I had a strop back & said I hadn't been out for 4 days. That shut her up + she said I should have phoned. Constant whinging about 'arm' – wants to have steroid injection. No heating on. Bloody freezing! Well, she's in a good mood now, so enjoy your soup". (L).

PM – "Strop back, eh? – is that the easy option? I still think she 'saves up' the anxiety, (whilst alone), and releases it when we appear. As she said to me, 'I'm not constantly phoning you, am I?' Soup lunch. Dosette done. Need new scrip before next Saturday. Usual Routine. Aldi – no real problems. Quick whizz to cemetery for [a bit of] 'timeout'. Mum Ok on return, but 'tired'. Wouldn't surprise me if she had anxiety attack or provoked an argument. 4-45 – [As predicted] 'funny turn' whilst trying to carry coat, hat & [roll of] tape upstairs, followed by 'I'm frightened', 'I don't know what to do'. Sat her down, made cuppa & then I made tea, whilst talking Reassuringly. I took her coat upstairs, and when I came down, she was on her feet again! She cannot sit & rest. Forgets what she's done, so doesn't realise she's overdone it. 5-30 I washed up. (Mum did eat her tea, so appetite OK), but Mum's back upstairs [faffing about], and has been out to bins 3 times. 6-00pm She's calm again. Now just 'tired', and needs sleep. Not Mum's best day, but I've had worse. Still, quite draining. 7/10".

There was much to re-visit and re-learn from that one Saturday's business. Firstly, from L's early visit, it was clear that Mum had been worrying because L had not contacted Mum for over 4 days; even by phone. (L had been beset by a cold, and hadn't wanted to worry Mum, unnecessarily). This suggested that, despite the Dementia, Mum still retained a sufficient degree of cognition, and therefore a reasonable concept of time, and of time lapsed, regarding the lack of contact from L. Secondly, it showed that, in the right circumstances, L too was quite capable of disregarding the 'easy option', and of 'taking the bait', and having 'a strop back'. Thirdly, it pointed up the winter 'heating' dilemma once again. Fourthly, the 'arm' pain didn't appear to be there all the time, and may just as easily be some sort of auto-response to felt *psychological* stress and strain as to a felt physical one; so, might a steroid injection for a potentially psychosomatic matter be a little OTT? Then, from my afternoon shift, there were other potential lessons and reminders for us. Firstly, there was further evidence of her seemingly entrenching bouts of OCD activity; these too, as I've said, probably a response to her fears, anxieties and decreasing confidence in coping with what had hitherto been 'second nature', 'everyday' matters for her. Secondly, Mum's assertion that she did not 'know what to do' suggested that we needed to try even harder to imagine just how scary such Dementia-lead moments might be for her. Thirdly, that we really did need to try *not* to take any of her 'bait', but, instead, to stay calm when 'under fire', to *expect* 'the flak', and, to that end, consider finding little pockets of 'time-out' for ourselves *during* a shift; here, refreshing my own faculties by popping up to visit Dad's grave *alone* for that precious few minutes of private reflection. Fourthly, that the OCD behaviour was probably here to stay, and that invoking the Routine element, in particular, of 'The 3 Rs', still remained our best, and core, source for providing consistency to her.

11th Feb. (Tues): "Mum OK on arrival. Soup lunch. Then L arrived & Mum had an 'audience'; so Mum started moaning and arguing. Once L left, & Mum was 1:1 with me, there was no more arguing. [When] Mum has an audience to 'play to', she does! Often having stored anxiety. Usual Routine. Opticians, Tesco, Argos, Aldi. Home again, home again, jiggety-jig. Cod-pieces (!) for tea. No anxiety attack today. Anyway, decent day. 7/10".

Coincidentally, in the local paper of that week was a report that the biggest (30-bed) Nursing Home in the area was to close. I drew Mum's attention to the article, and made reference to it in one of my logs, to show both Mum and my siblings that going in a home carried no absolute certainties. My twofold point was that, had Mum already given up the familiarity of her own home to take up this money-gobbling option, she would be amongst those vulnerable residents (some had, reportedly, lived there for more than 20 years) about to be unceremoniously uprooted and moved to God knows where, and that these homes were essentially commercial enterprises, and only functioned so long as they paid their way, and preferably made a profit.

On that same (Thurs) day, I had also drawn Mum's attention to (and logged) the fact that I had a cold of my own; in case she caught it and she (and my siblings), thought it was something more serious; not that, (like everything else), it wasn't potentially serious in these Dementia-ridden days. Nevertheless, we had pursued the 'Usual Routine' and apart from a couple of mild instances of her thriving hyperactive OCD stuff, we had enjoyed a 7/10 sort of day; but:

15th Feb. (Sat): "Mum not bad. Soup lunch. (She don't seem to do chicken dinners now). 1-00pm – Uh Uh Mum sniffling. Hope her 'flu jab offers some protection! 2-00pm - Uh Ooh, Mum coughing like me! Come on 'flu jab, do your job. [Usual Routine]. Aldi. All OK. Beware! Mum is talking in a croaking voice + coughing – but in a surprisingly decent mood. Salmon sarnies for tea. 4-40 – [mini hiccup] after I couldn't find TV book. Mum said it hadn't come [with her Sat paper]. I was getting ready to go paper-shop, but just thought to look in bin & there it was! Taped up. Mum got a little upset & said, 'I don't know what I'm doing'. I 'backed off' (easy option) and left her to [finish making] tea. 6pm - Last minute [toileting incident]. Mum struggling on toilet. 'Huffing, 'puffing' & crying. I sat at top of stairs and heard a couple of 'plops' – so she did something. Helped her down. Made [laxative]sachet. 6-45 – 2nd trip to toilet. Came down for Vaseline at her request. Sat [outside loo] advising her to 'relax'. Several 'plops'. Mum opened toilet door with several [solid] stools IN HER HANDS to show me!! Back to pot to redeposit. Helped her wash her hands. Escorted her down to chair. Made cuppa & 2 ginger nuts, to sit & relax for 20 mins. Mum much calmer, but ready for bed. Departed 8-15. Not entirely happy, but she's ready for [sleep, & constipation crisis over], so can't see benefit of me staying. 5/10".

The last thing we needed was something that affects *everybody* negatively, regardless of Dementia, (like a bad cold), to inflict Mum, along with all the other things she, and we, needed to manage. Yet, not only did Mum seem to be *acquiring* my cold, but I had been 'treated' to another tricky, technicolour, OCD-type, (perhaps 'winter-cold'-*associated*), toileting 'event'; in which Mum's behaviour had once again deteriorated to the point of 'basic'. Our 'real' Mum would never have *dreamt* of sharing the contents of her (albeit stable) faeces with me! Not *my* ideal moment to share!

Central to Monday the 17th of Feb was Mum's appointment back at the clinic for the steroid injection in her arm/frozen shoulder. My sister was on 'escort duty' that day, and logged, relatively positively, that Mum "did very well"; adding "review in 3 weeks", and "doesn't seem to be any reaction yet".

18th Feb. (Tues): AM – "Arrived 9-30. Mum in back garden. Tablets taken OK. No reaction from injection. No mention of arm at all. L rang. Said they gave 2 injections. 1 to numb the pain, and then the actual steroid. After the phone call Mum started to talk about the injection and then never stopped talking about it. Sue [T's partner] is doing Wed and L is doing Fri. She is on a course.

Not a bad morning. Mum seemed to go back 5 yrs - in a good way. (Will it last). 9 ½ /10". (T).

PM – "Mum crying as I arrived. Funny, after your morning score. She responded to Reassurance OK. Soup lunch. Mum went to toilet & came back saying, 'I did very well', & 'I've had a good road through me. Great!'. Usual Routine. Tesco – got extra groceries, 'cos have dog for next 2 weeks. Mum unpacked OK. No issues on return. Fish finger tea. I washed up & dried; Mum jumped up to 'put away'. Watched TV. Score 8/10.

NB [My] Sue away for 2 weeks from tomorrow. – ALL HANDS ON DECK!"

The new week was off to a pretty good start. Consolingly, amid Mum's steady deterioration, it was good to know that both she and we could still experience two nice days in a row. My partner was off on holiday, with her friend, (I felt in no position to take even 2 *days*, let alone 2 weeks, away from the 'front line' with Mum these days; and wouldn't have felt at ease if I had), and I would be obliged to bring my dog with me on *all* visits to Mum whilst my partner was away, so I was praying that the 'good run' might continue. Would my prayer be answered?

20ᵗʰ Feb. (Thurs): I'd had an e-mail from my cousin to say her equally-elderly, and dementing, Mum had been briefly admitted to hospital with pneumonia; but the key point of note from the missive was that she'd, "struggled the worse with memory issues whilst away from home". I'd discussed this with Mum, over lunch, and then logged it for my siblings; making the point for the latter that, "I think that's exactly what would happen if Mum 'went in a home'".

More practically, on that day, Mum seemed to have the sniffles again, so despite following the usual Relaxation & nap Routine, I decided, in the end, not to take her out either. Having been in all day, it was perhaps inevitable that the lack of distraction fuelled some partial return to her moans and groans, and, at one point, to her grumpy suggestion that I should "Go" and, late in the afternoon I logged:

"Offered Reassurance, & [suggestion that she try and] tackle the anxiety. She probably needs to get out a bit tomorrow if poss. – or else! She made [tea] @ 4pm – needed something to do. Looking for an argument. Some strong discussion around Mum saying WE don't care – spoke firmly [about] how lucky she is to have [all] 3 of her children living locally and visiting daily; then pulled out the [Nursing Home] closure article, when she said a 'Home would look after her.' Slowly, she came round, but it shows how much she turns in on herself if alone/ not distracted. A long day for Mum- all at home & hard work keeping her from slipping into anxiety; but score 7/10 'cos no real problems".

22nd Feb. (Sat): "When I walked in, Mum was ready to go into her 'whingy 6 yr old' routine, but I concentrated on [dog], and gave Mum the job of getting her food & water. Dosette done. Usual Routine. Mum woke 'cold'. Went in kitchen and radiator was turned off. Told her off! Crying followed. 'Go, Go' etc. VERY frustrating; but yes, I'm wrong again – to get sucked in. So much for relaxation! Anyway, we sat quietly for 10 mins. When calm, persuaded her to come out [with dog]. [We] went cemetery for walk with [dog] then general drive round for an hour. Checked round for essential shopping. I brought some from home [and] by planning ahead no shopping necessary. BUT – please check for Food Needs & top up as req'd. Further tea-time discussion of her obsessive need to DO, whilst saying she's 'tired' – a fundamental dilemma. Do not know how to get Mum to see it – anyway plenty of potential for argument, so 'easy option' for rest of day. Tiring day trying to manage both Mum and dog, but [ok]. 7/10".

24th Feb. (Mon): AM - "Oh dear. Not a good day. Aldi. Back home major panic attack, but ate dinner. Lot of pain in legs & cold. Cried. Worn out. Wants someone here 24 hours or [go in] home (again). Very tiring". (L).

PM – "Mum rang frightened etc. Tried to talk to her but she put phone down on me. Felt obliged to go up. Mum sat in kitchen crying. Said she tried to sleep but couldn't get off. Also legs felt weak & eye playing up. She eventually settled down and said I could go. No heating on in either room. Mum said it was summertime because the sun was out and she had turned them off. Kept talking about homes. When I said which one she backed down. Tried to get her to put another cardigan on, but she said

'Stop telling me what to do, it is my house'. There is no answer. Just stick with it. Over & out". (T).

25th Feb. (Tues): AM – "As the saying goes, what a difference a day makes. Mum OK on arrival apart from her cold. Heat on in both rooms. L cancelled Mum's hair appointment until next week. L called at Doc's. [for advice]. They said {Mum] may have water infection & asked for 'sample'. L took sample back to Doc's. L bought 'honey & lemon' for her chest. L said Mum may be drinking a lot of tea. She is going to replace teabags with decaffeinated [ones] on the advice of the chemist. Mum will not notice any difference so 'easy option'". (T).

PM – "Mum has cold but seems to be coping OK. Calm Reassurance + hot drinks. 'Usual Routine'. Gave Mum choice of 'fresh air' or not; she chose fresh air. Slowly got ready. Mum whingy, [and uncertain] saying, 'I won't fall, will I?' 'No, Mum'. Drove to paper-shop. Paid papers to end of March. Then gave Mum option to go to 'Birds'. 'Go on then, I'll try'. Walked round the little path [with Mum and dog]. Then 'Bernard' arrived – only person more depressed than Mum! Home for 3-15. Checked for shopping needs. [See list]. Fish finger tea. L rang. Gave update & food list. Otherwise OK & telly. 7/10".

We were working our way through another 'sticky' period; one where I was hamstrung for shopping/outing options because my dog would be with me each time I visited, until my partner returned, and one where Mum was not only struggling with the anxiety of being alone with her Dementia, (especially at night), but now with the added downside of dealing with that persistent cold as well. Not surprisingly, she was 'playing up' the more, and we needed all our patience and understanding to keep things on an even keel for her - and us; for it was anxiety-provoking for we siblings, too; especially when we weren't there. Further incapacitated by her cold, then, it was hardly surprising that the thought of 'going in a home' and of 'being looked after' was also finding fresh expression. Realistically, of course, for any serious consideration of a 'home' we would first need to see a *consistent* request for one, from Mum; and even then it could take a great deal of time to sort out. Given that she had consistently refused to even attend *day-care* in any of the potential establishments, it was hard for us to start taking more *permanent* options seriously; so, for the moment, it was a matter of 'keeping calm & carrying on'.

1st Mar. (Sat): "Arrived, as usual, to Mum looking to whinge. Small but controlled argument (about kitchen radiator being off), to stimulate the 'adult' (rather than the 'weak 7yr old'). She had made a full Saturday dinner for the first time in weeks. Dosette done. Relaxation Exercises + 35 mins nap. Choice offered [to go out or not]. Mum chose to take part, so:-

Drove to local Londis with suitable list prepared. SENT MUM ALONE INTO LONDIS! [I stayed outside with dog]. She was supposed to buy 2 x pints of milk, Flora margarine & polos. She came back with JUST THAT! [Wow!].

Drove to cemetery – 1st of Mar so Spring & pleasant walk. Mum 'tired' and [still] had 'cold', but generally OK. Salmon sarnies for tea. Keep check for basic grocery needs. Not a bad day given Mum's cold & [dog in tow]. 8/10".

Given that I *was* rather constrained by the dog, and that Mum needed those basic grocery items, I had decided to take a bit of a risk, by sending Mum, (albeit willingly), into the local mini-market on her own, but she had done incredibly well. I had not really expected her to get everything on the list, nor to arrive back without the likelihood of some sense of confusion, a wrong product or change, and a consequent loss of confidence, but she had truly 'trumped' me on both counts. It showed that, with Reassurance, the right support and due preparation, and despite the dreaded Dementia, she was still capable of functioning independently and well in the right circumstances. I was so proud of her, and just felt extraordinarily, if momentarily, uplifted. Really well done, Mum!

3rd Mar. (Mon): "Arrived to no heating on. Mum having sharp pains in her head. P. Off & Doc's. Good news - blood pressure OK and head pains not serious. Bad News - Did a memory test which she failed badly. Dr. R concerned about this. Would like to refer to [hospital] for further tests. Dr. R would like to speak to Keith about his reservations on tablets, when I told her

169

he doesn't agree with tablets. Dr. asked [if anyone has] Power of Attorney. Look out for rashes in her head in case of Shingles". (L).

4th Mar. (Tues): "I'm not against further memory tests; my reservations re further tablets are (a) who ensures she takes them; (b) What side effects – since nearly all involve some potential 'tiredness', dizziness', etc. I will try to talk to Dr., but I DO agree with proper Memory Tests, if Mum will GO! – at least then we know where we are. Water bill has arrived. [Usual Routine]. Mum still 'tired' & [had] 'cold'; decided not to 'push' it. Walked dog. Mum up & about on return. Beans on toast for tea. T/C from T. He's had T/c from A-care – Debbie off again tomorrow (Weds). 5 x since New Year. We're not asking for replacement. Mum Ok after tea. No major problems. 7/10".

Debbie, the A-care lady, had missed 5 visits since the New Year. Mum had accepted the various explanations offered by A-care, and had tended to take the loss in her stride, but when the need for *consistent* company, and for a *settled* Routine, had been specified, for someone with Dementia, *this* frequency of 'loss of service' was distinctly disquieting. (My own suspicion was that just *sitting* with Mum, as opposed to actually *doing* practical things for her, was perhaps starting to 'wear a bit thin' for Debbie). On a more positive note, my partner was back from her jollies.

8th Mar. (Sat): "No dog. (Very strange feeling). Mum not bad at all today. Casserole (tinned) for dinner. No kitchen heating. Put it on. Dosette done.

Ps I'm in the middle of composing a lengthy e-mail to Dr. R. Look for it in your inbox. [see Appendix 2].

Relaxation exercises + 25 mins nap & cuppa. Aldi service resumed. Went cemetery. Salmon sarnies for tea. 5- 20 – Mum up & faffing - upstairs, out back, plants. It is a nice evening. Generally OK & decent day. 8/10".

With some lovely Spring weather to savour, March was off to a pretty decent start. Mum seemed to be enjoying the nice sunshine, and, for now, a better, relatively settled, spell; and one thankfully free from too many traumas for her worn out offspring. Could it be that the cold, dark, days of winter had been getting her further 'down' than normal? How long might this fresh, and very welcome, 'Spring factor' last? At least it reminded us again of what was still possible, and that the Dementia didn't yet hold *total* sway. Hope sprang eternal.

12th Mar. (Weds): "Good start. Went to [next town]. Oh dear, [started] crying, saying nobody wants her. Came out of the blue. Anyway, managed a hotpot dinner. But felt very tired. Going to have a sleep before Debbie comes. I think it may have been 'out of her comfort zone'. Anyway, not bad at 1-30". (L).

14th Mar. (Fri): "Not the best day. Mind all over the place. Clinic done. [Re Frozen Shoulder]. No more visits. Just keep on with the exercises. Went market. Mum not interested in anything. Bought sandwiches and brought them home". (L).

18th Mar. (Tues): "Mum OK. Seems to be in a decent mood at present – lighter nights maybe? No reply from Dr. R yet. Have taken [latest] A-care bill. Soup dinner. (Without seeing the tin, I know it's Aldi's lamb & vegetable – might start a stage show guessing soups). [Usual Routine]. Tesco. Fish for tea. 8/10".

22nd Mar. (Sat): "Mum OK & 'proper' dinner + rice pud! Radiators ON – but low. Mum definitely seems a bit better to me. Relaxation + nap + cuppa - Aldi + High St amble. Hailstorm as we arrived home. Salmon Sarnies. Another decent day 8/10".

26th Mar. (Weds): "Good day today. Trip [over to town]. Pottered round Iceland. Got doughnuts. To church for dinner. Very nice. Packed today; even vicar. Hotpot + salad + choc cake. She's eaten the lot". (L).

March had been just about the best month that any of us could remember for some while. The light nights, and warmer Spring weather, seemed to have worked a treat. To sort of celebrate, and as yet another treat, on the 2nd of April we had arranged for Mum's beige living room carpet to be steam cleaned. This required my sister to take her out for a couple of hours in the morning, whilst my brother shifted the furniture around as necessary, and we were *all* well pleased with the fresh-looking result. It appeared that the 'good run' was still intact, and all seemed to be going pretty well, but was a potential crisis with A-Care about to interrupt this?

14th Apr. (Mon): "Tel. bill paid. Sandwiches for dinner. Not bad today. Asked about Debbie on Sunday. Can't remember, but doesn't want her to come anymore!" (L).

15th Apr. (Tues): AM - "Mum OK on arrival. Got worked up & agitated regarding Sunday's incident & the woman that came. 'Kylie' arrived. Tried to phone you on your mobile. Mum got worked up & cried, but calmed down when Kylie assured her Debbie would not get into trouble". (T).

PM – T here on arrival. 'Kylie' of no fixed surname or contact no. had been and gone. T had agreed a meeting for next Thurs. [Not convenient. I will e-mail A-Care]. T left. Soup lunch. [Usual Routine] + Tesco. Fish finger tea. 4-55pm – T/c from a Matt K @ A-care. Debbie has bad back & won't be coming tomorrow. (Weds). Kylie's surname [obtained]. Her mobile is apparently broken – sounds like the whole of A-care is broken! Matt actually rang here, but asked for T. Told him NOT to ring Mum's unless specifically agreed – but to ring our home numbers. Hopeless! And caused Mum to keep asking who rang. Otherwise a decent day. 7/10".

The nub of our 'carer' problem here was that (once again) Debbie was not available to keep to her visit, (this time on the Sunday), and, against everything we had agreed in such circumstances, (that we should be informed at our *own home* numbers, and not at Mum's, and that no-one should be sent in her stead without prior agreement), A-care *had* apparently taken a unilateral decision and simply sent an alternative carer! (A carer that Mum had never met!). Hence, a dispirited Mum had told my sister on the Monday that she did not want Debbie, or any other carer, to come any more. We had duly contacted A-care to complain, and they had further compounded their inefficiency by agreeing to send a 'Supervisor', (Kylie), to explain and discuss matters with me at Mum's on the Tuesday; yet, despite me informing them that I would not be there until lunchtime, Kylie had arrived *unannounced* at the house during the morning, and had been and gone before I got there. Luckily, my brother had still been on hand to speak to her, and to manage the situation. Otherwise, Mum would have been left 'home alone' to deal with yet another unfamiliar face from A-care. Talk about a shambles!

16th Apr. (Weds): "Not a good start. Very down & weepy. Anyway, went [to cafe] for dinner. Picked up after dinner. Anyway, she knows Debbie not coming today - but not bothered". (L).

We had made it to Easter, and beyond. My brother covered Good Friday and Easter Sunday, with home visits, and my sister Easter Monday; the latter taking Mum out to the Garden Centre; all without incident; and invoking the 'Usual Routine', I did similarly with Easter Saturday; the 19th. Indeed, with the good March 'run' extending well into April, and with my Saturday visit relatively unproblematic, I found time to log, topically and frivolously, thus:

"Did you hear about the Easter Bunny that died. It was sprayed with a mystery aerosol, and it got up and ran off, moving its hands in all directions. The aerosol was HARE restorer, that gave the HARE a permanent wave!".

On the Wednesday after Easter, the 23rd, we met at Mum's for the re-arranged meeting with 'Kylie' and another female 'manager' from A-Care. They had confirmed that Debbie had left, and so would not be coming again. We had discussed the possibility of introducing a new carer, and left it with the A-Care pair to identify any suitable replacement from amongst the workforce, for us to consider.

24th Apr. (Tues): "Mum OK still. Soup lunch – during which I asked what she remembered from [the meeting] yesterday. She remembered the 2 A-care women coming, and also that Debbie had left, & that we & A-Care are seeking a replacement. Good. I've added that it may take a week or two. She's taken it all pretty well. Window cleaner came. She took £2 off me for that – claiming she'd no change – they all say that! [Usual Routine]. Beans on toast for tea, followed by TV. No problems. 8/10. 4-30pm – T/c from T. A-Care plan from yesterday is 'under way'. 'Joan' say 'Yes'. Ps Haven't mentioned T's T/c to Mum – one small step for Mum-kind; no need for her to know the 'background' work".

27th Apr. (Sun): "OK on arrival. Mum greeted me with, 'I don't think I want them people'. I said, 'Shall I cancel them?'. She said, 'Alright then, let them come'. Did a bit more gardening. A good morning. Nothing else to report". (T).

It was clear that the potential arrival of a 'new' carer was playing on Mum's mind. Once again, her 'comfort zone' was being invaded, and tested, triggering anxiety, particularly at the thought of dealing with new change on her own, and, most worrying of all, posing a potential threat to her 'good run'.

29th Apr. (Tues): AM – "Mum all over the place on arrival. Crying, panicking etc. Calmed down after a while. Said she thought she was on her own. Told her there was never a day when she was on her own. Went through the times etc for the carer. Told her the name of the carer. Said she might know her. Finished the gardening. L arrived. Mum played up to her. Started to cry, feeling frightened etc. She stayed an hour. One of those mornings when Mum was on edge for some reason. Had better mornings". (T).

PM – "Woke Mum up from sleep, on arrival. (13-45) - not happy, a bit confused. Mum came round slowly & made soup. She does seem a bit confused today though. No Relaxation today. Already woke from nap. Tesco. Fish finger tea. Generally moany, and not quite as upbeat as recently. 7/10".

To add to our woes, Mum's central heating boiler went 'on the blink'. Luckily, my sister's husband did plumbing; but the wait for the 'part' still meant that Mum had only the limited heating from her front room gas fire, by way of core heating, for several days. Equally luckily, the weather wasn't too cold, either and, to be fair, Mum didn't make a fuss, and just carried on. And then came the arrival of Joan, the new the carer. I had arranged for the introductory visit to be made on a Tuesday afternoon, so that I could meet her, and offer 1-off support to Mum by being in attendance on this inaugural visit.

6th May. (Tues): "3-15pm Joan arrived on time. Mum quite anxious. Jabbered a lot. A lot of repetition. Anxiety decreased, and Joan OK with her. A good start. Joan coming Friday. Ps It was Joan's 59th birthday today. 3-45 – T/c to Boots Chemist. New prescription ready by Thurs. Boil-in-the-bag cod for tea. Mum now pretty tired, a long day for her. 7/10. Ps. My gran cycled 10 miles a day for ages in her 60s. Now we don't know WHERE she might be!".

For the record, Joan came complete with her own Daily Report Book to complete, and leave, (by the telephone table), by way of feedback, (typically with something nondescript like, "Nellie was fine. We had a nice cup of tea and a chat. All was well on leaving"); apparently, Debbie should have also!

8th May. (Thurs): AM- "OK on arrival; and we had heating on in both rooms. If she phoned once last night, she rang 4 times. Said she could not get her telly on. Tried to talk to her over the phone, but [came] up in the end. When I arrived, she was sat watching the telly! (T).

PM – "I think its horses for courses, 'cos no sign of upset for me. Shitty day weather-wise. Mini- argument over swollen fingers. It's all the hard labour that causes it. When I told her this, she still refused to say she'd rest them. Catch 22 – do a lot of physical labour with arthritic joints & they'll swell & hurt. Relaxation & 25 mins nap. Managed 20 mins round cemetery with her [and dog]. Picked up local paper and New Prescription. Beans on toast for tea. Also, looking for argument over 'medication' – wants her pills herself! Not her best day, but poor weather didn't help. 6/10".

10th May. (Sat): "Mum very weepy as soon as I arrived. It was like a 'release', because of 'quiet', 'nobody to talk to' – 'back hurts', 'arm hurts', 'fear', all part of getting anxious, tense & depressed - familiar stuff, but not something I'd seen for several weeks. Like a 'winter' session. She had made dinner though; and improved over lunch. And heating was on. [Usual Routine].6/10".

Due to my siblings having to be elsewhere, I then found myself on 'filling-in duty' on the following 2 days, too. On the Sunday, Mum kept asking when L was back, but the day passed passably; with my log's parting (tongue-in-cheek) comment reading: "Whoever's coming tomorrow, don't be late. Oh, it's me again!"; whilst the Monday was a working weekday, so trips to the Post Office, the Coop and the paper shop, and to the chippy to collect something for lunch, served to fill the day there. And, of course, Tuesday afternoon was my 'shift' anyway.

13th May. (Tues.): "Normality is restored. Mum OK on arrival – back to normal? She said Joan's visit was OK yesterday – 'she's nice'. Soup lunch. [Usual Routine]. Tesco. Fish finger tea. All OK 7/10".

14th May. (Weds): "Crying on arrival. Pain in hands. Won't take painkillers. Wants to go Doc's. Well, what a difference a trip out makes! Went [Garden Centre]. Nice lunch. Good day". (L).

15th May. (Thurs): "Mum OK on arrival. 'Tired'. Soup lunch. NB – did you get e-mail re Joan on holiday 16th to 30th June. Same as [my] Sue going Turkey! [Usual Routine] + cemetery walk with [dog]. Mum 'tired' on return. Looking for argument. Asked me 4 times in 2 mins 'is L back?' Asked her to sit & think – I said the words [Garden Centre] to her & she remembered going for lunch yesterday so answered her own question. Beans on toast for tea. 7/10".

17th. May. (Sat): "Mum would have cried if I'd let her; but 'distracted' her with 'nice weather', 'plants doing well, Mum' – so she was OK & got on with dinner - ham rather than chicken. She said she had no chicken. I checked. She HAD. Also, tablets not taken. Mum noticed I was checking. We agreed she need not take them this late in the day (12-45). Checked Joan's 'report'. She found Mum weeding. Got no answer @ front door, so came round the back. [Usual Routine]. Aldi – (Met Debbie, ex-carer outside! – she's gone to a different agency). Salmon sarnies for tea – with Cup Final. 8/10".

22nd May. (Thurs): "Mum grumpy on arrival, because she could not find her stockings. Went to pieces at 11-00am. Frightened, crying, etc. L called. Mum laid into her and me as well. She has been on-the-go since 11-15 [and] would not sit down or listen to me. A bit calmer as I left". (T).

23rd may. (Fri): "Been Doc's today – hand + wrist sore- New medication plan - No paracetamol, No Ibuprofen, No Olive Oil. New tablets – Co-codamol as per Doc's + cream to rub 2+3 times a day (contains chilli powder so wash hands after use). Blood tests done for Gout. X-ray booked next Wed at [hospital]. Picked up a lot now. Blood pressure checked. All OK". (L).

24th May. (Sat): "Mum upset on arrival – because 'confused' by new medication & cream. Seemed to think cream was for legs! and she HAD to take the Co-codamol. Spent some time trying to clarify all this. May be easier to go back to paracetamol if confusion persists. Dosette done. Mum improving now. Lunch – chicken cooked, but no spuds – added chicken to soup! [Usual Routine] + Aldi. Otherwise, all OK. 7/10".

27th May. (Wed): "Mum seems OK today. Hospital. Waited an hour [for X-ray]. Result – the swollen part doesn't show anything, but they are concerned about finger of same hand. She is going to see Doc at hospital. I have to phone our Doc's on Friday. Not sure what they saw. Cafe dinner. Done well today". (L).

"8-15pm – Mum phoned. Had rubbed her hand with the cream and touched her eye without washing her hands. The cream had burned her face & eye. We washed it with warm water and the burning sensation went. Mum kicked us out at 9pm". (T).

28th May. (Thurs): "Surprisingly, Mum OK on arrival after last night's incident. She remembered everything. She assured me that she put cream on this morning and then washed her hands. Mum fairly alert today. Not a bad morning". (T).

29th. (Fri): "4-15pm – called out. Mum got cream in her eyes again, whilst Joan was there. Joan wiped her eyes with warm water & a towel says Mum. After conversation with Keith, I have taken the cream away. Mum will use olive oil & take the Co-codamol". (T).

31st May. (Sat): "Mum OK on arrival. Soup lunch & rice pudd. Dosette done. Need new prescription by next Sat.

Relaxation +30 mins nap. Aldi. 20 mins 'time-out' @ cemetery, while Mum unpacked. 4pm. 'tired' & looking for argument. ('You don't care', 'never have done', 'all for yourself', 'no sympathy' stuff). Also 'frightened'. Not sure where it came from. Managed to avoid argument. Salmon sarnies for tea. TV. Mum more settled by 5-30pm. 7/10".

2nd Jun. (Mon): "Oh, dear. Bad on arrival. Crying, frightened. Didn't want to go out. Managed to get her out, but wobbly. Met friend in car park. Then, guess what - realised she didn't have her glasses on! Post Office & straight home - felt better when she put her specs on! Will phone doc's later for X-ray results". (L).

3rd Jun. (Tues): "Mum OK' if 'tired', and a bit chesty. Need to keep an eye on that. Sounds 'loose'. Mum says it's not troubling her/ keeping her awake. [Usual Routine]. All OK until I insisted on throwing 'out-of-date' eggs & ham away. Got upset. Said T & L 'don't boss me'. Told her the eggs & ham would make her ill. She told me to 'Go', 'Go', 'Go'. Wasted 20 mins waiting for her to calm. Eventually OK for Tesco + £1 shop for tape. Also, Mum still chesty. Fish finger tea. 7/10".

5th Jun. (Thurs): AM - "On arrival back door locked. Knocked on window. No answer. Knocked a couple of times. 'Oh dear', I thought. Went round front. Looked through window. Mum in chair. 'Is she still with us?' I wondered. Knocked on window. Mum jumped up and let me in. 'Why are you knocking on window'? she asked, 'You made me jump'. I said, 'You were having 40 winks and I could not get in'. Anyhow, everything OK apart from her being chesty. No mention of fingers or hand hurting". (T).

PM – "Bit scary for you T – to get no answer. Still, all's well that...? Mum OK on arrival. (Invoices for Joan in back of book). L rang – GP not available. Also, L on holiday Mon 9th to Fri 13th. 'Who was on the phone Keith?', Mum asked repeatedly. '[It was] L. She's on holiday next week', I said. 'What about my pension'? 'Where's she going', when, why, how? I assured her we'd cover all her needs. She soon calmed down. ALSO, [my] Sue away 16th to 30th June, so I'll have dog for 2 weeks. Shopping help needed."

The 'holiday season' was getting under way; what with Joan's, my partner's, L's & T's, (and rumours that both immediate neighbours also had plans), it could only mean the likelihood of more anxiety for Mum, as her Routine was disturbed yet again, and 'swaps' were being sought and traded as necessary; not to mention the extra anxiety for those 'covering', and unable to find time for holidays, given Mum's permanent needs. Even before anyone had departed, I was *already* longing for a return to Routine, and to 'normality'!

9th Jun. (Mon): "Arrived 11-00 am. Mum on point of crying. Quiet. Confused about who was coming. Reassurance worked. Went [Garden Centre] for lunch. Bought Geranium. NB Mum still chesty sometimes. 7/10".

12th Jun. (Thurs): "OK on arrival but not for long, 'cos the toastie loaf had green mould. Raised the issue of throwing out-of-date stuff away. Mum said, 'It's alright'. Argument about it, but I don't suppose anything will change. We need to regularly check any fresh stuff, 'cos she keeps it & eats it – will lead to food poisoning! [Usual Routine]. For paper + cemetery walk with [dog]. [We] sat in Rose Garden @ cemetery. Nice day. Beans on toast for tea. All OK. 7/10".

14th Jun. (Sat): "Mum OK on arrival. Soup. Had email from [A-Care] reminding me of Joan's holidays. Just another reminder that I've got [dog] until 30th Jun – so shopping will be limited after today. Do check sell-by dates on fresh stuff & replace as necessary. [Usual Routine]. Dosette done. Aldi done. All done. 7/10".

15th Jun (Sun): "Crying on arrival. Soon came round. Early warning of my 4-day break. Cover needed 27th to 30th June". (T).

19th Jun. (Thurs): "Mum OK on arrival, but quickly into moany 'No-one next door' etc. – like a split record these days, but you'd miss it if it wasn't here, wouldn't you? So patience, stay calm and relax. [Usual Routine}. Usual stuff around 'tired'. Could have argued, but what's the point most of the time – so easy option today. 7/10".

20th Jun. (Fri): "OK on arrival. Mum in backyard. General chit-chat. Fairly good morning. L rang. No car today. In garage for exhaust. She said Kate & Sarah [adult grandchildren] were visiting Mum on Sat. Have told Mum. She was looking forward to seeing them". (T).

21st Jun. (Sat): "Mum good on arrival – 'cos aware Kate & Sarah coming – obviously putting on her best. Also made full Sat. dinner, but only gave me 'small' rice pud, 'cos 'saving some for K & S'. Have taken A-Care bill. Dosette done. Short Relaxation & 20 mins nap before Kate & Sarah arrived. Spent 2 hours. I then went Cemetery with Mum and [dog]. Back for salmon sarnies. Mum responded well to the 'busy' company. Good day generally. 8/10".

28th Jun. Sat): "Last day with [dog in tow]. Mum OK; sounds a bit breathless at times. Still coughs [up phlegm] a lot. Worth mention to Dr. – why not suggest home visit – helps with [general]

Reassurance. Joan's back on Monday, too. Dosette done. Need new scrip by Friday!
Well, well, last page of Volume 2. [Usual Routine]. Salmon sarnie tea. All OK. 8/10".
29th Jun. (Sun): AM- "[Mum] a bit fed up today. Says she's missing T, [who usually does Sundays]. Sandwich & crisps for dinner. Didn't want a walk. Back to normal Mon". (L).
PM – "Rang Mum @ 4-00pm. Crying & upset. 'Unable to find Songs of Praise', 'Fear', 'No-one to talk to'. Decided to come up, as unable to calm her over phone. Arr. 5-20pm. Mum just generally fed up & depressed due to 'the quiet'. Neighbour away. T away. Songs of Praise not on until 5-30. Watched it together. Too much change in Routine at once + too quiet & alone = fear + depression. Dep. 7-15. All OK by then.
HERE ENDETH VOLUME 2!

The final log into Vol. 2. had fallen to me, and perhaps encapsulated our central concerns and ongoing dilemmas re Mum. Namely, that most of her efforts to combat the Dementia seemed to work best in the comfort and security of her own home, IF/WHEN one or more of we offspring were in close attendance. Then, the likes of the '3Rs', along with a bit of managed 'distraction', (especially via familiar local outings), worked well enough, and the 'fear' deposited by the Dementia could often be *offset* in that familiar company and setting. Alas, the sheer practicalities of being in full 24/7 attendance were just logistically impossible, and Mum would have to continue to self-manage at least *some* spells of time, (especially through the night), if she was to *remain* in her own home. Interestingly, (I suspect mainly to attract our attention, and in her more desperate 'hours of need', and most difficult moments), Mum was increasingly raising the spectre of 'going in a home' and 'being looked after' herself; though quickly choosing not to follow through (at least not consistently) whenever the possibility was 'seriously' raised with her; and *very* quick to 'poo-poo' any *suggestion* of an actual exploratory visit to a potential residence.
The inaugural entry into *Volume 3* was on the last day of June, and fell to my sister, who logged a relatively standard and

relatively uncontroversial Monday morning entry about their trip to the Post Office, and for some essential shopping, with a reminder that Joan was due later that day - and the first couple of days of July were similarly uncontroversial; that is relatively so, in that so many of Mum's age-related, and Dementia-lead, limitations, and associated, and more unpredictable, moods, behaviours, regularly required tasks, (e.g. re medication or toileting), and accompanying 'fears' etc. were now almost ingrained and taken as the 'new norm' by us these days. But at least the potential de-stabilising effect of the 'holiday season' was drawing to an end, and both Mum and I could look forward to a more settled return to established Routine.

In fact, the first entry of any real significance in Vol. 3 was 3 days into the new month, and didn't so much put *Mum* 'back in the frame', as the interminable inefficiencies, inconsistencies, constant rethinks and changes, (and invariably revisited prescriptions), blithely conjured up by the medical profession; in this first-up case, once again the GP.

3rd Jul. (Thurs): AM - "Mum Ok on arrival. L arrived. [Called at] Doc's regarding Mum's X- ray. Mum's got osteo-arthritis in all bones of her hands. Also, the cream she's been using is too strong. L has prescription for a cream that is only 1%. [The other] cream has been thinning her skin according to the doctor. Also, the Co-codamol makes you constipated, and the Doc had told her to stop taking them and has prescribed soluble paracetamol. L will get them on prescription. We have explained it all to Mum. Mum's mind is doing overtime with questions regarding L going to the Doc's. You may have your ear bent". (T).

PM – "Mum quite good on arrival. Soup lunch. GP's advice – didn't I tell you it was osteo-arthritis! Also, why did GP prescribe 10% strength in the first place – bloody hopeless – you really do have to check things out yourself for the best. Relaxation exercises + 25 mins nap. Rang A-care [re bill]. Mum [now] banging on about 'no Co-codamol' – I presume new scrip will have soluble paracetamol. Hurrah; Good News - £36 off electric bill. [Out] for paper + cemetery (again, but safe bet) [with Mum & dog]. Beans on toast for tea. Played 'fish' [card game] with Mum. All OK. 8/10".

4th Jul. (Fri): "Been chemist. Soluble paracetamol + low strength Ibuprofen. Scrip upstairs. Joan not coming today, she's busy! Mum has bad back. Yippee, [neighbour] is back. Mum does not want soluble paracetamol – tastes funny. I have taken them away. Just buy ordinary ones from Aldi". (L).

In my next day's log, and effectively rendering the latest trip to the GP redundant and a waste of time, I simply confirmed my sister's view, with "Let's just stick to Ibuprofen Gel & standard paracetamol, eh?", before describing a relatively trouble-free Saturday afternoon that followed 'the Usual Routine' - but then the medics decided to become intensely involved elsewhere and in a far more worrying scenario.

On the following Monday, my sister, and brother's partner, took Mum to the hospital for what we thought would be just an outstanding outpatient's appointment for some long-awaited, bog-standard 'tests' and 'checks', but something obviously wasn't to their satisfaction, and Mum was surprisingly kept in overnight, and not released until the following Tuesday afternoon. The same 'escort team' had then been required to present Mum for a scan early on the *Wednesday* morning. Consequently, our home visits had been thrown out of synch, and I agreed to put in a stint on the Wednesday afternoon; where I logged:

9th Jul. (Weds): "L & S took Mum for a scan today, which scared her. Outcome is likely to be blood clot on lung. Have told Mum it's just a 'slight infection' – that [may] need treatment. L here on arrival. Mum not bad. Some anxiety about treatment to come, but otherwise OK. Soup lunch. Relaxation + 45 mins nap. Interestingly, Mum cannot now remember staying O/n in hospital! I went Tesco's [alone] to top up essentials. On return, Mum took up option to come out - went 'Birds' – chat with Bernard. 4-25 – L rang. She's had 'all clear' from scan. So nothing to treat! Hurrah! (L to check why scores were high then). Fish finger tea. Mum settled again now. Good day from my point of view. 8/10".

11th Jul. (Fri): "Went [over to town]. Still a struggle breathing. Bit of cough. Gets upset 'cos can't walk fast. Worried about her legs bleeding. I think it could be the medication they gave her to thin the blood. Elec. bill paid. Assume Joan's coming today. Tablets not taken, so took about 10-30 – no problem". (L).

13th Jul. (Sun): "Mum all over the place at first, crying etc. Worried about the gas bill for some reason. I've checked it and it is not far out. Caught Mum rubbing her legs with the cream for her hands. Her legs were a mess this morning. After a bad start, not a bad morning". (T).

The latest personal and practical problem for us to get to grips with, and yet another that appeared 'here to stay', was that of the skin on the lower parts of Mum's legs getting worryingly thinner, and becoming increasingly susceptible to 'breaking' and bleeding at the slightest brush. It most certainly was *not* helped by Mum rubbing either too much, or even the *wrong*, or wrong strength, cream on them; and too frequently. I was, though, by way of consolation, pleased to have finally brought my hitherto sceptical sister 'on board', following her lately-logged acknowledgement that *tablets* prescribed to thin Mum's blood, and to help it flow better *internally*, *might* also be contributing, adversely, to that concurrent '*skin*-thinning', *ex*ternally; and to an associated bleeding that was becoming harder to staunch whenever such a 'breach' occurred; and often resulting, as I've said, in both Mum alone, and we, when to hand, struggling the more with the task. (Not that we had any proof to back up our 'tablet' suspicions; nor, then, did my sister's 'boarding' make any *practical* difference, at this late stage 'in the game').

Meanwhile, unsurprisingly, and following the old (Mark-Twain-attributed) adage that 'Life is just one damn thing after another', everyday practical problems continued apace in *all* our lives.

22nd Jul. (Tues):

AM – "OK on arrival. It would be £29.99 for a new [front door] lock. [It had been 'sticking']. Mum said to leave it until it breaks, as she is familiar with the one she has got. Also, L's car has broken down. Also, Mum rang me 8-10 times on Sun. to tell me she had no telly. WE had no telly. It was not just a fault with Mum's. Came back on at 4-30pm. Also, there was quite a bit of water in the fridge. Perhaps you could call at [dealer]. I [think] the warranty has expired and if they have to come out to it we will have to pay. Mum has bent my ear something shocking since we found the water in the fridge". (T).

PM – "Mum 'tired' on arrival. Soup lunch. Spoke to LEC direct who say its condensation due to hole blocked. When I got here NO water in fridge. Also, I think the new lock should be fitted asap – the old one is not reliable, and 'sticking'. NB the [fridge] warranty has NOT expired. [Found] receipt in cupboard with LEC instructions. Relaxation exercises + 25 mins nap + Tesco. The fridge IS working [in that it] chills stuff – just condensation? Fish finger tea. All OK. 8/10".

24th Jul. (Thurs): AM – "Ok on arrival. L rang. Engineer coming Sat. There was water in the fridge today". (T).

PM – "Mum just 'tired' on arrival. Soup lunch. On LEC man – OK for Sat. Relaxation exercises + 25 mins nap. Went [local shopping, 'cos had dog]. 1. Sent Mum in Boots for Ibuprofen Gel - she came out with - Ibuprofen Gel! 2. Sent Mum in newsagents for [local paper]. She came out with [local paper]! Hurrah! Beans on toast tea.

NB Late [tongue-in-cheek] discussion of things to put on Mum's gravestone – which Mum has approved:-

1. Mi speed's gone.
2. Go an' 'ave a shit!
3. Me, a don't moan.
4. These [neighbours] are a mystery. ['cos they were rarely at home].
5. Oh, I *am* tired; *absolutely* tired.
6. You'll be old yourself one day.
7. I don't think you realise how old I am.

All OK. 8/10".

26th Jul (Sat): "Started early with 9-45 call [to me at home] from Fridge Engineer – coming [to Mum's] between 12 & 2. Mum OK on arrival, but immediately got anxious [about] fridge man coming. Good Sat lunch & pud tho'. Relaxation Exercises; plus nap interrupted by Fridge Engineer @ 12-45 – here 10 mins.

Poked long wire down hole – got him to GIVE it to me; it's in cupboard near pills. Dosette done – need new scrip by FRI. Aldi. (Mum struggled to open lock to get in – says she'll have a new one – strike while the iron's hot!). Salmon butty tea & telly. All OK. 8/10".

On Monday, the 28th of July, my sister's log particularly asked, "Did Keith know Joan didn't come Friday – assume today is OK"; whilst my brother's next-day log included his asking me, "Did you get my e-mail on Fri regarding Joan not coming? She had an upset stomach, they said. Check the next bill". (The answer to my sister's question was, "No", as I hadn't had time to read the late-Friday e-mail before leaving home early on the Saturday).

Joan's 'miss' was only her second since taking over from Debbie; but I couldn't help wondering if it might be the start of a similar pattern. A-care were first and foremost providers of time-limited *practical* help, (making the client something to eat or assisting in washing them etc.), and they never claimed that providing constantly-renewed *mental* stimulation was the forte of any of their staff, so perhaps Joan, too, was finding her twice-weekly appointments with Mum a bit 'samey'; or maybe she was genuinely ill, or she too had issues in her life. Either way, the alarm bells were beginning to ring once more. Anyway, life went on. This was just another potential irritation to manage and re-manage, for and on behalf of Mum and on *we* went.

2nd Aug. (Sat)): "Mum OK at first, but got upset when she realised she's made soup and not Sat dinner; but soon sorted. Dosette done. Spent some time stemming blood flow after scab came off leg sore. Relaxation + 25 mins nap. Aldi. Called in at park for brief walk & sit. Mum unpacked while I popped to cemetery [for time-out]. Fridge has been dry every day last week for me. Seems OK now. Every time Mum tries to open front door from outside she struggles. Needs new lock. Starting to get darker. Dark @ 9-30 now. Need to think of 'distractions' for dark nights or you know what'll happen. Mum still wheezy on occasion when out of puff. Keep an eye on, with option of GP 'listening' if nec. Salmon butty tea. 7/10".

Yet still the household and maintenance jobs kept coming. Amongst a *variety* of outstanding one-off such jobs, and at some point in early August, my brother had manfully completed the promised task of painting Mum's small, wooden, fading and drab-looking, brown, picket, front fence, and between us, we had managed to source and fit a new front door lock, to replace the one that had been stiff and sticking, and a source of irritation, insecurity and potential of anxiety, for some time for Mum.

9th Aug. (Sat): "Nattering already started by Sarah [granddaughter, who] was there on arrival, so Mum OK. A-Care bill has arrived. Also found another bill in the letter rack. Dosette done. [Usual Routine]. Aldi + key- cutting. (Yours are in the wooden bowl).

I pronounce the Fridge officially DRY!

I pronounce the [new] Lock officially open!

I pronounce the Fence officially excellent!

Any more jobs? OK, stand at ease. Chicken sarnie tea. Ps Mum still 'phlegming' on occasion, but no pain there. 8/10".

On her visits (particularly of the 27th of July, and of the 7th and 11th of Aug., (and a few later ones), Joan the carer's reports had become unusually 'active', in that they had focused on Mum's latest leg pain. On the 27th, for example, she had noted that, following a visit by the District Nurse, (DN), Mum should no longer use the particular cream that she had been using on her legs, as it was burning her skin. (Oh, for goodness sake!) The DN had recommended a different one; whilst, for example, and respectively, on her visit of the 7th, Joan had 'reported' that, "Nellie was upset when I arrived. She said her legs are very sore. She seemed better when I was leaving", and on her visit of the 11th, that she had given Mum 2 x paracetamol for the pain in her legs. Hence my referral to these in my log of the:

12th Aug. (Sat): "Mum OK on arrival, but could have easily been upset; insecurity. Have read Joan's report, too; unfortunately [I think] it's the future. Over winter we still need to think of 'distractions'. Mum's again said 'NO' to library book [from mobile library], and to my suggestions of jigsaw or day-care. Soup lunch. 1-45 – whilst making cuppa I noticed Tues. pills not taken. Gave them to her. [Usual Routine] Tesco. Fish finger tea. 7/10".

Despite the ongoing and now ingrained, Dementia-lead, worries and more or less 24/7 management issues, we all felt that Mum had been coping well- enough, and that 2014 had not been too harsh to us thus far. Nonetheless, managing these issues still held the potential for regular and recurrent stresses and strains all round these days; whilst the level of supervision that Mum's deteriorated predicament required still left plenty of scope for potential disruption-and-tiredness-based tensions; both directly with Mum, and between we, (only human), carers and siblings.

17th Aug. (Sun): My brother had already completed his usual Sunday morning visit, and deemed it to be "not a bad morning", but his day was far from done.

"7pm – Mum rang. Frightened & confused. No telly. Put phone down on me. Felt obliged to come up. On arrival Mum was watching telly. Nothing wrong with telly. Started crying. Said she wanted to go in a home. When I challenged her, she said she did not want to leave her own home. She made comment that she had not seen L since Wednesday, and [L] had not phoned. That was one reason why she was upset. I was still here at 8pm". (T).

18th Aug. (Mon): "Mum in a state. Can't go toilet. I did phone Friday, but I don't come up again til Mon unless I'm passing. Didn't have a good Sunday myself. Not been too well. It's now 11-15. Mum still trying to go toilet. Been PO but Mum had chest pain so came straight back. Soup for dinner. Mum very tired". (L).

19th Aug. (Tues): AM - "Today's pills not taken, so I gave them to her. Water all over the kitchen floor where spinner is kept. Mopped it up. We presume Joan is coming on [Bank Holiday] Mon. Aft. Mum says she has got a bad stomach. There is a bug going round. Read L's notes about not calling after calling on Weds until Mon. Under the circumstances I would have a rethink. Mum says she has got a bad back as well". (T).

PM – "Not too bad for me. 'Tired'. She's clearly taken a depressive turn for the worse; maybe under the weather, or darkening nights; could be a long winter, left alone for too long. She hasn't the capacity to 'entertain' herself, and will fall more easily into introspection, self-pity and depression. [Usual Routine]. Mum went toilet. Came back 'weak', but OK for Tesco's. Fish finger tea. Definitely not at her best today – 'arm aches', 'it's mi mind', 'am tired' stuff. 6/10.

My main worry at this point was that Mum's Dementia-based 'forgetfulness' now appeared more frequent, and real, than ever. Give-away comments such as "it's mi mind", and "a don't know what am doin'", pointed persuasively to the probability that she *was* experiencing moments or periods when she could no longer 'think straight', or rely on her memory; and, even more importantly, *knew* it. And this now threatened to be at the heart of how the Dementia was likely to affect her, going forward. Teasingly, it was nowhere near a 24/7 issue at this stage; but it *was* sufficient for her to realise that she *had* the damn problem; and cause upset. My best guess was that some sort of short-lived 'brain freeze' was claiming such moments or periods from her, and that that, of course, was triggering her (all too understandable, but not so easily solved) bouts of 'fear'. From there, it wasn't too big a leap to see her behaviour becoming more erratic, and why she might, say, ring my brother, (who lived nearest), and try to get him round for company and Reassurance; but under the practical pretext of, say, the TV not working. Nor was it a big leap, say, to find this Dementia-lead forgetfulness triggered, and her anxieties and insecurities raised, and that same 'fear' triggered, by even minor disruptions in her familiar, relied-upon, *Routines*; including, of course, not seeing one of *us* for several days - say when on holiday, or not well ourselves. Within such a difficult dynamic, then, it wasn't too surprising to find that our *own* human anxieties and frailties surfaced on occasion. As both her offspring *and* main carers, then, we did sometimes see them emerge, (a shade defensively), in the logs between *us,* vis-a-vis our personal perspectives, family pressures and responsibilities, rostered visits and 'shifts', (and any 'extra' ones), etc. By and large, though, we usually managed to keep these things in check, to air differences considerately, and to continue to work well together in often difficult and discouraging circumstances on Mum's behalf; and on we went.

21st Aug. (Thurs): "Mum not at her best. Argument over nothing [lead to] her crying & 'Go', 'Stop Coming', '[T & L] never argue', etc. She's very vulnerable at present. May be under the weather, but I haven't heard 'Go', 'Go' etc. for quite a while. Soup lunch. Mum didn't want to do Relaxation today. Said she was too 'tired'. She slept for 45 mins & woke 'cold' – even though radiator on. I walked [dog]. Mum not keen; weather cold. Beans for tea. Bucked up a bit, but 'tired', 'legs' stuff all day today. 6/10".

25th Aug. (Mon): "Oh dear, Mum in a state. Day forgotten. Was asleep when I came. Started crying, but soon came round. PO done + Aldi + some new shoes from Aldi. Lunch out. Better now. Ready for sleep (& that's just me!)". (L).

27th Aug. (Weds): "Iffy start, as usual. Came round. Went [next town]. Mum bought jumper. Hotpot in cafe. Mum seemed much better. Went to Doc's. Saw a new one. Nice man. No problem with lungs – just hypertension. Talked about Mum's memory. Vascular Dementia is caused by the blood vessels narrowing in the brain (like her legs). This causes different part to shut down. He said eventually they will be too narrow for blood to pass thro'. He said, she knows what's happening; that's the worst part for her – hence the crying". (L).

28th Aug. (Thurs): "Mum OK. ('Tired' as always). Soup lunch. Good start. Read L's stuff re doctor:-

1. [Am] in general agreement – old age – vascular Dementia.
2. I take it GP has no hope/recommendations at all.
3. Do I take it the wheezing is via hypertension?
4. 'Eventually too narrow for blood to pass through' – does this imply stroke & death?
5. Altho' there's no rush, I would like 'new' GP to SEE Mum; and then pronounce again.

1-00pm – Relaxation Exercises + 30 mins nap. [Went] for [local paper] walk with Mum & dog. Beans on toast tea. Decent day. 8/10".

30th Aug. (Sat): AM – "Prescription upstairs. Mum been onto T – no paper, so brought one up. Bit weepy. Doc's have phoned re 'personal care plan'. We have appointment for Tues. 9th Sept. @ 9-30. Yes, eventually the narrowing of capillaries will narrow more, so her mind will go completely; but it is a slow process. Lovely soup for lunch". (L).

PM – "Mum knew L had been. Re Personal Care Plan (PCP):-

1. Remind them I have given a full(ish) social/medical history to cover recent years – it should be on file/computer. [see Appendix 2].
2. Ask if we get written copy of the PCP.
3. Ask if ANY 'options' re vascular Dementia – any new medicines or procedures.

Soup lunch + rice pud. Relaxation Exercises + 30 mins nap – Aldi. Dosette done. Went cemetery while Mum unpacked. Salmon sarnie tea [& chat]. ('I don't think u realise how old I am' – 'I do Mum, u never stop telling me'. Wrong reply but no big issue; still should have gone 'easy option'). Decent day though. 8/10".

The 'new' doctor's prognosis didn't really tell us anything we didn't know/suspect, but it was still pretty depressing to hear it confirmed officially, as it were; not least because the prognosis came with little or no hope. Still, at least they seemed to be taking up the cudgels in the form of something called a 'Personal Care Plan'. Given the foregoing prognosis, it was hard to see just what this might offer, but, despite Mum not doing too badly at present, this PCP did seem to offer the chance of a faint, perhaps final, opportunity to grasp another modicum of long overdue help, input and support from the medics.

Whilst we awaited that appointment and input, things plodded on well enough in that 'relativist' sort of way that we had come to accept of Mum's limitations now; a particular and poignant, if brief, 'new' upset occurring on my visit of Thursday, the 4th September, when I reminded her that it would have been Dad's 95th birthday. A compos mentis Mum would *never* have forgotten this, and she got predictably distressed and apologetic once she realised she had done so. Of course, *I* had remembered the occasion for us both, and to commemorate it, we bought flowers, took my dog for our familiar cemetery walk, and actually sang a chorus of 'Happy Birthday' together at his graveside. (Not including the dog, of course, since she had yet to learn the words!).

9th Sept. (Tues): AM – "No-one here on arrival. Mum & L arrived back from Doc's. Computer broke down. Nothing happened. Appt next Weds @ 9-30am. Mum's mind working o/ time as to why she did not see Doc. She may bend your ear about it". (T).

PM – "Whoops; what a disappointment. Bloody doctors. Bloody computers. They're about as [unreliable and] useless as each other! Anyway, Mum OK. Used the opportunity to remind her what a waste of time the anxiety about going to GP's was. [Usual Routine]. Mum went toilet. 'Weak'. Also, Mum still anxious about who she saw @ Doc's & about missing Sunday paper [which had failed to materialise]. Quite draining to keep explaining – but hey ho, that's the job. Tesco. Fish finger tea. Not Mum's best day. Constantly 'tired' & moaning; [esp. about} Doc's and lost paper. 7/10".

13th Sept. (Sat): "Mum crying when I arrived. 'Fear'; 'mi mind' stuff. Got worse – she'd made mash & chicken, but had no veg. She also had 2 tins of fruit with 'best before' dates of 2011 & 2012! Cried again when I threw them in the bin. 'Oh, Keith, don't do it'; 'Oh, Keith I am upset'. I didn't give in & she calmed down, but tough start. Have taken latest A-care bill. Dosette done. L arrived & Mum replayed [upset] to the 'new audience' for a while. Relaxation Exercises + 30 mins nap. She awoke much calmer. Cuppa. Aldi. Salmon butty tea. Not bad after dodgy start. 7/10".

17th Sept. (Weds): "Doc's. Half hour wait, then too busy, so saw nurse. Weight & blood pressure checked. All good. Put on 2lb. Waste of time really. She will be sending me a copy of the Care Plan, with a number to ring in case of emergency. Bit rubbish (but Keith knew that – know all!). Dinner at church. Usual memory & tiredness [issues]". (L).

18th Sept. (Thurs): AM – The only log of significance from my brother's morning visit and chat with Mum was his suspicion that

"Mum is hiding from [her brother] & Joan, as the only people she wants to see are the 3 of us".

PM – "Mum quite good on arrival. Baffles me how she can be so 'up & down'. Soup lunch. Can't make head nor tail of Dr's visit. She's been twice & still not seen by GP. How on earth can he make a valid Care Plan! (It's not the nurse's job). I told Mum I would complain, but too anxiety-provoking for Mum & now she needs 'Flu jab on 29th; but L away 'gallivanting' Any ideas? For T –shall I do Mon 29th [& Flu jab & PO], & you Weds. 1st Oct. & rest of week as normal? [Usual Routine]. Decent day. 8/10".

29th Sept. (Mon): "Mum a bit weepy & unsettled on arrival. Discussed whether to have 'flu jab. I felt the risk of her catching 'flu without the help of the jab could be life-threatening. Mum agreed to have it. 11-10am. Went surgery. Jab made Mum jump & briefly cry, but soon over. Mentioned 'wheezing' to nurse, but of course no sign of it at surgery; and Mum got upset when I asked her to 'wheeze' for the nurse – so didn't press it. Went P. Off. & [over to town]. Round shops. M&S for lunch. 1-00pm back home for cuppa. Mum nodding off. Left her to have sleep before Joan. Will ring later, as usual, in case of any effects of jab. But no issues on leaving".

30th Sept. (Tues): "Mum not happy. Talking like baby. Asked her to talk like adult. Conversation improved. It is possible 'flu jab is having small effect – something new in her bloodstream; also, jab was in her left arm though she hasn't mentioned any pain yet. Gas man called to read meter. Relaxation Exercises & 30 mins nap. Woke 'woozy', a bit 'dizzy' & 'fear'; & arm aching – anxiety? A bit reluctant to go out, but I persuaded her. Tesco. Went cemetery for 'space' walk. Not too bad on return, but generally negative today - could be wheeze, jab, L away, late taking of medication, or combination of. Worst day for over a month. 6/10.

2nd Oct. (Thurs): AM – "No problems on arrival. I have told Mum to leave radio on – acts as someone else in the house. Will she do it? No reaction to 'flu jab – bonus. Mum said L rang at tea-time last night, but still asking when she is home. Not a bad morning". (T).

PM – "Whingy. 'Oh dear, I am tired'. I was strong with her. There was potential for an argument, but [prospect of] 7 hrs of whinging was worth it and she rallied round. Soup lunch. Mum still wheezy. Not sure what to do about it. You can't hear it when she's sleeping, and she couldn't produce it for the nurse on Monday; and she's not hurting anywhere. [Usual Routine]".

Mum had definitely been more anxious and fretful whilst L had been away for a few days. This was quite noticeable whenever *any* of we 3 were away, and her Routine was disrupted. On the other hand, it showed that she still had enough awareness and cognition to know someone *was* away, or at least that something had changed in the visiting Routine. My sister's 'return to the fold', and her next, (Monday the 4th), log noted, "Back to Routine. Mum cried when I got here. Missed me last week. Usual PO - and sausage butty for dinner. Care Plan on side – waste of time"; whilst, and striking a similar tone, my brother's following-day return to his usual morning visit logged, "OK on arrival. Mum very chatty. Probably feels better because L is back"; but signed off worryingly (and very likely relievedly) with, "Mum has been on the toilet 3 times this morning, without success. You may have a problem".

7th Oct. (Tues): "Mum OK. Read Care Plan:-

1. Interesting to see 'list' of medical history.
2. Would it be useful to have T's & I's phone nos on Plan too – in case L is 'away'?
3. Under 'medication' it still says Carvedilol – take one twice daily. This is only once daily (morning) since previous Dr. OK'd it.
4. Otherwise, not much else to say; though Plan made without seeing Dr.!

Relaxation Exercises & 30 mins nap. Tesco. Drove to cemetery & down to dad's grave on way back. Fish finger tea. 7/10".

8th Oct. (Weds): "Rang L early to swap my Thurs.PM for *Weds* PM. Arr 1-40pm. Mum [had been] playing up to L again. Saying she was frightened of ME – cheeky sod! Within 10 mins of

L going Mum was OK & talking quite well (like an adult). She insisted on finishing off making my cheese on toast, then wanted sleep. Relaxation Exercises & 30 mins nap. I *asked* if she wanted to walk round cemetery with [dog] & me, and she chose 'Yes'. Beans on toast for tea. Mum generally OK. (see L –she's not frightened of me). 7/10".

9th Oct. (Thurs): [I was able to make my Thurs. after all].

"Mum would have cried at me if I'd let her. Even the 'easy option' for 7 hours is too much if it's 7 hours of rain & whinging, so I forced the argument, and she rallied within 15 mins.; after saying 'no sympathy', 'don't come', 'T & L don't shout at me', (it's not shouting, its 'calm assertive', like the dog whisperer recommends). I have to Routinise the day in a *'be positive'* fashion, [as per list on wall] – or I'd need psychiatric help myself [after 7 hours]; & Mum HAS to cope unless one of us is moving in. [Or she goes in a Home]. Anyway, sermon over. Mum improving as I write, so soup lunch & more or less normal. Mum talking like an adult again (not baby). Suggestion for U 2 – try [it] for 7 hours & see if 'easy option' is still OK! [Usual Routine]. Mum fine and keen to come out with [dog] & me. Cod in butter sauce for tea. Despite U 2 struggling AM, my afternoon was a good one (not counting first 20 mins). 7/10".

Both my siblings took the hint about 7 hour 'shifts', but rather than take up my challenge, they each acknowledged that it was a 'long time', and respectively suggested, in their next log, that I *shorten* it, by arriving a bit later. I was happy enough with the Routine that I had established for my 7-hour stay, and, reluctant to change it for either myself or Mum, simply pressed on regardless; but not before I took a rather sardonic, holier-than-thou, tone to respond and make my point one last time on the:

14th Oct. (Tues): "Thank you for your consideration. The 7 hours is OK. My point was I have to bring her out of her 'down' moods to *do* stuff, so the 'easy option' ain't that easy for 7 hours. Anyway, Mum OK on arrival. Soup lunch. 'Tired' & 'Legs'. [Usual Routine]. Tesco. Fish finger tea. Repetitive 'Tired' all day today; + looking for argument at times - so only 6/10".

The next potential 'new' flashpoint of anxiety was identified as 'the clocks going back'; which we had Reminded her of over the previous few days; and which I carried out for her before leaving on the 25th of Oct. It would, of course, bring the erstwhile problem of *darkening nights* back into play again - for the moment at about 5-30pm.

1st Nov. (Sat): "Mum actually OK when I arrived, but then got upset 'cos she hadn't made Sat dinner & had to open soup. (Though she had cooked chicken). Soon sorted. However, pills not taken – gave them to her 12-15. Dosette done. Have taken A-Care bill. Will send cheque Monday. [Usual Routine]. Aldi. 7/10".

3rd Nov. (Mon): "Oh dear, not a good day. Usual P/O & M&S. Pain in legs. Her ankles are swollen today. Mum got upset & wet herself in car! Encourage regular pain relief. 2 x paracetamol". (L).

4th Nov. (Tues): "Moaning from start ('Legs'). Heating off, so pointed it out. Usual 'row' about 'cooking', (warming up soup), 'so no heating needed'. Put it on – got threatened with 'won't let you in if you keep bossing me'. Stayed firm. She calmed down. Reassurance etc. Better by end of lunch. [Usual Routine]. Tesco. Generally OK after iffy start. Steady as you go, Cap'n. 7/10".

After the reasonably stable *Spring and Summer* of 2014, the colder, and ever-darkening, nights of autumn, and beyond, seemed to be pushing Mum, in an all to predictably SAD, (Seasonal Affective Disorder), way, inexorably back towards those prowling feelings of anxiety, loneliness, and 'fear', and those oft-accompanying tendencies to need to visit the toilet more frequently, or complain of the real or perceived worsening of her various 'pains', etc. that had tended to beset her throughout the same winter period of the previous year; and once again the issues and worries of 'heating and eating' already seemed to be firmly back on the agenda, too. Going off Mum's most recent moods and indicators, it looked like we were in for another long struggle (despite the addition of the relatively stable support visits from Joan), before the dawn of Spring returned to, hopefully, herald some practical and psychological upturn and relief once more - but, as ever, with my lovely Mum, there was always room for a smattering of more positive surprises, and a reminder that an active Routine, with suitable stimulation and distraction, could still be a very useful basis for, at least temporary, 'improvement', and therefore enjoyment, whatever the weather.

8th Nov. (Sat): "Well I never! Mum OK on arrival; but I am 'unbalanced' by Mum's bus trip to [town] with Sue [my brother's partner], @Fri. I didn't see that one coming! Hope springs eternal. Dosette done. Mum to toilet twice. [She] had made soup & chicken + rice pudd too, for lunch. Mum 'weak', 'cold' after toilet. Just wanted to sleep. No relaxation exercises; just 35 mins sleep. Woke still 'weak' & 'cold'. Didn't want to go out. Persuaded her. Worth doing, 'cos she got better whilst out & distracted; & OK by return home. Salmon butty tea. Good start & end to day. Slight hiccup in middle, after toilet 'weakness'. 7/10".

As she occasionally did, my brother's partner, Sue, had once again been good enough to provide 'cover' for us in our rare triple absence; this time for the morning of Friday the 7th; and to both her and our surprise, Mum had actually *accepted* Sue's casual suggestion that they catch the (once an hour) local bus over to the town for a 'change' and a cuppa. Moreover, Mum had then completed the trip without problem. We were all pretty flabbergasted. Of course, and alas, it would turn out to be but a 'one-off', and by the Saturday we were back to something more akin to the unpredictable 'normality'.

9th Nov. (Sun): "Mum in real bad mood on arrival. Commented that none of us do anything for her. 2 windows open, no heat on, and a cold morning. Watched some Sun telly. Mum calmed down. Still remembers Fri etc. Mum could not rest this morning. Doing silly jobs. Could not keep still. Trouble with eye this morning. Had better mornings". (T).

10th Nov. (Mon): "P.O. done. Went to cenotaph [To see wreaths, after Remembrance Sunday]. Pills not taken, so took about 10-30ish. Hair appointment made for Mum. Good day today. Must be the bus ride". (L).

11th Nov. (Tues): AM – "No pills taken. That's 2 days on the bounce. Gave them to her at 10-00am. No heat. Windows open. Same old story. Quite chatty today. Told her Chris W had died aged 66. She bent my ear all morning regarding [when and] where Chris will be buried. Read Joan's notes from yesterday. [Joan had commented that Mum had said her breathing 'wasn't very good', but that Mum 'seemed fine to me']. A good morning until 11-00am. Mum been to toilet 4 times up until 11-45am without success. 'Houston you may have a problem'". (T).

PM – "Mum sweeping leaves when I arrived. Mini argument straight away 'cos she threw them over [neighbour's] wall. When I pointed it out she said 'Don't boss me'. Soup. Chatted about cenotaph, PO, Chris W. Slowly came round. Then another mini-argument when I brought up the 'missed pills. How did I know? From this book. Mum going to tell U 2 off for 'telling lies'; 'cos she says she did/does take her pills. She was worried about her 'mind' today. Reassurance, cuppa & cake later & she settled again. Then another argument after she said I didn't care about her. Told her a few home truths, which upset her. (I know, got drawn in again, but, my God, I never STOP thinking about her needs). Anyway, relaxation exercises (I needed them!), & 35 mins nap. Awoke much better/ less confrontational, and ready for Tesco. Went cemetery while Mum unpacked. On return, kettle switch loose. Need new kettle? Fish finger tea. Funny day. Really up & down. 6/10".

Having read the above, and after posting that she had bought a new kettle, my sister's next (Weds) log (and cheekily offering me some of my own advice from the 'Be Positive' list), suggested I come with a [more] positive attitude, and then (and somewhat rashly and inconsiderately in my view), wrote that, at 89, "so what", if tablets forgotten, or if she wants to sweep leaves. Perhaps not too surprisingly, I took a little umbrage, and the bait, and once again there was a point of potential argument between siblings; and in *my* next log, I once again found myself taking on a rather holier-than-thou position to point out that it was I who spent by far the most, (and certainly most-at-one-go), hours in Mum's company, and to suggest to my sister that she too try a 7-hour stint or two; adding, for good measure, that I had, that very day, managed to persuade Mum to "positively" join me in a half-decent tea-time rendition of 2 verses of one of her favourite hymns, "How Great Thou Art". Luckily, with logs exchanged, and respective views respectfully aired, the matter didn't escalate further, and life carried on as cooperatively as ever.

That said, the *issues* responsible for any potential tensions, and for the likes of Mum's increasingly OCD behaviours, (and, always, of course, underpinned by the Dementia), hung around like a bad smell, in their ever- frustrating and unpredictable ways. For example, the taking of her medication was an issue rarely far from the 'front line', as we each, and variously, continued to log her missing it fairly regularly, (and had to decide whether to give it late or not), or occasionally suspected her of taking a *double* dose, when the next day's dosette compartment was found empty. As always, it was difficult to know just what effect on her moods (or the Dementia), these 'missed', or any 'doubled-up', intakes might be having. And alongside the medication issue, there was still the familiar pattern of arriving to find Mum in a decidedly downbeat mood, and/or beset by 'fear' and anxiety, after a long spell, (especially overnight), on her own; and of her steady improvement once the stabilising Reassurance of our in-house company had been in place for a while. For me, of course, 'the Usual Routine', (of those Relaxation exercises followed by a short nap, and then some sort of neutrally-distracting and stimulating local outing), was ever a central bedrock in the management of my 7-hour 'shifts' but, in differing personal circumstances, we each, inevitably, dealt with, and reacted to, things in our own way.

For instance, my brother's logs often described the fallout from his efforts to raise the issue of Mum leaving her windows open, whilst having no heating on, and in the coldness of late November, as "fighting WW3", and now we were staring the management of another *Christmas* squarely in the face and I was 'first to blink'.

22nd Nov. (Sat): "Mum OK on arrival, but no heat on in kitchen or front room. Put it on – easy option. Soup lunch & rice pudd. Christmas:-

Usually I cover Christmas Eve. (Weds 24th this year).
Usually T covers Christmas day. (Thurs).
Usually, L covers Boxing Day (Fri).

Are we OK with that again? Then me on Sat (27th) as usual and on to a Happy New Year 2015. Dosette done. [Usual Routine]. Aldi. Salmon sarnie tea. 7/10".

No sooner had we begun to consider the Year's *Festive* options though, than November decided to bequeath me its own particularly *un*festive, and most unwelcome, legacy, by drawing to a distinctly downbeat close with not only a further noticeable dip in *Mum's* morale, (with *its* associated need for additional input), but also, and at the very same time, in mine; by simultaneously requiring me to take my 'turn' at navigating some distinctly 'choppy health waters' on my *own* domestic front.

29th Nov. (Sat): "Very bad start! Mum too long alone at this time of year. She thought L was coming to take her for pension; was ready with bag & (light) coat. Obviously thought it was Monday! Also, tablets not taken. Gave them to her. No lunch ready. She got upset when she realised she'd got wrong day. She had cooked chicken & made rice pudding; but yesterday – so cold. Warmed it up. Lots of [anxiety-based] 'frightened', 'go in a home' stuff [followed]. We made soup together + cold chicken. It took a while, but she slowly came round. Lessons:-

1. We need to keep to settled Routines, (during dark nights & this time of year), as much as possible. (Even small changes confuse her).
2. Left too long alone (at this time of year) leaves her more vulnerable to confusion/upset. Also, Mum to toilet. Hot news! 'She's been!'

Update on [my] Sue's back – Big problem! More or less sofa-bound for a week now! Saw Dr. at [local] hospital on Thurs. He distinguished current back pain as Sciatica. Awaiting scan on this. Can't tackle hip [replacement] until Sciatica pain is sorted – looks like a long job. I feel like a Community Nurse covering 2 cases 17 miles apart! AM KNACKERED!

Relaxation Exercises + 30 min nap. Helped. Dosette done. (Seems to have forgotten she got wrong day now). Aldi. Complained of hip pain all way round Aldi - though not back at home. Salmon sarnie tea. Tough/poor day really. Got off to a bad start, (I arrived tired myself), and never fully recovered. I'll give it 6/10 'cos Mum didn't give up".

My partners own chronic, long-standing, but hitherto manageable, hip problems had taken their own decidedly serious 'turn for the worse'. The (bearable wait for a) hip-replacement operation that she was already down for had now been pushed off her more immediate agenda by the sudden acquisition of a severe bout of left-hip Sciatica that would see her increasingly unable to even mount the stairs to bed, and confined to sleeping on the lounge sofa. Worse still, as the pain confined her the more, we were required to purchase a downstairs commode for her basic toileting needs, during what would turn out to be a fully 3 MONTH, heavily-drug-prescribed, wait before the necessary, pain-relieving, operation could be carried out. (Even then it took all my persistence with the medics involved to persuade them that Sue's case was among the more urgent!). Trying to manage these two time-consuming 'cases' 17 miles apart would turn out to be the most wearing and stressful period in all of the 4 years since my retirement. For now, before each of my 'shift' days, I would have to attend to Sue's personal, and all our household, dog and shopping, needs before my midday departure to attend to Mum's; and then do exactly the same on my return - but there was no alternative; the 'show just had to go on' at both ends and then, as if to add insult to injury, my sister's first-day log of the new month of December included. "[Her husband's] van broke down. Starter motor. Bloody great"; but Mum's needs hadn't gone away, and *still* needed attending to.

2nd Dec. (Tues): AM - "Not good on arrival. Mum crying [ostensibly] because she had lost the station on the radio. Also, Tues/Weds pills missing. Presume she may have taken 2 lots. Either way, Weds missing. I have moved them all up one day, so there is none for Sat. You need to put some in. Mum settled down once someone (me) was here. Mum said mind wandering, fear, etc. No heat on. Once house warm Mum got better and had good conversation. NO mention of bad back or legs. Toilet twice. Mind is going worse. 89 in Jan. We plod on. L was talking to [Mum's surviving brother] at dentist. Has been in [hospital] with chest infection, but on the mend. Have not mentioned to Mum. Just something else to worry about". (T).

PM – "Mum not bad today. Heating on too. Some moans about 'legs' & 'back', but not much. RE Nails – will leave that to you L to contact Dr. re chiropody. Re Tablets – will wait til Thurs before putting new tablets in 'Sat'; she might 'miss' another. If so, let it go & swap tablets to Sat. Soup lunch. 12-30pm – T/c from Dr. M @ [GP] surgery. Looking for update for 'Care Plan'. Asked, 'Have there been any changes'? After a long conversation, he agreed he would do home visit to meet Mum (&us), to discuss all aspects of Care Plan. Told him L would be contacting re chiropody & nails. Dr. M is available Tuesdays & Wednesdays. I said one of us would get back to him asap. Dr. M says get chiropody form from Reception. Tesco. Bought tin of Qual. St. & tinsel for Xmas. Fish finger tea. 7/10".

My sister's subsequent, and succinct, next-day, log read, "Doc's arranged for Tues. between 1-2pm. Sorted podiatry form"; and whilst we awaited the arranged meeting with bated breath, the most distracting highlight of the next few, thankfully standard management, 'shifts' at Mum's was that of Mum and I purchasing the traditional Christmas wreaths, and then laying them on the graves of Dad and my maternal grandmother, respectively, on the Saturday *preceding* the meeting. Although, my brother excusing himself from actually attending the meeting, with the perceptively acerbic end to his log of the 7th, that read, "Don't give the Doc a hard time, otherwise he will move on", provided me with a wryly distracting moment of mirth. At last, then, the day of naively-rekindled medical hope and anticipation dawned. I was to meet the new man himself.

9th Dec. (Tues): "Mum moaning about 'legs'; otherwise not bad. L arrived 1-00pm. Dr. Do-Dah arr. 1-40pm. [His] main recommendation was to 'trial' an anti-depressant, (Sertoline I think – will check later online). I revisited [my worries here]; but L was keen. I felt T should be involved – bought time [to think]. I still disagree; as I 'fear' the side effects – and am not able to find [yet] more time @ present, should things go wrong. However,

I accept that I can be out-voted; but I would not be able to 'pick up' further issues relating at present. Left up in the air. He listened to Mum's lungs. Also looked at her legs. Seemed to be making note to refer surface sores to Di Nurse. No other advice re Mum's leg pains. He left in a rush – to catch surgery. Await further development/new Care Plan? No Relaxation or sleep today! Went Tesco. Mum OK & could not remember much of the meeting by then. [Indeed], she was asking if both Dr. and/or L had been! Fish tea".

The doctor's visit, and particularly his recommendation of an anti-depressant as his only offering for Mum's increasingly complex needs, provided another potentially pivotal point in Mum's 'treatment', going forward; and there certainly *wasn't* unanimity amongst we siblings on the matter. My own strongly-held views, (that neither Mum's existing, nor her long-standing, medication, had been *evidently beneficial* to date), were well known by both my siblings; and my opposition to the latest offering had strengthened further when my online checks turned up the anti-depressant as being Sertraline, and as carrying some 'common', and, in my view, serious, side-effects; especially for someone already suffering from Dementia. They included, for example, diarrhoea, constipation, fatigue, headache, and, ironically anxiety. With my own domestic situation currently claiming every 'non-Mum' moment of my time, and with us already having enough trouble getting Mum to take the few tablets that she was already prescribed, I was deeply anxious about Mum even 'trialling' that 'risky' anti-depressant. On the other hand, my sister, (she of the lesser cynicism about the medical profession in general, and of the more trusting of them to actually know what's best, medically), was broadly in favour. Whilst my brother's view was non-committal; though, from the outset, he had been keen to stress that, "it should be a joint decision". So, conveniently, his log of the 11th, that, "at 89 [an anti-depressant probably] would not benefit her", as "on a good day she is not too bad", handed me the vital edge in the argument; and, by dint of lack of further action on the subject, my insistence that online evidence suggested that the drug carried some potentially serious side-effects for someone with Dementia, and my firmly-restated declaration that, (due to my partner's own current health issues), I could not guarantee to be available to help *police* the taking of the extra drug, or its' likely effects, I eventually won the day and on we went; neither the GP's long-awaited home visit, nor his precious Care Plan, having really changed anything at all in terms of Mum's day to day care and needs.

On the other hand, there *was* effective unanimity for my sister's insistence that "regular pain relief in the form of paracetamol", (which was freely available from any chemist, and already formed part of Mum's medicine cupboard, anyway), should remain available *as necessary*. I say 'effective' because, during my afternoon visit of the 11th, I even logged a few 'qualifications' about *that*.

"Just a thought or 2 on pain relief:-

1. If Mum takes it too often she might get 'used to it' & need higher & higher doses for effect.
2. If it works, (paracetamol or whatever), she might take that as a sign that the problem as gone - & might DO even more and make the problem worse.
3. Can we get paracetamol off GP for free.

Ps GPs are Generalists, not Specialists, & don't always know best.

Mum is now asking 'How's Sue'?, so something is sticking in her mind [still]. Generally awful weather today. Generally poor day for moaning. (Have invited Cap'n of England Moaning Team to meet Mum. Pretty sure she'll get in!). Bean on toast tea. 7/10.

Ps Off to Nursing Home No 2".

13th Dec. (Sat): "Mum very upset & weepy on arrival. 'Don't know what I'm doing', 'mi legs', 'fed up with mi self', sort of stuff. (Too long alone). Told me to 'Go', 'Go'. Absolute rubbish start. Needed to confront those issues first. Got worse before it got better. (All I need right now!). Had to sort more soup, 'cos Mum hadn't enough in pan. House cold. No heat on. Anyway, 20 mins in & we'd worked through it. Mum calming; but more confused today than I've seen her for a while. No tablets taken – will leave it that way. Dosette done. New Scrip needed by Sat. Relaxation Exercises + 30 mins nap. Mum more relaxed now; cuppa. Aldi. By now Mum 'back to normal'. 6/10".

15th Dec. (Mon): "National moan day; Arghh. Lots of pain. [Have] booked Mum in at Clinic for ulcer on leg. I'm not happy with the redness. PO done, papers paid, dinner done, Xmas cards. Anything else? I have spare Valium should anyone need it over Xmas". (L).

16th Dec. (Tues): "Mum surprisingly OK & helpfully philosophical – 'Got to keep going 'til you drop', 'It's just old age', 'If you can eat & sleep, there's not much wrong with you & I can do both' - as you say, T, 'what a difference a day makes'. Wow, what a better attitude – and all without pills! L is taking Mum to [pub] on Boxing Day – I think we should take initiative & cancel Joan, [anyway]. Just to update u on my Sue - still awaiting date for scan. She's been sofa-bound & hasn't left the house for over 3 weeks now & no end in sight – so I'm busy sorting her out, too. Be patient with me. Oh, & I've got bad back myself! I think we're just going to have to 'write off' this Xmas. [Usual Routine}. Tesco. Some moans about 'legs', but generally best day for a week. 7/10".

17th Dec. (Weds): "Will phone with details. Not a good plan this boot! No [other] options. Appt booked for next Tues. for another dressing. This is not going to be easy. Coated in iodine, so a bit stingy at the moment, but that will get easier. Has to sleep with bandage on". (L).

Mum had now been seen by the District Nurse with regard to the sores/ulcers developing at some points on her leg(s). As the above log suggests, the District Nurse had applied iodine and a bandage to the actual sores, and required Mum to wear the dressing in bed, too. She had also supplied a sort of sponge 'boot'/ shoe for Mum to wear on the most-dressed foot when not abed. The potential for anxiety, irritability, and dressing removal, over the week, until the District Nurse next examined the sores, and therefore for trouble, was obvious.

18th Dec. (Thurs): "Mum OK. Seems happy enough with leg bandage at present. Less so with the 'shoe' – I must admit, I can't see the shoe's use inside or out – uneven with a normal shoe on other foot. Anyway, seems to be providing DISTRACTION. [Usual Routine]. Sang 'Away in a manger' together. Mum has coped well, so am giving her 8/10".

20th Dec. (Sat): "Improved quickly once she had company. Soup + chicken+ rice pud. Says leg 'jumping' – 'getting better'. She then noticed it was dirty under the plant stand in the outer place & obsessively set about moving the stuff, mopping & cleaning it – no matter how I tried to dissuade her. I had to let it happen. Nothing would stop her. Then 'tired' & wondered why! Shows she's fit though. Noticed pills not taken. Gave them 1-30pm. Later, short Relaxation + 20 mins nap + Aldi. 7/10".

22nd Dec. (Mon): "What a bloody mess. Bandage cut off. She said she hasn't done it. Couldn't get appointment today. No D Nurse available. I shouted at her today & she was upset. Told her we can't look after her if she keeps messing with things. PO & dinner done. Going home". (L).

Our worst fears had materialised regarding the bandaged leg. Mum had cut off the itching bandage, and left the sores open to the air. In the absence of the imminent availability of any District Nurse, my overwrought sister had had to carry out a 'DIY repair' as best she could; but a repeat episode seemed highly likely.

23rd Dec. (Tues): "Eventually arrived [with dog] @ 4-20pm, after horrible day @ Infirmary, with Sue screaming in pain on scanner; and [then] terrible drive thro heavy wet traffic. Mum moany; mainly about 'leg'. (Says it's worse since new bandage; but looks better/lighter).

NB need to be at home for [Sue's] GP home visit @ lunchtime tomorrow (Weds), so may not be at Mum's til mid-afternoon. Can calls on my time, by the needy, get any worse! Still, keep calm, and carry on. Be Positive".

24th Dec. (Weds/Christmas Eve): "Arr. 12-30pm with [dog]. Mum moany but OK. Relaxation Exercises + 25 mins nap. (1st time for a week). Brought Mum groceries from home. Managed brief trip to cemetery, but weather foul. Beans on Toast tea. Nice sing-a- long to 'Carols from Kings'. Yes, Mum singing too. Merry Christmas. 7/10".

25th Dec. Thurs/ Christmas Day): "Picked Mum up at 11-15am. At first she said she wasn't coming. Eventually went cemetery and down to our house for 12. Not bad until all 9 people came. Then seemed to become too much for her. Ate all her [Xmas] dinner, but then went to pieces, fear etc. Spoke to Keith @ 4-30ish. Told him what was happening. Would not speak to him on phone. Took her home at 5-15pm. Seemed to come round when it was quiet and 1:1, instead of a crowd. Stayed until 6pm". (T).

My sister met with a similar reluctance and initial lack of enthusiasm for the pub meal they had booked for Boxing Day, but Mum eventually went, and apparently "did well"; but, for all of us, the strain and emotion of Christmas had been competently negotiated, and was now safely back in its' box for another year. (I was doubly glad, as my drugged-up partner had never left the sofa, except for the commode, and had eaten only the smallest portion of the most 'essential' Christmas dinner that I had prepared, for her and our daughter).

My visit to Mum of Saturday the 27th, (with dog), had come with a thin covering of snow on the ground, but saw us essentially 'back to normal' and the [Usual Routine]; not least because Mum had already taken down all her Christmas cards, and the few decorations and strands of tinsel that she had allowed us to put up. Meanwhile, my sister took her to keep the 'legs' appointment back at the clinic, on the last Weds. and day of 2014. She reported Mum's 'legs' as, "Healing well. One is nearly completely healed. Doesn't need bandage, thank God! Back next Wed. Appt made for feet for Thurs. 29th of Jan. Happy New Year". (L).

2015

As well as the 'usual suspects', (moans, anxiety, pills), the New Year, and its inaugural day got off to a dodgy start with 2 new 'Mum' worries to potentially manage; one *personal* (her legs), and one vital *household*, at this time of year. Irritatingly, the Central heating was now 'on the blink'.

1st Jan. (Thurs): AM - "Mum all worked up on arrival. She had lost the station on the radio. Pills taken, heating on. Phone call from L, asking me to check Mum's leg. When I checked, she had put masking tape all over the edges of the plasters, because she said 'they were coming off'. L told me to take it off, because it would irritate the skin. I have taken most off, but Mum got all worked up, and would not let me take off any more. L arrived to look at Mum's leg and take off rest of tape. She said she could not rest, [and] told Mum not to put any more on. Will she obey?". (T).

PM – "Soup lunch, [and] New Year joke: Mum: 'Arthritis'. Me: 'Arthur who'? Mum: 'Arthur Itis'. Me: 'Where does he live'? Mum: 'In my legs"! (Bum Bum!). Relaxation Exercises + 40 mins nap. Shocking weather, but went for drive. Returned 3-40pm to find Central Heating had gone off. [Again]. Check of the boiler showed pressure had dropped to ZERO. Let water in and pressed triangle sign [button] and the heating returned; but needs checking, 'cos [this is second time], and Mum wouldn't know what to do – AND ITS WINTER. Sandwich tea. Given the lousy weather, and dog limitations, decent day. 7/10".

3rd Jan. (Sat): "Mum not bad ('legs' excepted). Soup lunch & [tinned] rice pudd. [Brought groceries from home]. Another wet & weary day; and, with dog, that restricts what we can do. Update on Sue. Now on her 6th different pain-killer; with no noticeable change [so far]. Has appt with Spinal Specialist @ 12th Jan.

Ps Central heating ON @ 12-30pm – let's see if it stays on. Dosette done. [Usual Routine].

Pps Oven signs [are now badly worn]. Managed brief cemetery walk, and drive. (C H still on, but I dare not [meddle with it] in case C H cuts out again). Chicken sandwich tea. Despite constant moans – about 'leg', 'hip', 'tired' etc. I'll give her 7/10".

Whilst my partner remained confined to our sofa, my own patterns and Routines remained much more ad hoc. Usually, I was now finding it easiest to shop early at my large *home* Tesco's, (for both her and for Mum's needs), on 'shift' days, and to bring Mum's grocery items, plus our dog, with me on my visits; which made my options more limited and less varied (and, in consequence, of course, less distracting and that bit more pressured), at Mum's end...but on we went.

Tuesday the 6th of Jan was the 19th anniversary of *Dad's* passing, (although the actual date fell on a Saturday, on the year he died - 1996), but Mum tended not to remember such events nowadays, and would probably have allowed it to pass unacknowledged had I not decided to remind her. In the event, (and dog in tow), we managed a brief cemetery walk for the purpose, followed by a general drive round by way of additional and time-consuming distraction.

Meanwhile, the very next day, (the 7th), and like a small 'light at the end of a darkening tunnel', saw my sister logging, "Clinic done. Healing well. Should be last visit next week".

10th Jan. (Sat): "Tough start. Lots of weeping & wailing. 'On mi own', 'don't know where I am' stuff. (All I need, but keep calm and carry on). [Offered plenty of Reassurance, but] didn't 'reward' by giving too much attention, & she slowly 'came round' – now company's here. I'd brought plenty of foodstuff [from home]. Soup lunch. Relaxation Exercises + 30 mins nap. Woke just as moany – 'Oh dear', Oh, mi legs' etc. Managed brief walk round cemetery. (You just have to get out when you're here 7 hours). Salmon butty tea. Hard work today. 6/10".

The 13th brought a few issues too. Firstly, A-Care had rung the house to say Joan was going to Dublin for the weekend. (So wouldn't be visiting Friday). Then, my latest unproductive update on my *partner's* lack of progress read, "Seen Spinal Specialist @ Mon. He said her slipped disc was bad enough for surgery; but she's chosen the Steroid (Cortisone) injection as 1st option; if that don't work then its surgery; and if that doesn't work then it's 'curtains' & Sue disabled". Then, to cap it all, it started to snow, leaving a light covering on the day, (and showering 'reinforcements', on and off, over several others), and again limiting our chances of getting out. And all the while, Mum's *main* moan was that of the continuing (worsening?) chronic pain in her lower 'legs'. On the 'every little helps' *upside*, my sister's log of the 14th noted, "Clinic done now. All healed well. Finished". Hurrah. Well, at least it was *one* thing less to worry about.

That said, among the assorted 'logs of note' around those days was my brother's of the 15th, telling us, "Mum thought she was going out with L", my sister's of the 16th, advising us that "Mum burned her hand on the oven – keep an eye on it", my brother arriving on the 18th, to find her "at the top of the b/yard, no coat on, in her slippers, feeding the birds, (I ask you)", after a fresh fall of snow, and that of the latter's on the 20th,, noting from "the A-Care log [that] Joan did not attend, but a young girl called Naomi came". (It later turned out that Joan had rung in sick, and despite our all previous discussions, someone at A-care had still, unilaterally, sent a 'replacement'; luckily with no noticeably negative effects on Mum).

The "pain" in Mum's (lower) legs also seemed intent on continuing to make its presence fully felt; prompting my sister to visit the local chemist to ask, somewhat in desperation, if Mum would benefit from the wearing of special (surgical) support tights; and to then log (on the 21st), that she would be making further contact with Mum's GP, after the chemist advised that such tights were only available via the latter, and on *prescription*. And all of the above, plus the other well-established issues with her medication, her heating, the cold, dark, drabness of the winter season, and more, predictably contributing to Mum regularly re-visiting her moments of "fear", of thinking she ought to "go in a home", because, "I'm getting worse", and, of course, of feeling further confused and isolated in the face of the unforgiving Dementia.

Another worrying factor, in consequence, was Mum's New Year tendency towards depression, and, through that, to a yet poorer and more forgetful attention to personal hygiene, and, perhaps inevitably, to an associated dip in her household standards and upkeep in general. For example, my sister's log of the 22nd noted that she "made [Mum] change her clothes", (after watching her wear the same ones for several days in a row), whilst my brother logged, on the 30th, (the day before Mum's 89th birthday), that he had felt the need to "change Mum's bedding"; advising that he had also "taken her bedding [home]to wash".

31st Jan. (Saturday, and Mum's 89th Birthday): "Mum OK. L had been. Soup lunch. Sarah [grand-daughter] arrived. Good chat etc. Dosette done. Groceries [brought] for Mum. Relaxation + 30 mins nap. Brief drive out. Chicken sarnies. 8/10".

Mum had reached the ripe old age of 89. Her birthday, largely at her own request, but partly due to ongoing pressures and limitations at my own end, had been kept 'no fuss' and low-key, with our respective visits, simple personal and essential household presents, and minimal celebration; and therefore relatively 'normal' for these strange days. Falling on a Saturday, then, the bulk of that 'normality' fell, willingly, within *my* remit, and (essentially following the 'Usual Routine'), we enjoyed a pretty decent day. Happy 89th Birthday, Mum.

Apart from the hope, and hint of Spring, that came with the lightening nights, and first sightings of snowdrops, the new month of February brought little positive change; and, alas, that included with my own partner's difficult and draining situation. My more upbeat and hopeful log of the 3rd of Feb, that, "tomorrow, my 'nightmare' may be over/reduced – Sue going for steroid jab @ 7-30am", was roundly trumped, just two days later, by my decidedly down-in-the-dumps log of the 5th, that read, "The light at the end of the tunnel has not come on yet, re Sue. Jab done, but no difference so far. Also, my oven's packed up so I'm looking for a working gas oven to PUT MY HEAD IN! When your luck's out...". Thankfully, Mum wasn't adding anything exceptional to my predicament at that time but it couldn't last.

9th Feb. (Mon): "Mum hysterical with pain in legs. Didn't want to go out. Phoned Doc's. Booked appt for Weds for legs – I don't think we understand how much pain she's in. I will ask for a referral to hospital; though she is now saying she doesn't want to go". (L).

I was pretty sure that Mum's 'legs' were still essentially a problem of poor blood flow, and aging, and that the 'Doc' would have no 'magic answers' beyond more pain-killers; I wasn't disappointed.

11th Feb. (Weds): "Been Docs. This is the Plan:–

Mon – Docs for leg scan – 10am.

Weds - back to Docs for results.

Change to Co-codamol – she must be given them at dinner time and bedtime. There is little blood flow in the right ankle. Bottom line [could be] blood clot/lose foot. Encourage raised legs". (L).

Interestingly, part of my brother's next day log included the observation that, Mum had been "Quite chirpy [and] did not mention her legs much today. Yes, they may hurt, but is it attention-seeking sometimes? I told her to put her feet up, but she told me she had hoovered and polished even with her bad legs". (T); whilst I too had a few questions and observations to log.

12th Feb. (Thurs): "Mum quite good, 'legs' notwithstanding. Soup lunch. Not entirely clear on the 'Plan'. Is she having scan @ GP's? Will she take Co-codamol regularly? What is she changing to Co-codamol from? Presumably from 'parrots-eat-em-all'? [paracetamol]. Getting Mum to rest is not easy – whether it's with feet up or not!

Went for [local paper] & cemetery walk [with Mum & dog] – during which I asked Mum several times, at 10 mins intervals, WHERE her legs hurt most – She consistently pointed to her LEFT HIP!! Don't know if Doc is scanning that? Could it be sciatic – like [my] Sue? Beans on toast tea. 8/10".

Worryingly, it looked like Mum was acquiring a *new* and chronic (this time left *hip*) pain; and a further potential restriction to her mobility and independence. Meanwhile, and more socially, the local paper that we had bought on the Saturday had apparently carried news of the death of Annie O, (another long-standing old villager that Mum knew, and the wife of *Billy* O, who had preceded her just a year or so ago). This was apparently Mum's main topic of conversation on my brother's Sunday visit, but, thankfully, it had not 'thrown' Mum unduly.

16th Feb. (Mon): "Scan day. Results Weds. They have to calculate the results of both legs – called Doppler Test. Def. poor circulation. Left worse than right leg – hence hip problem? P/O & M&S for dinner. Podiatry appt booked. Not til March! "(L).

17th Feb. (Tues): "Mum OK if you don't count 'legs'. [Usual Routine]. Cemetery walk & drive with Mum & [dog]. Mum did struggle with walk today, re 'legs', and when I asked her where the pain was worst, she again cited the left HIP. Also, another potential problem – Mum says she can't get wedding ring off her finger. It won't go past the [swollen] knuckle. L- if you read this before you

211

go Dr's tomorrow, you could 'run it past' Dr or nurse you see. 7/10"

18th Feb. (Weds): "Doctor's report printed off to read. She has ref. to [hospital]. She feels it's an urgent case. Done it electronically, so expect to hear next week. Mum had a 'little accident' in Tesco – quick dash to toilets – not nice". (L).

19th Feb. (Thurs): AM - "Mum ready to go out on arrival. Thought she was going to Doc's with L. Soon calmed down. No pills taken, then 'Oh mi legs'. On the go all morning, doing silly jobs. If you read the notes, it states that Mum's legs are an *old age* problem. [My Sue] says, on a [previous] visit to [hospital] with L & Mum, regarding her legs, a doctor said eventually Mum would need a w/chair. Hope not". (T).

PM – "Mum OK on arrival, Soup lunch. Usual 'legs' stuff. Read the PAD stuff. [Peripheral Arterial Disease, where the arteries have become narrowed, restricting blood flow]. I guess the diagnosis IS accurate. (Hardening of the Arteries); but:-

1. Mum consistently mentions LEFT HIP [more than calf or ankle] pain as the worst. Little mention of that in the 'bumf'.
2. Apart from dietary improvements on Fruit & Veg., Mum is already 'positive' on the risk factors.
3. The 'bumf' repeatedly recommends REGULAR EXERCISE for PAD – Well, Mum gets loads – and it makes pain *worse*.
4. I think an MRI scan IS a good idea. It will give a more detailed view of her leg 'innards'. Update on Sue – taking her for 'pre-op tests' tomorrow (Fri), so hopefully, back surgery not far off – and my nightmare will end! Managed short cemetery walk + drive to 'Birds'. Beans on toast for tea. 7/10".

Mum's leg pains, in their various ankle, calf and hip guises, really did seem to be restricting her mobility nowadays; especially outdoors; adding to the already significant restrictions that had been imposed on *me*; especially since my own partner had ceded

212

her own mobility to serious sciatica. Hopefully, the end, (or at least help), might be near on both, for I was so very drained by the never-ending, 'dual' care role that had been my desperate 'lot' for nearly 3 months now.

24th Feb. (Tues.): "Mum Ok; except 'legs'. L, letter has arrived today from [hospital] – appt for 9-15am next Monday for Mum. Talking of appts – [my] Sue was contacted yesterday to be offered back 'op' @ Weds 4th March. However, further T/C today saying [her] urine sample showed 'infection' – she has to take antibiotic & infection has to clear – otherwise 'op' may not go ahead on 4th. Brought groceries. Relaxation Exercises + 30 mins nap. Short cemetery walk. (Mum can't do full 'round' at present) + drive round. Sausage rolls & beans for tea. 7/10".

The last few days of February were very much 'holding' and 'waiting' days, as these respective early- March appointments, and their teasing hope of some sort of relief, were dangled before me. At least my brother managed to use the time productively, online; to sort out some acceptably-priced house and contents insurance for Mum's property for another year; letting us mentally 'cross off' one more outstanding task from a list of so many.

2nd Mar. (Mon): "Nice doc. Scanned Mum's legs again. Good examination. Result: Nothing can be done. It's the left leg, behind the knee [that] has [poorest] circulation. At Mum's age, too old. Stents too invasive. He said, if it was his Mum [he'd] do nothing. Encourage paracetamol. He thinks she has a low pain threshold, [Throughout her life, Mum had never given in to 'cheap' pain, so one thing Mum had NEVER had was a low pain threshold!] + arthritis pain. Cafe for fish & chips. Then had panic attack. Soon came round. New pill box. Mum doesn't remember hospital now – but she is discharged". (L).

On the following day's visit, (Tues the 3rd), I was able to log that, with a 7am start, my own partner's date with her medical destiny was to go ahead on the 4th. as planned; and it did. In consequence, I was obliged to miss, and seek 'cover' for, my usual *Thursday* visit to Mum. However, on my next visit, with my partner's 'op' completed, I was able to log, somewhat relievedly:

7th Mar. (Sat): "Arrived OK. Mum OK. 'Legs' still an issue. [My] Sue 'hobbling' on a stick to kitchen. Still too sore for stairs. Clips/stitches out next Weds. No medication to take now. Hurrah! Slow progress! Brought groceries. Soup lunch & [tinned] rice pud. No heat on. Put it on. No relaxation exercises, as Mum fell asleep before we got started. Walk round cemetery. Some leg pain, but she did it. Nice weather. Nice walk. Drive round [town]. Chicken bap tea. Last minute issue – CH 'cool'. Checked boiler. Pressure drop. Reset pressure as before. Heat returning. Not had this for some time. Decent day. 8/10".

On my own home 'front', my partner's sciatic hip 'op' had finally been realised! The sciatic pain had been newly, but hopefully once and for all, banished to the far reaches of memory and posterity, and it already felt like a dead weight had been lifted from my shoulders. My general mood and patience both felt much improved. The end of my 3-month, 'dual care', nightmare felt noticeably within reach, just because one of my 'patients' now had a tiny degree of independent mobility again; albeit still very awkwardly, and with a pair of sticks, for the time being. Alas, there was no such relief, and, indeed, only steadily-increasing worry for me, at Mum's 'end'.

8th Mar. (Sun): "Called out early at 8-30am. Mum said there was a noise coming from the phone, and it would not stop. When I arrived, it was the smoke alarm, as there was a slice of toast under the grill. It was as black as coal. Mum tensed up when she realised what she had done. She eventually calmed down. Phoned Keith with update. [Mum] would not let the incident drop. Reassured her everything was OK. She said it had frightened her and would always check in future. Hope so, otherwise Fireman Sam will be coming. Soup lunch. (Don't mention the 'toast'. She has forgotten about it). (T).

Mum's forgetfulness, and therefore level of functioning, was getting ever more worrying. On that 'score', we'd also noted that some of the signs on her oven were getting hard to *read*, but had so far found no suitable solution; and now the potential threat from leaving some part of the oven *on* had materialised in the form of toast under the grill. Yet again, (for she gave the shortest shrift to the idea of an unfamiliar *new* oven), the only readily-available options seemed to be Repeated advice to Mum, and *our* further vigilance; but some unavoidable risk (from say a fall, or, as here, with use of 'apparatus'), seemed inevitable given that an 89 year old with creeping Dementia was effectively living alone for significant hours of each day. In the *absence* of obvious solutions, (from anywhere), we were simply 'running with' this problem, despite the in-built unease. For what it's worth, though, and thankfully, the 'toast' incident was, so far, a 'one-off', and, for the moment, on we went.

14th Mar. (Sat): "On the home front *downside*, we've no oven, and now no C. Heating or hot water. (Back to Dickens' times). On the upside, Sue is doing OK on stick. At Mum's all OK. Usual moans. Dosette done. Brought groceries. Soup lunch. Brought Mum a Viola plant, and new [kitchen] 'runner' for Mother's Day. [Sunday]. Relaxation Exercises + 30 mins nap. Cemetery walk [with dog] + drive round. Not quite so much moaning today. Chicken Bap tea. Decent day. Ps the 'patch' next to Mum's bed is still damp, but there's nothing to dry it with. [We suspected that Mum was 'missing' the chamber-pot that she was increasingly using in the night]; otherwise] 8/10".

17th Mar. (Tues): AM - "Received call at 8-30am. Mum had burned the toast again, and smoke alarm was going off. Arrived 9-30am. Mum all over the place. No pills taken. No heating on. Windows open. [She] said she was going to a solicitors to stop us all coming. She thought she was going out, so was ready with coat on etc.

[As agreed], have cleaned the carpets as best I can. Not a bad job. Most of the stains have come out. As I was doing the carpets, Mum was walking all over them. Cannot keep still. I have put 5 days on the calendar that need covering. Shit morning, but kept my cool". (T).

PM – "Mum OK. T must have taken the brunt this morning. Brought groceries [and dog, from home]. Took latest A-care bill. Soup lunch, as always [these days]. Notes from the Home Front:-

1. The C. Heating is working again. Aaah, warm.

2. New oven bought @ internet – coming on Friday; incl fitting – Aaah, pizza again.
3. Voyager Sue now steady on stick; esp round house. Have also taken her to Tesco [pre CH 'fix'] – we didn't need anything – just to keep warm!

Relaxation Exercises + 35 mins nap. Cemetery walk & drive round. (Mum's hip hurting on walk). Fish finger tea. 7/10".

19th Mar. (Thurs.): "No heat on. No pills taken. Windows open wide. I think there has been some kind of accident. Sheet on [clothes]line, smell of pee in same spot in b/room". (T).

Anyway, our Routines with Mum went on much the same for the latter days of March. Of note, on my [Usual Routine] visit of Sat. the 21st, I was able to log, with relish, "let me know re T's hols – I have a little more flexibility now Sue's up & about on stick & driving; + we have heat, hot water & new oven heaven"!; whilst the highlight of my sister's log of the 24th read, "All done at [foot] clinic – nails cut;. [Adding ridiculously], she can't go again [though] cos she's not poorly enough"; and on the 28th of the month we received a "letter from the hospital [that] I can't make head nor tail of", where I concluded, "sounds like Dr couldn't find anything worth treating". Then:

31st Mar. (Tues): "[Dogless] after 4 months. Trial to see if Sue can cope. Strange now though. Mum has a cold. Soup lunch. Relaxation Exercises & 35 mins nap. 'Oh mi legs - they do hurt'. Stop press – went to Tesco with Mum! First time since early Nov. Met Cousin. Fish finger tea. Interesting day renewing old Tesco routine. I'll give it 8/10 for novelty".

Early April brought no great changes, (certainly no noticeable Mum-based *improvements*), to the now standard and established pattern of issues that we routinely managed with, and for, her. With the first and unwelcome signs of a 'cold' in evidence, my log of the 2nd was typical of the early days, and of a pretty unremarkable Easter that year, for all 3 of us:

2nd Apr. (Thurs.): "Arr. 11-50am [with dog]. Poor start. Mum on toilet when I arrived. Came down weepy, saying she was 'cold'. Radiator not on in kitchen. Mini-argument, that stopped her crying as she reverted to 'Well, don't come then'. Mum went back to toilet, leaving grill turned on, but unlit! [Turned it off]. She came back saying she had 'been', & [now] felt 'weak'. Finally [managed] soup lunch, whilst constantly 'on the go' – talk about St. Vitas Dance. Relaxation Exercises + 35 mins nap. Mum woke [claiming] she has cold – I think she maybe IS under the weather today, & has sniffles. Persuaded her to go out [for distraction] for [local] paper + short version of cemetery walk. (She struggles on long version now). Beans on toast tea. 7/10".

7th Apr. (Tues): AM - "Heating on, but 3 windows open. There were numerous phone calls to L & me between 9-9-30am. Generally, she was 'frightened' & 'confused'. I am away this w-end". (T).

PM – "Mum continued the crying, 'fear', theme on arrival. Didn't give it *too* much attention, & she soon came round. Still moaning about her 'legs' & 'cold' though. Soup lunch. Mum's cold does seem persistent – a week now. [Usual Routine]. Met Gill O outside PO. Mum asked 'How's your Mum!'. [Gill's Mum, Annie, had actually *died* in early Feb!; and Mum heard me having to make hasty and embarrassed apologies on her behalf!; the incident affecting Mum negatively for several days; whilst, on the 'flip' side, reminding us that her deteriorating memory did still function well enough, on most occasions, to note *something*]. Tesco. Met cousin [again] who had a cold. Chicken & beans for tea. Decent day. 7/10".

The faux pas with Gill O, along with news of the death, just days later, of Richard S, another old villager, would (as I've said, and somewhat surprisingly) take root in Mum's mind, and affect her adversely for several days hence; showing that her memory did still retain stuff for the most part. (Though not *necessarily* in the right order). Perhaps the saddest, and most revealing, consequence here, was that logged by my sister on the 12th, when she described Mum as "crying because of Gill O. Scared Mum is next to die"; whilst on the morning of the 14th my brother logged, "The incident(s) with Gill O & Richard S are still on Mum's mind".

Physically too, new issues continued to arise. Along with her low-key, yet persistent 'cold', another recurring physical problem began to stake its claim over the same April days - that of swollen ankles. My sister had made a first brief referral to the problem on the 8th, and then returned to the matter on several later occasions, including the 17th, where she logged, "[Mum] struggling with legs swelling again – shoes a bit tight. May have to go back to docs".

At least my *afternoon* visit of the 14th brought some distraction, in the form of a visit from my adult daughter, who was home on leave from her teaching post abroad. She joined us round Tesco, and the day went relatively smoothly, earning a 7/10 from me. It also carried first mention, and my keen recommendation, of a specialist Dementia Clock that I had found online. It was relatively costly, at £72, but it came with good reviews, and a specification that showed the individual day, date and time in clear, large, black and white displays that Mum would be able to see easily from any distance if strategically placed – say, in the kitchen. My hope, of course, was that it might limit the increasing frequency of her 'confusions', over such basics as what day it was, where she was expecting to go, and with whom; and thereby give some sort of boost to her cognition, and therefore to her flagging confidence.

16th Apr. (Thurs): "Rang 8-55am. Weepy. Decided to come up and 'cover' T's absence. [Away]. Door locked. Mum crying again. Improved after a few minutes + cuppa. Complaining of sore left hand & middle finger. Probably arthritis. Can't see anything unusual. Suggested she wear rubber gloves when doing work in water – u can guess the answer! Soup lunch. Told me 2 x "I saw [Richard S] funeral go down". It, [and through it her *own* mortality] was definitely [still] on her mind. Reassurance to settle her. Relaxation Exercises + 35 mins nap. Woke 'woozy' & 'frightened'. Sat it out [with more] Reassurance. She agreed to go for cemetery walk. Beans on toast tea. A long & tiring day for us both. Mum definitely 'unsettled' at present. Ps Mum struggled to get left shoe on – swollen ankle. 6/10".

Joan then missed her usual Fri visit, and I arrived on the Saturday to much of the same. In the end, I did manage to persuade her out to Aldi, but, both for my own benefit and clarification, and hopefully for others, I decided to attempt some sort of logged précis of where we were.

18th Apr. (Sat): "Another difficult day to assess, really:-

1. Still seems to have [remnants of] chesty cough/phlegm.
2. Different aches today – 'back', (left) 'side', left arm; and never stopped saying she was 'tired'.
3. On positive side, coped OK with [distractions of] Aldi + cemetery, & still on-the-go most of the day.
4. Couldn't get 'tight' shoe on left foot.
5. Could still have the cold, which others have said causes varied aches.
6. Memory 'all over the shop' at present.
7. Not sure if there's any benefits to/from Dr. Apart from a weepy arrival, I've had worse days, so I'll give it 7/10".

One very obvious omission from my impromptu pseudo-assessment, a clear and ever unfailing contributor to any sudden downward shifts in Mum's mental functioning, was immediately picked up on once more on my brother's return from his 'away-days', when his first-day-back log of the 19th read, "Mum glad I'm back. Will have been on her mind. When L is away in June we will [probably] have the same problem. No crying this morning. Just 'tired'. If you watch Mum, her mind is thinking all the time. Hence she thinks silly things and gets frightened etc. Anyhow, a good morning. No aggro".

The point that Mum was unsettled by any break in Routine, and especially if that break involved one of we three going 'AWOL' for any length of time, (including overnight), was well worth restating and bringing to our conscious attention once more, for it was now central to absolutely everything in the support, well-being and management of Mum's (slowly dementing) life; hence the regularity of her upset on our arrival, and her invariably improved demeanour soon after we were re-established in her company. On the surface, the logical conclusion was that her demeanour would benefit from 24/7 cover; ideally from us, but possibly from a Care Home. A-care certainly didn't offer that sort of option; alas, neither option was *immediately* or practically viable anywhere so, on we went. And the next problem to take its turn at the 'head of the queue' for our management would be her worsening incidents of incontinence 'leaks'. My sister was first to raise this afresh.

20th Apr. (Mon): "Bit better. No mention of Gill O. P/Office & hairdresser. Chippy dinner – Mum had a wee accident in cafe – bit embarrassing. Pain with legs & swelling. Might speak to GP, though don't know what can be done". (At least Mum seemed to have got over her hang-ups surrounding the recent demise of two other villagers).

Alas, the very next day, my brother's log drew our attention to a same-day incident logged by Joan, Mum's A-care visitor, regarding incontinence; who, as well as informing us that Mum had told her "my mind wanders", had also written, "I think she is incontinent of urine. Her skirt looks a bit damp at the back". My brother's reactive suggestion was that "incontinence pads" were required; and that my sister should take on that responsibility. However, in my log of the 26th, I felt obliged to add that we ALL take our share of this problem; not least because future incidents, and the need for the pads' utilisation might well occur when my sister was absent. I also added that I had received and installed her new Dementia Clock in the kitchen.

22nd Apr. (Weds): "Good start. Mum happy with clock. Looks good. Tesco for [incontinence] pads. OK at first, but couldn't understand what to do. They are next to her knickers in drawer. I will ask her to put one on when we go out and see how she gets on. Have said Keith will ask her to put one on too. Nothing to be embarrassed about". (L).

24th Apr. (Fri): "Doc came Friday AM. All arthritis related. Got gel to rub in twice daily. Chest OK, just the usual". (L).

According to my sister's brief log, and for whatever reason, Mum qualified for a GP home visit on the Friday; resulting in a prescription of Voltarol, a strong gel for rubbing into arthritic joints etc.; but no mention appeared to have been productively made of Mum's recent tendency to her incontinence of urine so, on we went on our own here.

I think we all knew that her wearing of such a pad would meet with some resentment, and *I* first met with it on the following (Satur)day, when I logged, "Mum not keen to put on incontinence pad so 'easy option' I'm afraid – I've not had the problem when I'm with her yet". On the other hand, my visit of that afternoon (the 25th) saw my first attempt to put the Dementia Clock to the test, when I asked Mum, as we finished lunch, what day it was [and] pointed to the clock. She correctly said "Saturday". It already appeared to be doing its' job, and, clutching at straws, I repeated the exercise whenever the opportunity arose, during the last few days of April, in my unceasing search for even the smallest sign of a way out of the trough that Mum seemed to have slipped slowly into via her diverse collection of age and Dementia-related problems.

Alas, we entered May with little change in the gradual, but undeniable, downward trend. By now, Mum was nearly always feeling some degree of pain whenever she moved; but especially when attempting any significant *out-of-house* mobility. It was a state that so often tugged at the heart- strings of we carers, and put us under pretty regular pressure, emotionally, both *with* Mum, and *between us*, as we each tried to 'back-up' our individual perspective on the best way forward.

1st May. (Fri): "Started crying as soon as I arrived, so I told her off. Said, 'You only do it with me'. Soon stopped. [Out for] chippy dinner – hip pain. Is it only me that's doing pain relief? Her body is full of arthritis. Keith, if you remember Sue's pain, this is probably worse, and [Sue] was on morphine and tramadol, so every little helps – tablets & gel. When I'm old I hope someone cares enough to help me through it". (L).

From just those few words, it was clear that my sister's emotions were weighing heavy on her. I felt the need to 'steady the ship', and balance that patently emotional perspective with a renewed dash of objectivity and realism.

2nd May. (Sat): "Crying a little on arrival. Soup lunch. (Thank goodness for Heinz Big Soup!). On pain relief – see my notes, L. [In the margin by my sister's May-day logs I had added, 'L, U cannot solve all her problems now, no matter how much you want

221

to', and then gone on to add in my own log] - 'You need to take a more objective view of the situation [too]. Support her, of course, but both she and we have to live with the reality of her aging. [Also], *she's* rubbing on the Voltarol about 4 x daily – too much – she forgets. Same can happen with medication in general. [And it's something to do]'. Relaxation Exercises + 40 mins nap. She woke 'cold'. Argument with Mum. Usual stuff – 'You're no help', 'All for yourself', 'You try to boss me', 'Go, Go'. Mum said she wasn't going shopping. Drove to cemetery for 20 mins alone; to plant Begonias, and calm down - and let Mum calm down. Mum agreed to go out [when I got back]. Aldi. Had to take her back to car half-way round, 'cos of 'hip' and 'legs'. Salmon butty tea. Mum took Co-codamol [but only] at my insistence. She improved a bit. Tough day, poor weather. 6/10" - and on we went - some days still bucking the 'troubled' trend, but most, sadly, not doing so.

9th May. (Sat): "Mum a bit self-pitying, but I've had worse. Yes, she uses the Voltarol 3-4 times during my 7-hour stay, when its only meant for twice daily. Mum forgets she's used it. Soup lunch. Dosette done. Relaxation Exercises & 35 mins nap. Aldi/ Superdrug/Cem. Chicken Bap tea. I'll take the opportunity to give her 8/10, 'cos she walked round Aldi, up to Superdrug, and short version of cemetery walk - ain't done that for a while".

19th May. (Tues): "Received phone call @ 8-20am. Mum crying and all mixed up. Did not know what day it was etc. Arrived early. Mum still mixed up. [Despite new clock]. Water over kitchen floor through washing sheet. Have told her to give me sheet in future. Had it all this morn, get out etc. Eventually calmed down. Said sorry. Tries to do everything and gets worked up. Reassurance paid off and she got better". (T).

As we entered June, the pattern of Mum's mental *and* physical abilities remained very much up and (mostly) down, and, for the most part, tended to confirm, (as if we didn't know it), that real and permanent improvements probably *were* now beyond attainment, given Mum's long-standing range and level of difficulties. Ironically, at *my* end, however, things *had* now improved to the point where my partner felt comfortable accepting a friend's invitation to spend the first 2 weeks of the month continuing her steady recuperation in the sun and warmth of Turkey; so once again I would be dog-tied, and facing a fortnight of limited options, in relation to likely shopping, social outing, and other distractions with Mum. That said, we did enjoy a couple of warm sunny, and (despite the continuing limitations of her various 'leg' complaints), pleasantly distracting sits in, and potters round, a local park, and its lovely Summer flowerbeds and well-tended gardens and lawns, with the dog. It made for a welcome and refreshing change of setting. (On the matter of her leg pains and limitations, we had managed to acquire an old wooden walking stick, from goodness knows where, but, as the first to tentatively 'offer' it, my sister had met with a predictably affronted response, and therefore immediate resistance, from Mum, when she logged, on the 5th, Mum's "legs very swollen. Mum upset. It's water retention. [A] little argument over using stick. No chance!").

6th Jun. (Sat): "Arr. [with dog] to moans, but I've had worse. Soup lunch. Brought full load of groceries [with me]. Taken latest A-care bill. Dosette done. Anxieties sharply raised when Mum [was]sent Times instead of Mirror. Then when white bread had turned green [in her breadbin]. Significant argument. Said I was "no help to her", just as I was carrying 3 bags of shopping in from the car! We ALL [still] need to check for any fresh food going off. Relaxation Ex. + 30 mins nap. Paper shop to swap, short cemetery walk (windy) + drive round. By now Mum continually 'tired'; but no recollection of getting worked up by arguing. Ham & tomato baps for tea. Apart from 'argument', OK day. 7/10".

8th Jun. (Mon): "Usual start. PO & M&S. Mum complained about legs non-stop. Eventually I'd had enough [and] told her to stop moaning & get a stick. It shocked her & upset me. She then wouldn't hold my arm. Anyway, soon forgot about. Note to self – Be patient. She's old". (L).

Then, as if it wasn't hard enough, and whilst dealing with all that, the 'holiday season' got into full swing.

On the very same day that my own partner arrived *back* from her Turkey trek, (the 15th), one of my Mum's immediate neighbours set off on *their* annual escape; followed barely one week later by my sister and her spouse also heading off to Turkey, for a week that incorporated an 'immediate family only' beach wedding ceremony for their daughter (my niece), and her intended. Mum would surely notice these absences, and when Joan first went 'AWOL' on the preceding Monday, and then we found out that she had booked *official* leave on Fri the 26th and Mon. the 29th of June, it seemed like my brother and I would need to be at our absolute best, and provide exceptionally good 'cover', during these 'non-appearances' - or else! It had the potential to be a tougher-than-usual week or two - though, my brother's wife kindly took up the cudgels on a couple of those occasions, by filling in directly for my sister. Nevertheless, a cautionary example of the kind of anxiety-triggered 'activity' that we feared might rear its head was laid before my brother in good time, in the form of a foul and unwanted 'old friend'.

18th Jun. (Thurs): AM - "What a start. Had to clean No. 2s up off kitchen floor. Mum caught short. Could not get to toilet in time, [and had tried to use an old plastic bowl]. Mum crying because of what she had done. There may be a smell of disinfectant in the kitchen, as I had to mop the floor, as the smell lingered. L called in. She flies out [to Turkey] on Sun. She asked what the smell was. I explained. A smelly morning". (T).

My phlegmatic, and low-key, response, on a 'Usual Routine' afternoon visit, was to log that it had, "not been a frequent issue in recent months", and that Mum had made "no mention of No. 2s – already forgot, I guess" and on we went.

In the event, (the usual suspects notwithstanding), we needn't have worried quite so much, for, luckily, that was about as bad as it got during the various 'absentees' jollies, as far as Mum's misdemeanours were concerned. With those promised contributions from my brother's wife, and good communication between us, Mum survived well enough. Indeed, (despite the potentially de-stabilising 'wedding-day phone call' to her, midweek, from my sister in Turkey), the worst, and most annoying, source of increased anxiety, during such absences, was the practical return of spasmodic problems with the reliability of the Central

Heating system; and with my sister back home and 'in the saddle' on Mon. the 29th June, normal 'shifts' and services were able to resume until the next, and most obviously outstanding, 'holiday season' tripper, (my brother), wanted to claim time off from *his* supervisory duties, for a week cruising between selected ports of Northern Europe, just a fortnight later.

The (Gas) Central Heating, on the other hand, took a little longer to be returned to 'normality', but, after a few days additional wait, and with professional input, eventually, it was; but not before it had caused Mum significant upset, after she got it into her head that there was *gas* actually *in* the gas central heating radiators, and in the whole (currently capricious) system, that might somehow leak out in the night and "gas" her. It took absolutely ages, and eons of patience and gentle Reassurance, including using the radiator valve key on several occasions to 'prove' that there was only *water* in there, to convince her that she was not at risk! (Hard enough with *any* uninitiated or elderly person, I guess, but made all the harder for one struggling with Dementia).

The next problem to present was again an 'old friend', when my sister noticed that another sore on one of Mum's legs appeared to be infected. This prompted my sister to acquire a further appointment at the local clinic, on Weds. the 8th of July. It resulted in a diagnosis that the sore was not 'ulcerated', but quite 'deep', and would require a dressing, "that must not be taken off"; with a further clinic visit, inspection, and re-dressing made for the Friday. My sister obliged once more. Meanwhile, my main observation of note, on a fairly standard, dog-tied, 'Usual Routine' visit of the following day, (Thurs. the 9th of July), was that, "the window cleaner came. Interestingly, Mum gave him the £3 automatically. i.e. she *knew* it was £3, so she does [still] know stuff".

12th Jul (Sun): "OK on arrival. Pills taken. No mention of legs [today]. Explained I was going away and phone calls [might] be limited. Don't think it registered. A steady as you go morning. Nautical/Cruise saying – get it?". (T).

My brother was off on his jollies the following day, and would miss just two routine shifts; both on mornings where I visited in the afternoons; so we were hopeful that there would be minimal hassle, but, like all breaks in Routine, you just never knew, and remained wary. I was first to face one of his absences.

14th Jul (Tues): "Arrived 11-30. Door locked. Rang bell. Mum woke 'frightened'. 'Don't know where I am' stuff. Had been asleep in T's absence. Soon OK with Reassurance. Also, Mum's plaster had come unstuck. We had to put microtape on it. Also, it seems to be showing leakage from wound. Anyway, she's being seen tomorrow. Soup lunch. [Usual Routine]. Cemetery walk – nice day. Fish finger tea. 8/10.

Ps Mum let slip this evening that *she* had loosened one side of the plaster, to 'have a look at it'(!), & then stuck it back with [masking] tape".

My sister's distinctly irritated next day log, especially following the clinic visit, read, "There might be murder this week. Mum lifting heavy [plant] pots, [then] crying with back pain! Clinic knew she had taken the dressing off – that's a 1-week setback! Told her she must not touch it. That's why it leaks. Next week – clinic Tues @ 10-40". (L).

Like so many issues that might present as trivial to you or I, (the average compos mentis 'Man or woman on the Clapham Omnibus'), but to an elderly Dementia-sufferer can take on an irrationally disproportionate, even OCD, significance, a couple of fresh and relatively small and innocuous practical issues did raise disproportionate bouts of anxiety in Mum in the week that T was away.

Firstly, she noticed (rightly) a slight but consistent, drop in the pressure of water coming from her kitchen cold tap, (and for no obvious reason), and secondly, whilst trying to help, I managed to actually, and alas irreparably, break the clasp on her tried and trusted old purse, (the Routine, go-to, safe holding place for her ready cash, PO card, bus pass, etc), and thereby to disrupt another small but significant, much-relied-upon, part of her daily Routine.

Reassurance, that I would sort out both problems pronto, (the tap with a new washer, and of course a new purse as similar to the last as possible), just about 'held the day', but here were yet another couple of examples of how much Mum was now reliant on a well- established Routine, (especially in the 'comfort-zone' of her home), and just how easily she could now become de-stabilised and quite worked up, with the minimum of ado. And in due course, my brother made it back.

19th Jul (Sun): "Had not seen me for a week but started WW3 regarding messing with her plaster. No pills taken.

Told Mum about our trip, [how] it rained all day in Ostend & Bruges. Just our luck. Not bad for first morning back". (T).

Anyway, Mum couldn't have been doing too much harm to her (un)dressed leg, because my sister's log of the following Tues. (the 21st), read, simply, "Clinic done. All OK". (The dressing had simply been changed for another week without ado). To cap a "decent day", but in the afternoon, *I* was able to log, "Gave Mum her new purse, AND SHE LIKES IT! We swapped over her stuff. [Usual Routine]. 8/10"; my sister's Weds.log confirming that Mum still liked the purse 24 hours later. Hurrah! However, further and significant *domestic* problems soon beckoned.

25th July. (Sat): "[Usual Routine]. Aldi.

Ps. Advance warning – [my] Sue has pre-op appointment @ Thurs. next, the 30th July, for Hip-op. Likely to be early August. She won't be able to drive for at least 6 weeks, and will be hobbling generally. Restrictive all round".

Meanwhile, the *end* of July saw a 'signature instance' of another worsening 'management issue' at *Mum's* end. Yet another trivial issue, in non-Dementia circles, would henceforth find its way onto *our* 'needing *regular* time and attention' list. Insignificant in itself, and perhaps a reaction to a further deterioration in her eyesight, or, of course down to the worsening Dementia, but perhaps, and most likely, down to the worsening arthritis in her fingers, it soon began to further affect her everyday level of functioning and independence, and therefore to further affect her levels of frustration, anxiety and confidence and thus to consume plenty of our downtime.

26th July. (Sun): "Called out. No telly. Mum [consistently] pressing the wrong button. Telly back in 10 secs. She said, 'I think I want to go in a home', etc. Mum was all over the place with her mind & comments. She said she had phoned Keith first, and he had said to phone me. Do I believe this?" (T).

There was an *element* of truth in the incriminating accusation, and to assuage my guilt after reading T's Sunday log, I immediately felt obliged to provide an explanatory note in *my* very next log. Regardless, the TV *channel-changing* problem had also joined the list of regular, here-to-stay, time-consuming, trivia that, sadly, took on a disproportionate influence in the life of an elderly Dementia sufferer.

28th July. (Tues): "I rang Mum @ 3-30pm on Sunday, as usual, and spent a half hour on the phone trying to get her back to BBC1 & gave up. She was obviously pressing Channel 1 for too long and registering Channel 11. I did say I can't come all the [17 mile] way to [there, just now]. So I presume she rang you instead. [Usual Routine]. Ps [my] Sue now has date of 26th Aug. for Hip-replacement Op. (All hands on deck)". And on we went.

For, of course, Mum's now increasingly chronic and complex, no-way-back, Dementia-lead, problems (be they physical, mental or emotional), carried on largely unabated in spite of her stoic efforts to try and maintain her independence. And, *de*spite significant issues cropping up in the lives of all 3 of we carers (my brother, in particular, had recently posted that his partner's adult son was to undergo hospital re-tests for a long-awaited kidney transplant), we now had no option but to just carry on regardless in our day-by-day care of Mum. For there was no-one else to look after her, at least not properly, and at the level we had committed to, (either in her own home or out), if *we* didn't; or suddenly found that we couldn't.

29th July. (Wed): "[Latest 'leg'] clinic day. [Dressed] leg healing slowly, but its deep. She has bad rash on other leg. Nurse says it's due to Sudacrem – [too much of it] burns the skin – so that's gone. We [now] have E45 cream for rash. Keep up with Voltarol [for arthritic finger joints]. Dinner out. [Husband's] van finally blew up – the engine's [done], so he has hired one". (L). My sister summing up her weary-sounding log with the very witty, laughter-raising, (at least to me), and somehow classically-appropriate line, "If it's not one thing it's your mother!"

2nd Aug. (Sun): "Extra, Extra, T/c to Mum @ 4pm [as usual, and following my brother's usual Sunday morning visit]. Mum just crying down the phone. I could not [tease out] what the problem was. Decided to come up. Arr. 4-55pm. Mum on phone to T. Spoke with him. 5-25, persuaded Mum to walk round [block, for distraction]. It worked. Mum less weepy. The loneliness and fear gets to her – especially with [neighbours] away, & she struggles to fill the time/talk to someone/remember if anyone's been today. Anyway, Mum OK again [for now]".

Mum had been experiencing a particularly damp, quiet, and therefore depressed and lonely Sunday afternoon. I had felt the need to respond in person. August too was off to a (predictably) dispiriting start.

4th Aug. (Tues): "Mum OK. Neighbours back from their holidays too. Soup. Relaxation Exercises & 35 mins nap. Tesco. Mum's other leg also needs Nurse's attention. Late argument, 'cos taking tights off caused right leg [sore] to bleed. I needed to cover with lint. Mum upset 'cos she couldn't understand the cause of the problem/unwilling NOT to wear tights".

5th Aug. (Wed): "Clinic. Bloody hell. One leg healed good – the other [now] a mess! Nurse thinks she may have put wrong cream on – or olive oil. Needs to keep bandage on at all times. Even in bed. Tried to talk her into [wearing] trousers, but no chance! Dinner at M&S. All for now". (L).

So now both legs were receiving the attention of the clinic's nurse, and both would need our close supervision at home if the leg sores were to get better any time soon. Moreover, Mum would need to play her part, and to heed the clinic's advice, and not try out other, home-made, remedies of her own; just because she had forgotten what she should do, or was just curious, or simply looking for 'something to do'. Treading carefully with her, we continued to do our best here, as in all the other 'plate-spinning' areas of her life that still required our input and attention but it wasn't easy.

9th Aug. (Sun): "Walked straight into a row with Mum regarding leg. Mum rubbing right leg with cream, & sticking bandage with masking tape. She said Keith told her to do it.

(I don't think so). Am sure clinic will comment about it. A morning to keep calm & easy option. [Her] mind working o/time today. Had better mornings". (T).

10th Aug. (Mon): "Arrggh! What a morning. Bandage off – taped up. Shouted at her. Made her cry. Now feel bad. Had to get Emerg appt. at Doc's. The smell was sickening. Re-dressed. All oils & creams gone. Just painkillers now. She can't be trusted. New tights and knickers bought. Old ones thrown out. Another row! I don't hold out much hope for this leg to heal. Will see what DN says on Weds. Keith, please renew Mum's Blue Badge. It's expired". (L).

The GP had advised that we remove all the creams, oils, and powders, to keep the sores dry, and my sister had acted swiftly in accordance with that advice. Would that improve Mum's 'leg' matters?

11th Aug. (Tues): "Mum OK, but soon into argument when I [reiterated GP's advice]. She denied ever taking any bandages off. (Could have genuinely forgot). Soup. Sleep. (Mum fell asleep before exercises). On Blue Badge - Will get forms. Will need new photo. Criteria may have tightened. Will take some weeks anyhow. Tesco. Fish finger tea. 7/10".

12th Aug. (Wed): "[Clinic]. Mum's leg pretty bad. Nurse took photos. Def. Burns, so it's the Voltarol. Nurse said encourage painkillers [as necessary]. I think it will be a long job. Dinner out". (L).

13th Aug. (Thurs): "Mum crying when I arrived. 'Frightened'. Saying T had taken 'creams & pills'. Reassured her pills still [in dosette]. Explained [again] Dr. had said to remove creams. She said T 'too bossy'. (Just same as me). Further quiet Reassurance calmed her down. Soup. [Usual Routine]. For local paper [with dog, too]. Collected stamp and envelope etc [for Blue Badge Application]. Short cemetery walk + drive round. Blue Badge – form is complete – just needs photo of Mum & can then be posted. Beans on toast tea. After iffy start, OK day. 7/10".

15th Aug. (Sat): "Arr. 12-05. Mum on edge with 'fear', 'cos 'quiet'. Latest A-Care bill taken. Dosette done. Soup & rice pudd. Relaxation exercises & 35 mins nap. Interestingly, Mum chose the rocker to sit in & woke up saying she'd seen Dad through the window! At first, she feared he'd 'come to fetch her'. Reassurance that she was dreaming sorted it out. Aldi. Ps Mum struggling to get shoes on. May need some more 'flexible' ones. Ham baps for tea. 7/10".

18th Aug. (Tues.): "Sue's Hip- op moved forward 1 day. Now next Tues. 25th Aug. I will drop her off @ 7-30am & will be bringing dog that day & for a couple of weeks at least. Shopping will be difficult. May have to shorten visits to Mum a bit, if necessary, post-op. I'm not looking forward to it! Usual weepy start. Soup. Relaxation & nap. Tesco + photo-stop next door. Have completed Blue Badge [now]. Will post. Await outcome. Fish finger tea. Decent day. 8/10".

Mum's next day's clinic visit with my sister revealed nothing new. They simply redressed the sores where necessary, and repeated more or less the same advice, apparently adding that it may be a 'long job'. In its way, the clinic too was now becoming something of a predictable part of her weekly Routine.

20th Aug. (Thurs): AM - "Mum all over the place on arrival. Said I wanted her in a home. [I had] never brought the subject up. Her slippers were wet. [Suspect] she had just peed in the bowl. [Cleaned and] dried them on radiator. Mum eventually settled down, but remained on edge. Not the best morning". (T). PM – As an instance of OCD behaviour, I noted, "1-20pm – window cleaner came. Mum went [straight] out & cleaned the front-bottom one again! [Usual Routine]. Beans on toast. 7/10".

25th Aug. (Tues): "7am – delivered Sue to hospital for [hip] surgery. (3rd on, of 5). Arr. Mum 12-10pm [with dog]to crying. This time 'cos oven lighter had packed up. I had another in the car! Soup. Mum soon OK [with Reassurance]. Relaxation Exercises & 35 mins nap. Cemetery walk & drive round. Fish finger tea. Early departure @ 6pm, to drop off dog [at home] before visiting time @ hospital. 7/10".

Luckily, Mum's needs remained relatively stable for a few days. My sister's log of the following Friday, (the 28th) providing the only slight (though soon-to-be-repeated) worry, (including on the 31st of the month), when she wrote that, whilst out with her,

Mum was "not eating much these days". On the upside, though, she had also logged (like a welcome ray of sunshine) that the new *Blue Badge* application had at least been successful; the new one having arrived that same day, in the morning post; whilst, predating that by a couple of days, another most welcome 'ray of light', in that 'dark tunnel', had already 'shone' on Mum's sore legs, when, on the 26th of Aug. I had met with my sister at the house, following the latest clinic visit, and she had reported that Mum's legs were "improving. Left leg now has no bandage. Right leg is [apparently] better too". And so it was logged. And so, conveniently, we were able to end Vol. 3 of these diaries, *and* enter the new month of September, with the following hopeful, end-in-sight, log on the sore legs saga - if not on the eating worries.

2nd Sept. (Wed):

"Clinic day. [Legs] doing OK now. Should be last visit next week. Dinner at [Garden Centre]. Not eating much now, so [we] share everything. Mum tired, but not bad today". (L).

Here endeth Vol.3.

New 'diary', same old wad of Dementia-lead issues and problems to manage. The pattern was well entrenched now, and all the more depressingly familiar for that; with Mum definitely stuck *in* quite a depressed, not to mention teary, and generally 'down-cycled', frame of mind at present. Left alone for too long, she increasingly seemed to be meeting with the sort of Dementia-lead experiences that resulted in confusion and failure to function 'normally', (whatever that was these days); leading (quite understandably) to what she knew as "Fear".

Yet mostly, bless her, her innate stoicism meant that she tried, (and indeed managed) to cope alone with much of that loss of cognition, around what had previously been second-nature to her; until someone duly arrived to bolster and shore up her sagging resistance, in the form of a rebooted Routine and, of course, oodles of Reassurance. Sometimes, alas, the 'Fear' did get the better of her though, and she instinctively felt the need to pre-empt things; most often by initiating those well-established phone-calls to we offspring; and so often on the pretext (or perhaps genuine belief) that something, (for example, her TV, or maybe her heating), had gone 'on the blink'.

Following a recent spate of the latter calls, to my siblings, (sometimes one after the other), and still typical of the genre, came my log of the:

15th Sept. (Tues): "Yes, I too arrived to 'fear', & 'help me Keith'; even though T had only recently left. I think her Dementia [now] limits her memory, so that she quickly slips back into 'feeling alone'. Have taken latest A-care bill. Mum OK within 10 mins. Once someone's here with her, and offering a firm Reassuring 'line', she usually comes round. Soup & cake for dinner. Mum then fell asleep. Ps I think Mum may need a new downstairs front window – there's a touch of condensation between the glass – which Mum [keeps] trying to clean. She'll be ringing you! Short cemetery walk & drive round. Fish finger tea. Decent day, after poor start; especially as dog [still] limits our options. 7/10"

Inevitably, and on a 'life goes on' basis, real, time-consuming, everyday *practical* problems, both old and new, still continued to arise; both in Mum's life, and ours; and to impinge significantly on all our efforts to cope with the situation(s). For example, I was still dog-tied, and still trying to support my partner's physical needs, on the home front, as she attempted to walk herself back to some sort of 'hippy' normality, whilst my sister was trying to hold down her part-time dental-receptionist job, and support her partner in trying to find a new van. Then, in early September, and early on in Vol. 4, my brother's upsetting and out-of-the-blue log bluntly informed us that "Our dog has had a stroke. The vet said he has had a seizure of the nervous system to the brain [a bit like Mum with her Dementia}. His head is [now] listing to the left. [Any] recovery may take weeks".

Meanwhile, that onset of condensation between the glass panes of the double-glazing unit in Mum's front, downstairs, window (the one that she usually sat next to, in her favourite chair, and therefore looked through on a daily basis), began to cause her (and therefore us) some real, disproportionate, OCD, irritation. Unable to understand (between her ears), that the problem was *between* the panes, Mum began to regularly try and clean the said window, both inside and out, in a frustrated attempt to rid the window of its semi-permanent clarity 'disfigurement'. (The eventual solution, of course, was the fitting of a new unit; but that took a little time to organise).

So, the inaugural first entries into Vol. 4 were virtually indistinguishable from those at the end of Vol. 3, as we continued to manage and, as a matter of dated course, record, the steady and everyday flow of what, to most people, was such relative trivia. That is, there was little sign of positive change for Mum, or therefore for us, and just very similar 'loggings' from the 'off'.

17th Sept. (Thurs): "Arrived to 'fear' etc. No pills taken & WW3 because windows open & Mum said she was 'cold'. She [also] thinks her [cross and] chain is broken. She just hasn't got the hands to put it on anymore. Latest on [dog] – still not eating, but drinking. Head still to one side, but gets excited when we take him out. Slight improvement". (T).

20th Sept. (Sun): "Bad start. 'Fear' etc. Pills taken. 'Oh mi legs' has arisen again. [Dog still] a sorry sight at the moment. A bit like Mum". (T). "Called out at 4-45pm. 'No telly'. Arrived. Nothing wrong with telly. Just a ploy to get someone up. Maybe as last Sun, when L was called out. Annoying. Keith's turn [next] Sun". (T). Yet there was still the odd 'good' day.

24th Sept. (Thurs): AM - "Good start. No crying. Received phone call Wed @ 3-45pm. 'My telly is all green'. It was the rugby she had on! A fair morning". (T).

PM – "Mum best she's been for ages on arrival. No crying, and [stoically] saying, 'You've gotta keep trying'. Praised her positive attitude. Have taken A-Care bill. Soup. Relaxation Ex & nap. [Out] for local paper, then short cemetery walk. Put new artificial flowers on Dad's grave. Beans on toast. Good day, given [dog] restrictions. 8/10".

1st Oct. (Thurs): "Mum took ages to let me in. (On toilet). As there are keys in the door(s), we will not be able to get in if something happens. What is the answer? Anyhow, [Mum] not too bad. Pills taken. General conversation. Same old topics. All quiet of the western front.

Ps Spent most of the morning unblocking the Hoover.

Pps. Your soup has been warmed up 3 times since 11pm". (T).

Responding to my brother's morning log, and in trying to allay his reasonable worries in relation to any such 'key- bound' circumstance, I reminded him, in a postscript to that afternoon's brief log, thus:

"Mum OK again. (having a good spell for me). Soup warmed up a 4th time. Relaxation & nap. Cemetery walk, and drive. Beans on toast. Another good day. 8/10.

Ps If you push your key in [firmly] you can [eventually] push Mum's out the other side. However, that still leaves the problem of the chain. With the door [partially] open, on the chain, it might be possible to get a screwdriver and prise off the bracket on the door jamb".

Such were the many and varied, including emergency 'breaking and entering', possibilities that we had to prepare for in these uncertain days. My log was also intended as a subtle reminder to my brother that the 'same old topics' were almost an inevitability if you didn't succeed in distracting oneself *and* one's mother, whilst in-house, or, alternatively, by distracting Mum, by taking her *out* whenever possible. My log also provided a handy opportunity to remind *myself* that Mum was still *capable* of having 'better days', but it was soon 'business as usual'; especially when the routine was changed, and I was covering for my sister, as on;

5th Oct. (Mon): AM - "Extra", "Extra". "Arr. 10-20am. Mum crying, and 'full of fear'. Had gas bill & money out, but unable to 'sort it'. Confused & upset. Reassurance & cuppa solved the problem [once more]. Tablets not taken. Taken 10-45am. [Mum] took a while to get ready. Anxiety about going out. Lost confidence. Dep. 11-15. for Post office. Paid gas bill. Tesco for shopping. M&S for lunch. Treated us to some Percy Pigs on way out! (Yum). Home for 1-00pm. Dep 1-30 for Nursing Home No 2".

And then, later that same PM, a first minor instance of something we had all been half-expecting, and dreading, for ages.

"Responded to a phone call from Joan. Mum fell over in the backyard, noseying up by side of [old] coalhouse. Phone call to

Keith to put him in the picture. Stayed until 5-15pm, when I had to go and pick up dog. [Gave] her some tea. Which she ate. Mum not too bad on leaving". (T).

6th Oct. (Tues.): AM - "Arrived to WW3. As you will see, Keith, Mum has taken both bandages off her 2 cuts, and will not have any more put on. Advised her that her tights will stick to [the cut on] her leg, and she may have to go to clinic. All to no avail. I went to have a look between the [old] coal house and garage and there is every chance that she tripped over the [loose] bricks. At the moment things are normal, but there may be a reaction. She cannot remember the incident. Pills taken. Quite chatty. Same old topics. Challenging morning". (T).

PM – "Mum OK. Soup lunch. Mum unable to recall falling. Yes, both 'arm' & 'leg' cut were uncovered – but dry – and occasionally 'sore'. Checked her arms and hands. No obvious acute pain when I touched them, so nothing broken – but she was lucky! Need to keep an eye on her. Ask if any pain? Look for new bruising. [Usual Routine]. Fish finger tea. Can't complain really. 7/10".

13th Oct. (Tues): "Arrived to 'Oh, mi legs'. Pills taken. Mum's mind all over the place today. Fear etc. General chit-chat. The heating is a problem. Mum not putting it on. There was none on on Sun, and the cold weather has only just started. As I am writing this Mum has peed in the bowl and wet herself. Mum on the move most of the morning". (T).

Another intermittent aspect of our 'Mum management' that we particularly dreaded (for both her sake and ours) were those occasional, but obviously worrying, incidents that signalled a significant deterioration in her personal hygiene - and they had clearly *not* gone away; indeed there was the constant worry that their frequency might be increasing.

17th Oct. (Sat): "Arr. 11-50. Mum not bad. Usual anxieties. Put groceries [that I'd brought] away. Have taken latest A-Care bill. Soup. Dosette done. Clean round in bathroom, [after noting] some shit-stains on bath, rail and sink. Ps bought Mum a new toilet brush. Prescription due by Friday. [Usual Routine]. Baps for tea. Oi'll give it 7/10".

WHERE DID YOU GO TO, MY LOVELY? DEMENTIA DAYS

24th Oct. (Sat): "Arr. Noon. Mum started to cry. Soup. Brought tinned pudding. No dog today! 1st time since Aug. Mum OK with Reassurance. Dark nights won't help, but keep calm and carry on. Dosette done. Not sure paying window cleaner at his home will help. She may just think she 'owes' him if [he comes and] *she* doesn't pay. See how it goes. Relaxation Exercises + 30 mins sleep. Tesco. (Yes, Tesco, 'cos dog-less at last). Salmon butty tea. Not bad after early moans. Put all clocks back 1 hr. 8/10".

The clocks had gone back, the nights were 'drawing in', and our only new diversion of note was the late October arrival of an edge of town branch of 'value' supermarket Netto. (My logged 'opening' judgement being that it was "not bad for basics"). Then, with the new month of November came yet another potential problem.

3rd Nov. (Tues): "Not bad on arrival. Pills taken. Informed Mum that Joan was not coming again [ever]. Went with easy option and told her she had found another job. Anyway, Mum said she was not bothered, and she 'only sat there'. When A-care ring, I will inform them that we no longer need their services. Save us some money. See how it goes. I will make a phone call on Mon & Fri to compensate for Joan not coming. We can't do much more. Good morning.

Ps Window cleaner came. She offered him £3. I had to explain [new] payment method. Mum cried because she can't understand it". (T).

My initial response to the loss of Joan, after so many months, and after Mum had taken the time to get to know her, was that it definitely had the potential to cause 'trouble'. After listening to Mum, though, (typically, for example, my brother had logged that Mum had repeatedly said, "I don't need anybody"), and monitoring her reaction, we had decided not to put her through the potential trauma of having to try and remake a close relationship with any immediate replacement, and to see how things went. Obviously, that had 'implications'. It would mean that 'Joan's time' would once again have to be managed or covered by *us* in some way. That said, and despite a couple of early occasions where Mum did indeed ask, "Is Joan coming today?" she did not seem unduly phased by the practical loss of her carer's visits, or by our quietly-repeated explanation that Joan had simply left the job, and so we allowed our involvement with A-Care to just lapse naturally.

8th Nov. (Sun): "[Despite having done my standard Sunday morning visit], received 6 phone calls between 1-30 & 2-00pm. 'No telly'. 'Frightened', etc. Felt obliged to come up. Nothing wrong with telly. Mum said, 'Why have you come up?' Took a load of abuse. Said I was no use to her, and did not care. Left @ 3-00pm. Mum just sat in chair, no telly on". (T).

This was another good example of how Mum's mind could be fuddled by the Dementia; especially when left alone; and of how she might act instinctively, by taking up our oft-repeated offer to 'ring at any time' if she needed immediate help and support from us; and of how she might actually couch the problem in a very practical, more easily explained way, when, perhaps, she did not know how to express her true concern over what the hell was going on in her head at a particular time. It was also typical of how she might not even *remember* making each, or indeed any, in a *previous*, and often consecutive, number of calls on such occasions; and why, perhaps in sheer frustration, she might end up forcing an argument during some of them. In truth, even at this point, *we* still did not really understand how the Dementia actually did its' stuff, or what Mum was *actually* going through, or struggling with, mentally, on any of the occasions when it 'struck'; and, tired and under pressure, ourselves, we were well capable of responding with our own felt irritation, instead of with further gentle Reassurance, at being called out for a (practical) problem that appeared not to actually exist once we got there. A slightly different example of the sort of advancing confusion and 'forgetfulness' that we would often come across was logged by me on the:

14th Nov. (Sat): "A bit weepy on seeing me. Relief valve? Usual stuff about 'legs' etc. Otherwise OK. Soup + tinned rice pudd + cake. (Yum!). Dosette done. Prescription due by Friday! Relaxation Exercises & 35 mins nap. Tesco. [Pre] argument over tea towels. [It could just as easily have been about some other bog-standard in-house commodity]. Mum said, 'I've got plenty upstairs', when I [challenged] her over the one grotty tea towel she [keeps using]. Asked her to show me where 'spares' were. We looked high and low. None found. I said we were buying some at Tesco's. Argument actually re-surfaced IN Tesco's, but [I] stayed strong & won the day. They're in the bottom drawer near sink, if she hasn't moved them! Ham & cheese baps for tea. Given the dull, rainy afternoon it was, it's been hard work keeping her mood up, but the bright, Christmassy, lights of Tesco distracted her well, so still worth 7/10 in the circumstances". That's not to say the same *old* problems weren't still rife.

17th Nov. (Tues): "Mum OK, if 'moany'. (I take moany as standard these days). Soup. Tinned pudd - on a Tues. Tues. pills not taken. However, the Sat pills had disappeared, so she may well have taken [them]. I decided to transfer the Tues. pills to Sat. next, & let her go without today; 'cos she must have taken 2 lots somewhere between Sat. & Monday. Relaxation Exercises & 35 mins nap. [Sing], 'We've all been to Netto, we've all been to Netto, la laa la laa'. Fish steaks for tea. Can't complain. Be Positive! 8/10.

Ps late mini-argument over cooking tea. Mum took over an hour to do 'boil-in-the-bag' fish, insisting on ignoring the pack advice & doing it 'my way'. 'You're not bossing me, none of you'. Alright in the end, [but] you godda laugh".

19th Nov. (Thurs.): AM - "Not bad on arrival. Heat on, but windows [wide] open. Pills taken. Dulcet tones of 'Oh, mi legs' ringing in my ears. 'Have you taken paracetamol?', I asked. 'They are no bloody good', was the reply. [Otherwise] good morning". (T).

PM – "Mum OK. Usual moans. Soup. 'I don't moan', says Mum. U godda laugh. 'HA HA HA HAAA', I went [instinctively]. Mum saw the funny side and laughed too! Window cleaner came. Mum worked up 'cos she couldn't find £3. I sent her to ask, 'Has my daughter' paid u?'. Window cleaner went round front. Mum [again] said, 'I've no change to pay him'. I repeated that L had paid him. Slowly filtered through. U godda laugh! [Usual Routine]. Beans on toast for tea.

Ps Mum asking for olive oil. Should I give it to her? 7/10".

20th Nov. (Fri): "Dropped in. Mum watching TV. Came to door crying. No cardigan. No heat. Pan burning on stove with chicken burnt black. Threw it away. Mum cold. Bloody hell, Joan, come back!" (L).

22nd Nov. (Sun):

"4-45pm - [Despite having been up that morning], received numerous phone calls from Mum. On the last [one] she said she had no telly & no lights. Felt obliged to come up. Found Mum in kitchen. She had pulled the blind down, and was hysterical. Stood on chair to put [it] back and, in temper, [Mum] took a swing at me. Missed by a mile. Told me to get out. She had not switched lights on in any room. There was nothing wrong with anything [except] the blind. Mum tried to ring L, but to no avail. Eventually, she rang Keith, who would not come up. [I] relayed to him all that had happened. [He] had no answer [beyond] calm Reassurance. I cannot keep coming up on a Sun aft. I have a life & family. Mum eventually calmed down. I stayed until 6-30pm. Mum shut the telly off and said she was going to bed. Things don't get any easier. Keith said he would start coming on Sun aft. as well as Sat. I told him not to, as he too has a life, but he said she was always there for us when we were growing up. Don't know what the answer is". (T).

That was now typical of the sort of predicament that we found ourselves in on a regular basis - pills, bills, mending, shopping, personal hygiene and safety, cooking and heating, deteriorating physicality and accompanying chronic pain, home alone concerns, etc; and all underpinned, of course, by her 'fear' - essentially of the 'unknown', and generated by the damned Dementia.

As we approached the year end, then, we were all too aware of how Mum had been struggling with the kind of everyday domestic matters that were once 'second nature' to her; and of how she could quickly become drained, anxious and beset by that 'fear', during any extended periods alone; and of how little it was now taking to de-stabilise her - such as the window blind falling down - and to trigger panic attacks during what, for my poor Mum, must have been pretty scary episodes.

When these incidents repeated frequently, and over time, alas, *we* were prone to becoming drained by them, too; and the knock-on effect was to put *us* under pressure and to test both our individual patience and our emotional resilience; and, at those times, of course, there was plenty of potential for our own domestic relationships, plans and situations to be affected. As my brother had rather forlornly logged, on a couple of occasions when we'd found ourselves confronting such difficult, energy-sapping and unscheduled episodes, "Don't know what the answer is".

24ᵗʰ Nov. (Tues): AM – "Arrived to torrent of abuse. Mum was ready to go out. Started to cry. Told me to get out and never come again. Went with easy option. Sat in chair and wrote this. Did not speak for 15 mins. Eventually calmed down. Spoke about same old topics. I agree with L's point, that Mum is clever to a [manipulative] point. She will not have anyone from volunteer bureau, either. [L's suggestion]. She only wants us, but we all have lives outside. At the end of the day, it is mostly old age (89). Also there is a lot of boredom. As I am writing this, she has put 2 lots of Voltarol on in 15 mins. Challenged her about it. She said, 'This is my house and I will do what I want'.

Ps about 11-15 I felt the house going cold. Checked the rad, and Mum had turned it off. She must have done it when I went to the toilet. Going for a lie down". (T).

PM – "Spoke with T about all of the above, so arrived late. Mum struggling to light oven [with gas lighter]. Started crying with frustration. Luckily, I had a 'spare' [lighter] in the boot. (My boot is full of 'spares' – gas lighters, cans of soup, olive oil, plasters, batteries – all stuff I've arrived to find her short of in the past). Soup. Asked Mum how morning had gone. 'OK'. (No recollection of T's view of things). Soon calm with Reassurance. Relaxation Exercises & 40 mins nap. [Then] toileting time. Mum struggling to 'go'. Then weak, but 'went'. Reluctant to go out. Reassurance. Aldi. Fish fingers and peas for tea. A bit of a slog [today]. Dark nights don't help. Because she trots out the mantra 'I keep trying', still worth 7/10".

The dull, damp, autumn days of November, and, of course, the ever-darkening nights that now accompanied them, certainly didn't help us to cope with, or motivate, Mum. She still appeared to be stuck in a definite 'down' cycle, and to be functioning as poorly as at any time to date, and we were struggling to find many positives, or new 'avenues' to go down. My brother, in particular, (perhaps because of his lack of confidence about taking Mum out, and his effective 'self-confinement to barracks' when he visited), seemed to be taking the brunt of Mum's depressed and (so easily) disturbed state of mind just now; and to be encountering much of the attendant frustration being wrought on Mum by the Dementia. On the other hand, my sister had been keen to remind us about the significant 'pain' that she feared Mum was having to endure, and would regularly add suitable 'riders' for us in *her* logs around that time. They were obviously added to try and ensure that Mum did actually imbibe the appropriate dose of (paracetamol/ Solpadol) painkillers for her hip and legs, (as well her *long-established* prescription pills, of course), whilst applying the appropriate (Voltarol) cream to several arthritic finger joints; even though, or perhaps because, we had already met with instances of Mum taking too many of the former, and too often putting the latter on the wrong sore, when we weren't there to supervise. (Like the time she put the arthritic cream on a cold sore on her lip, for instance and it jolly well stung!). Yet, we felt that we had few choices but to remain vigilant, to continue doing our best, to live with some risk, and to just keep calm and 'chip away'.

Accordingly, and following Mum's recent rash of anxious phone-calls, regarding her apparently unruly telly, and its operation, I was positively euphoric when I thought that I'd found a potential solution to at least one problem. Through a diligent search of the internet, I had come across a 'new' TV remote. The maker was claiming that his device worked on any TV and had been 'purposely-designed' for the elderly, with fewer, and bigger, buttons. I was hopeful that my 'find' might help with Mum's increasingly arthritic fingers, and negate the increasing 'fiddliness' of her existing TV remote, and *its* rather small buttons; and, through its' introduction, of trying to counterbalance Mum's increasingly unscheduled calls to my siblings at inconvenient times. With a naive degree of optimism, I ordered one.

Yet, and despite my carefully constructed two-week 'training plan', and its patient introduction on the 26th, it was destined to remind us of just more wasted time, and of another good and well-intentioned attempt to solve a bothersome problem that floundered on the 'rocks' of the skulking Dementia; and on Mum's slowly declining cognition, and ability to deal with anything new or unfamiliar.

Typical of my logs, as I pressed on, (more in hope than expectation), was one that read, "Spent some time [tuning into, and] labelling BBC 1 & ITV1 on the new remote. Then tried Mum with it. She immediately started to talk 'fear' & started fretting. Too much too soon, so it's back in the box ['til next time]"; whilst, on a different occasion, my brother revealingly logged her telling him, "It's not for me. I can't think the same". (Once again, Mum had provided a telling insight into just how the Dementia was affecting her; not least by confirming that she actually *knew* she was losing her ability to rely on reason and to 'think straight'; and therefore to work things out on her own. Such insights made it hard *not* to sympathise the more with her feelings of 'fear', bless her. And I guess I was only kidding myself, anyway, in looking for some kind of simple and *practical* solution to what were essentially anxiety-based calls for help with far more complex *mental, emotional,* and essentially Dementia-lead *psychological* issues).

So, (and despite the new remote actually working OK), after trying to re- introduce my 'training' regime on a handful of occasions, with not a shred of a sign of any significant progress, it eventually went "back in the box" and stayed there - and the unscheduled phone calls carried on - as my brother, for example, logged, enlighteningly, on his visit of the:

6th Dec. (Sun): "3 phone calls [on Sat morning]. On each occasion she said, 'Just ringing to see if there is anyone there, in case something happens'. Keith, you need to liaise with L regarding Boxing Day cover".

So now it was time to turn our attentions to the emotions, practicalities, and planning that came with yet another *Christmas* approaching at speed. Always amongst the early Christmas traditions that (a compos mentis) Mum would ask me to help with, in late November, was the acquiring and then laying of wreaths on the graves of Dad, her mother, and that of one of her sister's who had no-one to tend it. Ordinarily, she liked them to be in place by the first week of December. However, such had been the creeping but perceptible deterioration in Mum's cognitive awareness, (and recent general morale), that she had taken no such initiative, or even made mention of the ritual, this year; and had I not taken the initiative *for* her, and brought wreaths with me on Sat. the 5th of Dec. I very much doubt whether she would have raised the matter herself this time around. Once reminded, though, she was both enthusiastic and grateful, and, keen to make up for her oversight, readily accompanied me to the cemetery that same afternoon, to lay the wreaths for yet another year.

Meanwhile, the usual plans to 'cover' Christmas for Mum were taking (a familiar) shape. The pattern of previous years was that I would cover/visit her for most of the day on Christmas Eve, Mum would spend the bulk of Christmas Day at my brother's, and my sister would usually take her out to eat somewhere with her family on Boxing Day. The only potential 'fly in the ointment' this year, was that Boxing Day fell on a Saturday, which was normally one of *my* main visiting days. The matter was easily resolved by agreeing that my sister stick to her usual Boxing Day 'gig'. And, of course, ordinary life went on regardless.

9th Dec. (Weds): Received phone call from L. Mum rang her at 10-30pm. She had obviously woken up and did not know what was happening. She asked L why she had woken up at that time. L talked to her, and told her to make a cup of tea, and that everything was OK, and [then] go back to bed. Stayed up 'til 12, but no further contact". (T).

My logged, and cautionary, comment of the following Thursday, was simply that, "I'm surprised Mum sleeps so well/ soundly @ night, and hasn't rung before. It's the future! We've been lucky".

11th Dec. (Fri): "Doc's [latest] tests show some slight less circulation on R side. Mainly arthritis. [Stressed] importance of pain relief". (L).

17th Dec. (Thurs): "Arr. 12-05. Decent start. Soup. 1 issue – smelled gas. 'Grill' knob turned on [but not lit]. Obviously turned it off. It's still a 'sight' issue. Can't think of an [easy] practical solution. [Usual Routine]. 8/10". And then it was here:

24th Dec. (Thurs. & Christmas Eve): "Arr. 11-35, damp & dirty with dog. At least the rain's stopped. Mum not bad considering she'd seen no-one today. 'Oh, mi legs'. Calm Reassurance. Soup, tinned rice pud + cake. Reminder to L – do dosette for week on Sat (Boxing Day), or Mum will have no pills to take! Hope to come up with Kate on Sunday for a couple of hours. 12-45pm – carol singing together (Away in a Manger, Holy Night, While Shepherds Watch). Yes, she did sing; couldn't shut her up once started. Relaxation Exercises & 30 mins. nap. Short cemetery walk, drive to Birds. Gave Mum her Xmas prezzies. Opened some, left some for tomorrow. Beans on toast tea. [Some anxiety]. She can't cope with change (of Routine), unless done with patience and Reassurance. OK day. Happy Christmas. 8/10".

25th Dec. (Fri and Christmas Day): "Not ready on arrival. Found decent clothes. No pills taken. No heat on. Got ready. Off we go. Anything can happen. Not bad, apart from Mum had accident. Piddled on hall floor as she went to toilet. Cried a little, as there were people in the house. Soon forgot about it. Ate soup, turkey dinner & trifle and later a cup of tea and mince pie. Brought her back at 5-30pm. Left her at 6pm, watching telly. Seemed OK". (T).

26th Dec. (Sat & Boxing Day): "Good meal at [local pub]. Sarah [grand-daughter] came up. Mum soon settled down, but tired. Pills done. Tiring Christmas". (L).

27th Dec. (Sun – 'Extra'): "Arr. 3-10pm with [my daughter] Kate, & dog. Short walk @ cemetery. Nice weather. Back for cheese on toast. No real problems. Dep. 6pm. I conclude – 'quite a successful Xmas' – to be repeated".

So another emotional and draining Christmas had been (relatively) successfully negotiated; and on we headed to another New Year.

New Year's Eve was a Thursday this time around, so I visited Mum as usual, with the dog, and followed the [Usual Routine].

There were no real issues, and the old year was ending on quite a reasonable note. It only remained for me to log, "Happy New Year", and see Mum off the bed but what would the New Year hold for us?

2016

With hindsight, we would remember 2016 as a year of major change for Mum; and change that, for me, spelled the 'beginning of the end' for her; but we entered the year still clinging to (false?) hope, even though, from Mum's longstanding myriad of problems, the pain in her [left] hip was first and fastest back to the fore.

1st Jan. (Fri. & New Year's Day): "No heat on. Pills taken. Mum's leg/hip giving pain. [Otherwise] not a bad morning". (T).

2nd Jan. (Sat): "Not a great start. Hip pain today + legs. Reassurance, but seemed more pained than usual. Still wouldn't let me make dinner. Yet, 'frightened something going to happen'. 'Oh, mi hip'. Soup. Pills not taken. Taken @ noon + Solpadol. [Somewhere along the line her usual *paracetamol* painkiller prescription had been replaced with this stronger, paracetamol + codeine, alternative]. Dosette done. Relaxation Exercises + 40 mins nap. Seemed to improve her mood. Tesco. Moaned a lot, but [kept saying] 'I keep trying', so hard to criticise. Salmon baps for tea. 7/10".

4th Jan. (Mon): "[Mum] won't wear warm jumper or gloves. Hip hurting. Bloody freezing in here. P/O & Tesco. Mum struggling with hip, so came home". (L).

For now, the hip pain seemed both chronic and consistent, regularly raising its 'head' in the presence of all 3 of we carers, (both at home, but especially abroad), and genuinely appearing to restrict Mum's mobility. We could only hope that this was to be temporary, and that perhaps the cold wintry weather was a key, (and therefore passing, arthritic), factor here; whilst just the routine arrival of the latest, if sizable, gas and electric bills, as well as the equally-sizable house insurance quote, plus the prospect of a couple of dates for standard health checks, somehow had the capacity to combine and 'sizably' raise her anxieties.

8th Jan. (Fri): "Usual aches and pains. Short trip to garden centre. Cold today. {Mum] couldn't walk far. Mum has 2 appointments - 1. Podiatry Clinic – [on Thurs. the 14th]. 2. Annual check-up at Doc's [on Mon. the 18th]. Will put on calendar". (L).

In the event, neither she nor we need have fretted here, as both appointments passed without real incident on their respective day. "Feet done for a few months. Keep an eye on plaster on leg", was all that my sister had logged following the Podiatry Clinic 'Gig'; whilst, "Doc's done. Everything OK", was her even more succinct, (and surely to be taken as relative rather than literal), input following the Annual Check-up at the GP's; before adding belatedly, "blood sugars a bit high".

Pre-Podiatry morning, however, one of my sister's logs must have asked if I too had noted Mum complaining of a lot more leg pain these days, when out and about, because my afternoon log *following* the podiatry visit included:

14th Jan. (Thurs): PM – "Arr. 12-05. Cleaned dog. All reasonably OK with Mum. For L, re Tesco. Yes, Mum *does* complain of leg pain! I get her to stand still & rest on trolley, 'til pain passes. Then I say, 'Would you like to sit in cafe, whilst I finish shopping'? She always says 'No, I'll carry on', so we carry on, & repeat as necessary. p s if I remember, I get her to take 1 or 2 Solpadol before setting out. Soup. [Usual Routine]. Beans on toast for tea. Decent day. 8/10".

On the month-end horizon now was Mum's 90th birthday. We had considered taking her out somewhere, but whenever we mentioned it, (from mid-month onwards), her consistent, and entirely predictable response to us all was that she didn't want to go out to eat, or indeed any fuss at all, and preferred to see it as, "just another day". So, we agreed to just visit her at home on the day, with our individually-chosen presents.

Meanwhile, the now 'standard' range of problems continued largely unabated. One in particular then suddenly returned to the 'front burner' as it were. Mum was suddenly back to her repeated (OCD) attempts to clean the condensation from inside the sealed unit of her double-glazed front room window, by continually trying to clean the *outside* faces. She just could not accept that it wouldn't 'go'. In the end, there *was* nothing for it but to have a new unit fitted; which, (eventually), we did. One practical problem down, umpteen still to tackle - and one that was far less easily solved was that of the ever-fading markings on her old oven. These, along with Mum's fading eyesight, still carried a risk of her turning on, or getting frustrated at trying to light, the wrong burner. Luckily, she'd used the same oven for so many years now that she could usually be relied upon to get it right through the 'auto-pilot' routine that she'd honed to perfection by 'custom and practice'; but it remained a potentially serious problem to which we had no easy answer beyond a new oven; which, (a) she still refused, and (b) would have presented its own potential 'learning' problems, lack of familiarity, and therefore risk, anyway. Effectively, then, we simply lived with the lesser and existing risk; and so on to Mum's 90th birthday, which actually fell on the Sunday; so I would be visiting 'back-to-back' *this* weekend.

30th Jan. (Sat, and day before her 90th birthday): "Arr. 11-55. Usual 'Oh, mi legs', and a bit of a cry, then, 'I don't know what I'm doing'. Usual Reassurance eventually brought her round. Soup + rice pudd. Nice roses L. Opened prezzies - new mat is by sink, and new cutlery is in kitchen drawer, ready for use. Relaxation Exercises & 35 mins nap. Tesco. Salmon baps for tea. All OK. 8/10".

31st Jan. (Sunday and Mum's 90th birthday): "OK on arrival, apart from no heat on. Your 2 cards were upstairs on bedding box, with [masking] tape round them. Brought them back down. [Gave Mum flowers]. Told Mum not to throw them away for at least a week. Just another day for Mum. 'Oh, mi legs' the only problem today. Not a bad 90th morning. (T).

"Called with Sarah [granddaughter] and cakes for Mum. T just left. A bit weepy". (L).

"Arr. 2-55pm. Mum half-asleep. Doors locked. Pushed her key out with mine and opened lock. Mum had been disturbed, and was disorientated. Distracted her with nice bowl of crocii [extra prezzie on the day], and resettled her with Relaxation Exercises + 40 mins nap. Whilst she was sleeping, found all birthday cards were [again] taped up & in stairs, ready for 'going up'. [Tellingly], Mum says they remind her she's 90, and she'd prefer not to be. I agreed she put them where *she* wants - upstairs [in drawer]. Soup for *tea* today. Can't complain (that's Mum's job). Happy Birthday @ 90, Mum. 8/10".

Somewhat eccentrically, Mum's latest Obsessive-Compulsive idiosyncrasy, (almost like a New Year's Resolution, and doing no obvious harm as far as we could see), was to 'dress' and compact anything 'loose' (say, paper, plastic, cardboard or cloth, but not tins, for example), with a tightly-bound band of masking tape before allowing said items to reach their 'dusty' end in the outside bin.

Anyway, we had all visited her on the day, albeit individually, for her 90th birthday, bringing presents that we'd thought appropriate. The day had duly passed without real incident, but, of course, the most telling action of the day had been that of Mum taping up the birthday cards we'd brought her as soon as she was left alone. Eventually, she'd confessed that seeing them on permanent display only reminded her, negatively, of just *how* old she was. Similar thoughts, (even allowing for her physical and mental limitations) had probably been behind her earlier reluctance to mark her special day with an outing or a nice meal celebration - and on we went. Alas, Mum had soon applied the same negative reasoning to some of her prezzies but my brother had failed to absorb the 'message', so I felt obliged to try and 'bat' for her once more.

2nd Feb. (Tues):

AM - "Usual things on arrival. No pills taken. Had words with Mum as to what she has done to the flowers I bought her. I pushed the boat out as it was her 90th. Very annoying. Limited chit-chat. Had better mornings". (T).

PM – "Arr. 12-05. Mum OK. Pea & Ham soup. Yum! For T, she is 90 you know! Don't expect gratitude. She's [often] a 'shell' now [thanks to the Dementia]. You will get [annoyed]. I know I do, but don't take any of it seriously/personally. The initiatives have to come from US. If you want interesting conversation YOU have to initiate it & don't expect grand responses. Repetition

helps + patience! Relaxation Exercises + 40 mins nap. Netto &
Aldi. Fish finger tea. (Used new forks!). 8/10".

Then, in the search for her valued quota of winter-sun, my
partner was off on the first of the new year's jollies, (I had long
since given up hope of going on foreign holidays myself, because
of my commitment to Mum, so my partner had taken to holidaying
with her friend), and a key 'fore- warning' in my log of the 13th of
Feb. read, "[Usual Routine]. Tesco. Biggish shop, 'cos have dog
for next two weeks"; with all the limitations on choices for
distracting Mum that that entailed, but we (dog and I) got off to a
reasonable start.

16th Feb. (Tues): "Sue left me (@5-15am) today, for Goa!
(Hurrah for freedom!). Means I have dog for 2 weeks. Nice walk
[with dog] round Reservoir this am. Lovely winter's day. Arr.
Mum's 12-03. OK. (Although I've put in her application for the
England Moaning Team again – I think she'll get an offer this
time!) Soup. Relaxation Exercises & 35 mins nap. Short cemetery
walk & drive round. Fish fingers & peas for tea. 8/10".

20th Feb. (Sat): "Arr. 11-45. Brought Mother's day card &
plant + bag of groceries. Mum OK [She was having a reasonable
'run']. No heat on in the kitchen – because she calls making me
soup 'cooking', [and thinks that's also warming the kitchen].
[Usual Routine]. I'll come up about 3pm tomorrow". However, it
seemed that the pressures were getting to me.

21st Feb. (Sun):AM – "Not Mother's Day. Mum banged her
leg. Stopped it bleeding. Not too much 'Oh mi legs' 2 day. Incident
free morning. Keith, Mother's day is Sun. 6th March! Fair
morning". (T).

PM – "Extra, Extra + dog day + 'Not Mother's Day' Day.
This morning someone left a telephone message trying to convince
me it WASN'T Mother's Day. How cruel. Anyway, I didn't [fall
for] the message, and came anyway. Happy Mother's Day, Mum.
Mum was OK. Short nap. No major issues. 7/10".

Yes, (and for reasons I couldn't explain), I'd got the wrong
Sunday, (by a fortnight!); but because I'd told Mum that I was
coming, I kept my promise. Sue was away anyway, and the dog
and I had no specific plans, so what better than to offer Mum

some extra Sunday company; but might the change of Routine have knock-on effects?

23rd Feb. (Tues):AM – "Mum must have waited for me coming. I got both barrels. 'Get out', 'Don't come again', etc. [She had been] ready for going out with L. Calmed down. Said she was sorry. Usual other things – No heat etc. Slightest thing got on her nerves this morning. 12 days to Mother's Day. Had better visits". (T).

PM – Arr. 12-10. Mum OK. Lovely day, if cold. Soup + cake+ Mum's crocuses are out – lovely. Full (if slow) cemetery walk [& occasional sit] - lovely crisp Feb. Day. Fish fingers & peas for tea. What more could you ask. 8/10".

3rd Mar. (Thurs): AM – "WW3 on arrival. Mum complaining of being cold, but no heat on in either room, & 2 windows open. Took flack. Brought Mum's bedding back. [T had found it damp and stained]. Mum said to stop taking it; she will do her own. After a bad start Mum calmed down". (T).

PM – "Dog day, without dog! Strange. [My partner had returned from her Goa 'gig']. Mum had pulled top kitchen drawer out & couldn't get it back. Took half hour to fix, so soup @ 12-40. Relaxation Exercises + 30 mins nap. Netto. Paid papers to 16th Apr. Beans on toast. 8/10".

5th Mar. (Sat): "Arr. 11- 55. Still a lot of snow [in village]. Mum quite good seeing she's seen no-one since Thurs. night. Heating on. Soup &rice pudd. Dosette done. Prescription due by Friday, the 11th. Relaxation Exercises + 35 mins nap. Tesco. Decent day. 8/10. Ps 'cos it really IS Mother's Day tomorrow, I've decided to pop up late afternoon, after I've had Sunday lunch with Sue".

6th Mar. (Sun. + Mother's Day): AM - "Good on arrival. Heat on. Pills taken. Brought biscuits & choco for M/Day. No incidents today. Reminded her Keith is coming at 3pm. ps L called in".(T).

PM – "Extra, Extra. Happy Mother's Day. Arr. 3-10pm. Cuppa. (Brought my present 2 full weeks ago! Although I brought her a new smelly thing today). Relaxation Exercises. Beans on toast tea. All OK".

8th Mar. (Tues): "Arr. 12-10. Door on chain. Mum a bit confused. Didn't know anyone was coming today. [Due to car trouble, T had not been able to make his usual Tues. AM visit]. Mum had had boiled ham butty for lunch already. Soup. Seen water bill. 'Oh, mi legs'. Oh, it does hurt'. 'They're getting worse'. So seen better starts. (I blame T for not getting bus up!). Anyway, soon OK [with Reassurance].

Ps if you ask Mum if both legs hurt, she nearly always says it's just the LEFT one so 'Oh mi legs' [may be] a bit of a habit in the plural. Relaxation Exercises + 30 mins nap. Aldi & drive round. Fish fingers & peas for tea. 8/10".

12ᵗʰ Mar. (Sat): "Arr. 11-50. Mum moany, but not bad. Soup. Dosette done. Notes for L.

1. Make sure you put scrip in case. Otherwise (like when T sent her to get black bag), she will see the packets, if she goes in the cupboard and ask questions!

2. No Solpadol with scrip, which is getting low. 1-00pm - Mum saying she couldn't 'go out' today, 'cos of leg pain. I said, 'OK, I'll go alone'. She said I didn't care about anyone except myself! Mum went in front room. I stayed in kitchen, drinking my tea. 10 mins later, Mum came back & said, 'I'll try'. (Potential argument managed). Relaxation Exercises & 35 mins nap. Tesco, & (briefly) cemetery. Not bad round Tesco, but [even the] short cemetery walk probably too much today. Salmon butties for tea. 7/10. Ps 6-30pm - Mum has a scabbed sore under her forearm. Doesn't remember how she got it. Only noticed it late on. Not immediate problem, but needs watching". The next problem to (disproportionately) tax us was Mum's kettle, a problem that had been 'brewing' for a while!

18ᵗʰ Mar. (Fri.): "6-45pm – Mum rang. Said she had no telly or lamps working. Arrived to no lamps or telly SWITCHED ON. Just a ploy to get me up here. Already had 5 phone calls between 1-00pm & 3-30pm. Asking where kettle was and fear factor". (T).

Mum's kettle had ceased to function. It was now a 'late' kettle. We suspected that it had 'given up the ghost' because Mum had been obsessively over-filling it to the very top, for even a single cuppa, 'in case it boiled dry'; only to then find she couldn't lift it. So my brother had brought her a 'spare' from home, (to use whilst I tried to source a brand new, slightly smaller, and therefore less heavy, replacement, to bring on the Saturday). Mum, alas, had refused his 'spare', so he had taken it back, and where the old kettle once stood was, currently, just an empty space.

19th Mar. (Sat): "Arr. 12-10. Mum not bad, given she'd seen no-one today; but briefly got worse (raised anxiety) when I [produced] new kettle. Showed Mum how to use it. Firstly, not happy with lid. (Not a flip-up, but can be filled via spout). Secondly, [still] insisted on filling it to max; then still too heavy. Long argument about filling it to '3 cups' mark. [max]. Will she remember? Eventually used it OK & made [cuppa]. Dosette done. Note for T – maybe called you out 'cos raised anxiety with *no* kettle. [Usual Routine]. Tesco. Salmon sarnies. 7/10".

Alas, my 'kettle training' worked little better than my 'new remote training'. Despite my regular reminders about only filling it to the '3-cup' mark, Mum had quickly reverted to her obsessive 'over-filling' of the *new* (if a tad lighter) kettle, when left unsupervised. Even so, I felt that I had a foothold, and, like a dog with a bone, continued to see it as something to 'chew over' with her.

Then, in the blink of an eye it was Easter, but we didn't do anything special to mark the occasion. Once again, Mum didn't want to, so we simply carried on 'as normal'.

With commercial outlets open as usual, my sister kept her (Good) Friday visit of the 25th to her usual trips to the usual shops. Similarly, on the Saturday, *I* kept to my 'Usual Routine'; whilst taking every opportunity to repeat my ongoing, but still largely ineffective, advice on not overfilling the new kettle. My brother, too, held fast to his usual Sunday, home-based, visit on Easter Day; the one obvious common factor, (and echoing down our respective visits), being, 'Oh, mi legs', as the chronic pain seemed unwilling to relent even for Easter. Then, slow-forward to post-Easter 'normality'.

5th Apr. (Tues): "Arr. 12-10. Mum OK, [but] 'Oh, mi legs'. Asked if she had pain in both legs. She said, 'Yes'. Unusual; she usually says it's only the left leg. Asked if she had pain anywhere else. She said, 'No'. So no pain under breast. Soup. Search for Sunday paper - found in bin, and taped up. Relaxation Exercises + 40 mins nap. Netto & Aldi + roadside stop to see new-born lambs [in field] - aaah. Fish finger tea. Ps No Solpadol left & prescription due! All OK today. 8/10".

On the previous day, (the 4th), Mum had mentioned to my sister that she had a slight pain under her left breast. My sister had logged this accordingly. Thankfully, though, Mum did not mention it at all during my visit of the 5th, nor later, so, hopefully, it had been some sort of temporary and passing indigestion-like issue, and nothing serious.

On the next day's (*Wednesday*), outing, my sister had arranged to call at my brother's house to drop off some gardening materials, and, of course, had taken Mum with her. My brother's log of the day after, (Thurs.), noted, "Mum remembered coming round with L yesterday"; confirming once again that, on most occasions, Mum's mind wasn't so much forgetting everything, but more likely finding that her thoughts (like the 'musical notes' in the now infamous comic sketch from the 1971 Morecambe & Wise Christmas Show with Andre Previn), were just not *necessarily*, 'in the right order'!

Alas, part of my brother's log of Sunday the 10th of April had reminded us of yet another awkward and embarrassing problem that hadn't gone away... that of Mum's increasingly-occurring blips in her personal hygiene, when he logged, "Took Mum's bed-sheet. It was soiled. Oh, dear. Put clean one on".

Chronic problems seemed to be everywhere just now, for Mum; not least because of the mobility issues stemming from those various leg-based pains.

16th Apr. (Sat): "Arr. 11-45. Mum OK, apart from usual moans. No heat on. Soup. Dosette done. Relaxation Exercises + 30 mins nap+ [more] moans. Tesco. Half way round, Mum complained of leg pain. I suggested she sit in the car. Usually it's a bluff, & she carries on. Today she agreed to sit in the car &

I finished doing the shopping on my own. On way home went to cemetery to see if she could manage short walk to Dad's grave. She did it, but more stopping and moaning. Generally, her moaning is constant at present. Is another visit to Doc's appropriate? (Ps she'd had 2 Solpadol before going to Tesco). Chicken muffins for tea. (Pps I've seen a fold-up wheelchair on-line for £99.99). 7/10".

Mum's chronic leg and hip pain had been pretty unrelenting in recent days/weeks, (in fact since the turn of the year), and the Solpadol pain-killers, prescribed to reduce it, currently seemed relatively ineffective, and to be offering little release from the pains whenever she was out and trying to remain mobile for any length of time. So, for the first time ever, and as a sign of the times and direction we seemed to be heading in, I had actually taken to looking on-line at *wheelchairs*. (Of course, *looking* was one thing, but we all knew that getting a proud Mum to actually consider *using* one would be a pretty herculean task!). Moreover, on this occasion, and in a rather ironic role-reversal, neither of my siblings felt there was any real benefit in re-consulting a GP who had simply put Mum's pain down to 'old age' on previous occasions, and prescribed nothing more than the existing painkillers; not that Mum was asking for, or would even agree to, such a re-referral. Indeed, when my brother 'chanced his arm', and put the option to her on his visit of the 17th of April, he was soon fobbed off, and logged, "I again received a load of abuse. [Mum] saying she only went last week". (Which, of course, wasn't true).

In consequence, his parting shot that day, was a cautionary log that included, "on your own heads be it if you mention the w/ chair"; my sister concurring wholeheartedly with that sentiment in her log of the following day, with, "wheelchair – no chance"

19th Apr. (Tues): "Arr. 12-10. Soup & rice pudd (on a Tuesday). Mum OK [beyond] 'Oh, mi legs' – mainly *left* one. Can we get stronger painkillers? Is physio out of the question? Any other 'aids'? Relaxation Exercises & 35 mins nap. Paid papers 'til 28th of May. Netto. Short cemetery walk. [Bit of a struggle]. Lovely day weatherwise. Shepherd's Pie tea. 7/10".

21st. Apr. (Thurs): "Arr. 12-10. Glass everywhere. Mum had minor bleed from 'nick'. She had dropped a glass. It was all over the cooker hob, kitchen top, and kitchen floor. Mum was busy cleaning it up. [Usual Routine]. (Ps Mum had no memory of breaking the glass later)".

And so we came to the end of Vol.4.

My brother had brought that volume to an end in pretty much the same vein as he had started it, back on the 13 of September 2015, with a fairly modest, nondescript, now almost predictable, log.

28th Apr. (2016 – Thurs.): AM - "No heat on arrival. Windows open. 'Oh, mi legs' ringing in my ears. [Otherwise] no incidents this morning. Last entry for me in this book. Not a bad morning". (T).

Vol. 5

And once again, the *new* 'diary' (to no-one's surprise) was characterised by much the same sort of *early* entries as characterised the *final* entries of the *old* one, (a bit like the arrival of a birthday that actually feels little different from the day before), and it was *I* who made the first foray there - and hot on the heels of my brother's closing contribution to Vol. 4.

28th Apr. (Thurs.): PM – "Arr. 12-10. [With dog]. Mum OK. Usual moans. Soup & Rice pudd. Mini-argument about overfilling kettle (again). Called me 'Bossy' & 'Only for yourself'. [Usual Routine]. 8/10".

Yes, the new 'diary' had qualified for a relatively mundane, and uncontroversial first log' - but *this* 'diary', alas, (like Schubert's 8th) would eventually recall a 'symphony' that was destined to remain unfinished, and the last of its line, because things would take a significant 'turn for the worse' long before its pages could be fully filled. In truth, I guess the signs were already there, and had been so for some time. Ironically, however, it would be the steady but continuous deterioration in her basic physicality (particularly through the pain in her legs) that would finally 'tip the balance', and move Mum beyond the 'point of no return', and on to an irretrievable change of circumstances. For now though, on we went.

30th Apr. Sat): "Arr. 11-50. Mum very upset, shivering & crying. She was not sure why. She thought the heating was off, but it was on. [Plenty of] Reassurance over 10-20 mins brought her round. It's when something /anything goes wrong (or appears to) that Mum gets anxious/frightened. This causes tension all over [leading to] tiredness, further leg pain etc. When Routine is disrupted [it leads to] confusion 'cos of memory loss. Doesn't then know what to do/how to respond [leading to] anxiety, panic attack – [which I think] was happening when I arrived. All settled again [for now].

Soup. Rice pudd. Mum calming down. Dosette done. Prescription due by Fri. Relaxation Exercises + 35 mins nap. Tesco. I introduced her to a Tesco wheelchair at the entrance. Invited her to sit in it. She declined!, and then 'managed'. Salmon baps for tea. 7/10 'cos of 'dodgy beginning".'

2nd May (Mon): "Good start didn't last long [once] she started walking. Managed to cash point & Aldi. Had some dinner. Didn't stay out long though. Wet through". (L).

3rd May (Tues): "Arrived to find Mum trying to wash sheet, (full of sh-t) & crying because of what she had done. Took sheet to wash. No heat. Cold house. Windows open. No pills taken. Probably all to do with the sheet problem. Anyway, after bad start, no other incidents to report. Mum's belt broke on Hoover. She said carpet in hall got caught in it. I will have to buy new belt". (T).

5th May. (Thurs): "No probs on arrival. Only 'Oh, mi legs'. Brought [washed] sheet & Hoover back (repaired). Said I would Hoover up. Mum said, 'I've done it'. I said, 'Funny, you've had no Hoover for 2 days'. No reply. No incidents today. Had walk in backyard". (T).

14th May. (Sat): "Arr. 11-50. Poor start. 'Not well'; 'Frightened'; 'Legs won't go'. Asked Mum to sit down, & advised I could do *everything*. Mum insisted on carrying on. Made soup/ pudd etc. I [still] think she gets 'down' when left alone for too long. 3Rs employed. Kept calm. [Mum] slowly came round. Relaxation Exercises (cut short when Mum fell asleep). Tesco. Salmon butties for tea. OK day. 8/10".

The week beginning Mon. the *23rd* already held the unappetising prospect of another potential challenge (or two) for the 'remainers'; for that was the day when my sister was scheduled to head off on her latest 'restorative' break; but that 'prospect' was thrown into somewhat sharper relief when an early indication of the *possibilities* arrived within hours of my latest post.

Following his usual Sunday visit of the 15th, my brother logged, "She panicked when I explained that L was not coming [tomorrow either, due to a work-related 'training day'], and that I [will be the one] covering the Monday; but having a rest Tues. morning. Mum complained of bad eyesight in both eyes today & [of pain in] legs". (T). So, when the next day dawned:

16th May. (Mon): "Mum ready to go out [with L] on arrival. Explained why I was here [on a Monday]. Had conversation regarding 'a Home', w/chair, stick. Mum looking for a row. I explained she was 90, and her whole body was 90. [Had] put soup out for dinner on Sun and rest in fridge in a bowl. It was not there Mon morning. Did she eat it or throw it away? We will never know". (T).

19th May. (Thurs): "Arr. 12-15. [With dog]. Brought Mum new planter; its outside with others. [In keeping with recent days], Mum pretty 'negative' again. Focus on 'Oh, mi legs'. Asked if both legs hurt – once again only left leg – hip & lower leg. Soup. [Usual Routine]. Beans on toast tea. Plenty of moans & I was going to give her 6/10, but because she joined in singing '1 man went to mow' after tea, oi'll give her 7/10".

20th May. (Fri): "Mum a bit down. Keeps asking about my hols & who's taking her to the P/O. Think it might be a struggle next week. Sarah [coming] 10-30 on Mon". (L).

Once again, there were signs that both Mum's memory and her cognition *were* still capable of working well enough on lots of occasions. Firstly, for example, she had been able to tell me, (and consistent with the last time I enquired), just where the worst of her leg pain was centred. Secondly, she had done well to remember, and indeed had enjoyed singing, most of the words to '1 man went to mow'; and thirdly, the news that my sister was due to go on holiday had clearly stuck somewhere in Mum's brain; if only in relation to the practical consequences for her with regard to their weekly trip to the Post Office, in order to attend to that week's monetary needs. And yet, that chronic leg pain, and the (more solitary) moments when the Dementia kicked in, and confusion reigned, (and she *knew* it), more or less guaranteed that her mood remained generally 'in the doldrums', and extraordinarily hard to shift.

My current 'bottom line' was that I was very wary of a break in Routine, (this one stemming from my sister's jollies), having the potential to add to our week's management issues, but cometh the moment:

23rd May. (Mon): "Hello, it's Sarah! Took Grandma for pension to Post Office. Complained of pain to legs. Went [Garden Centre] for lunch. She had cheese and ham toastie, and shared Victoria Sponge. Not one complaint of any pain while we were there. All in all a v. good day".

Late in the day, my sister had arranged for her adult daughter, (and one of Mum's much-loved grand-daughters) to 'step into the breach' on the first day of her holiday absence. And to our surprise, the (Mon)day had gone really well. Having a familiar and trusted 'replacement' visitor from within the extended family appeared to have provided the ideal, one-off, antidote and distraction. It was certainly interesting to note Sarah's brief but pertinent log, telling of Mum eating well, and of not complaining of *any* leg pain whilst they were at the garden centre; which tended to support my brother's view that Mum did sometimes use the leg-pain claim to garner additional attention. Anyway, well done, Sarah. Alas, it was 'business as usual' by the following day.

24th May. (Tues): AM – "Arrived to Mum's leg bleeding. Scab knocked off. Put plaster on. Washed tights – full of blood. 'Oh, mi legs'. Keeps asking where L is. Explained, but still kept asking. Asked Mum if she wanted ride to Post Office. The answer was, 'No, I can't walk far'. Went on my own. A better morning". (T).

26th May. (Thurs.): "Arr. 11-25 – [with dog] - early 'cos no T. Mum not too bad. Usual leg moans of course. Soup. Relaxation Exercises + 30 mins. nap. Went for [local] paper then cemetery for short walk; but Mum no sooner set off than saying leg pain too much. Put her back in car & walked dog. Drive to 'Birds'. No sooner got there than Mum said 'I feel sick'. Came back. Cuppa improved things a bit; but now saying 'I'm frightened' by [her various] complaints. Reassurance. Slow going but still Mum would not sit still. Insisted on making brew, then mopping kitchen floor after tiny dog spill [of water]. Beans on toast tea; but a hard shift. I do think Mum needs to see GP soon – both for continuing/ worsening leg pains – where she sometimes cannot complete even short walks, [but] also for 'feel sick' moans – which are becoming more frequent too. 7/10 'cos Mum joined in our 5pm communal reprise of '1 man went to mow'.

Ps 6-15 cry of 'Oh, it does hurt' & said leg felt 'numb'. Gentle massage & paracetamol seemed to help. Was up & about again by 6-45, definitely need updated view of GP, I think".

Not that I knew it at the time, (indeed, like everyone else involved, and at every stage, my intentions were ever good), but the die was now cast and, for my sins, initially by *me*, for it was I who was first to 'blink', and to trumpet the latest need to involve the GP again. Fate was about to step in. As 'Health-Matters-Manager-in-Chief', my sister had read my log, and, crucially, had heeded my call.

28th May. (Sat): AM - "Called for brew. Mum OK. Made appt. for Thurs. for eyes – but she said they don't bother her. Made Doc's appt. for Mon 6th June, 'cos not emergency. Says she doesn't want to go – we'll see". (L).

PM – "Arr. 11-50; 'cos expected Mum to have been alone. Turned out L had been! Have noted Doc's appt. – if only to Reassure both Mum and US that things are much the same - or are they? Soup & Rice pudd. Dosette done. Prescription due by Friday. Relaxation Exercises + 35 mins nap. Tesco. No sooner entered store than, 'Oh, God, Keith, mi legs". I noticed a Tesco wheelchair & took her over, & got her to sit in it! [When] I began to 'wheel' her she insisted on getting out! Oddly, she barely moaned going round. Home for salmon baps. I'm going to give her 8/10 'cos she did try".

A decisive, but almost 'throw-away' update in my sister's otherwise insignificant log of Mon the 30th read, "Think I will keep [next] Mon. appt at Doc's. [Even though Mum's first reaction, as usual when it came to the 'crunch', was to avoid it]. Can always ask for another Doppler Test".

So, the fateful appointment with the GP for the 6th was still set to go ahead. Indeed, at this point, Mum's continued, arguably worsening, mobility difficulties suggested it was the logical, and therefore right, course of action; but had we known where it would lead, would we still have kept the appointment?

1st Jun. (Weds): "[Mum] tired today. Tesco, but couldn't walk, so back to car. Cafe for dinner. Prescription ordered. Eyes tomorrow. Doc's and hair on Mon." (L).

My sister's positive log of the 2nd, and following the day's appointment at the optician's, read simply, "All OK with eyes. No change". So, in theory, that just left us with what we assumed would be yet another pretty unproductive trip to the Doc's, and just more painkillers, on the 6th but, Oh, No! Yet, and despite particularly chronic and persistent lower leg and (left) hip pain on the day, my *next* log gave not the slightest indication of what was about to unfold; or even that anything might change; let alone that this log would be the last one for fully 2 *weeks*.

4th Jun. (Sat): "Standard moans [on arrival]. Told Mum to tell GP on Monday! She said I didn't care. [Now eternally regretful, I then logged], There's only so much care you can supply to incessant, 'Oh, mi legs'; although hip again giving pain today. Soup & rice pudd. Relaxation Exercises & nap. Not completed due to [ongoing] leg pain. Gave her 2 Solpadol, & @ 2-45 we managed to get ready and go out. Drove to cemetery 'circle'. Got Mum and dog out, but Mum had barely taken half-a-dozen steps before, 'Oh, mi leg does hurt' rang out. Sat on bench for 10 mins. She then decided to try again, despite my suggestion to sit in car. Managed to reach Dad's grave, [via] 3 different benches. Same on way back. Drive round. Back home for salmon butties. Hard slog today. [Leg pain] does seem to be getting worse, & her walking getting less. Will be helpful to know GP's latest thinking. 7/10 for trying today".

In fact, and to the shock of us all, on the day of the appointment, (the 6th), the GP of the day got it into his head, and on the very flimsiest of evidence, that Mum's worsening hip pain may well be the result of a fall; and perhaps of something having *broken*. So he took the (arguably) life-changing and totally unexpected decision to contact the hospital, and to then send Mum directly home to await an ambulance that (along with my sister) would take her there, to be seen in A & E! Sadly, events would then conspire to ensure that she would not leave the place for 2 *whole weeks* - and even then, and even more sadly, she would emerge much the 'worse for wear', and for its' supposed care!

I am convinced to this day that this (essentially *first*) lengthy hospitalisation, coming at this late stage in her life, (at 90, it was probably the first time in her life that she'd been away from her own home for so long *on her own*), was far more traumatic than we thought possible in such a supposedly 'safe place'; and that the medics involved hadn't made sufficient allowances for someone they knew had been diagnosed with significant Dementia. Just having to *leave* her own home, (and at such short notice), would probably have been traumatic enough, after so many years, in *any* circumstances, for such an elderly, homespun Mum; but having to do so with the added burden of both her chronic physical limitations and the Dementia, and for the clinical, unfamiliar, impersonal 'illness' setting of a hospital *medical* ward, almost certainly lead to her further mental deterioration - and to the fact that she was never really settled, or the same, again.

At this point let me refer you back to Chapter 4, a. 'The Medics & The Hospital' when, towards the end of her fortnight's stay, Mum, and we, had been visited bedside by a social worker, to agree a statutorily-required Discharge Plan. That Plan was essentially for Mum to return to her own home, with her newly prescribed, morphine-based, pain-killer 'patches', and with our ongoing close support, of course, but now with some additional practical 'aids', (for the 'short term', Mum had eventually been persuaded to accept the social worker's recommendation of a bed-pull, walking frame, and that long-overdue commode), and with a few weeks of half-hour visits at 4pm on each Weds & Fri, from a local social services 'carer', supposedly to help and support her 'rehabilitation'. In addition, and at our specific request, the social worker had also agreed to at least *look into* the potentially attractive 'possibility' of a referral to the 'very busy' physiotherapy department but, in truth, we held no great expectations here.

Anyway, the social worker was required to see Mum one last time, before discharge, to ascertain that Mum still 'fitted' the Plan, and vice versa, and thereafter to officially ratify it. This eventually took place early on the mid-summer morning of the 21st of June, and Mum was deemed 'ready for discharge'. I was then contacted by the Ward Sister, and I arranged to collect Mum later that same morning.

The next (and lengthy) log to appear in this (final) 'diary', then, *followed* Mum's eventual discharge from the hospital, and her uneasy return to her own home. *Prior* to her return, and in line with the Discharge Plan, a walking frame, and a bed-pull 'fitting' that was there to limit the chances of her falling out of bed, had been pre-delivered and put in place in-house, as agreed, by the local social services; with a commode to follow.

21st Jun. (Tues): "Longest Day, after longest 2 weeks [I can remember!]. Nothing about Mum's hospital stay has run smoothly; but the K-Bee [me] is logging on. 'The Eagle has landed' – Mum is Home. Collected Mum about 11-40am & drove her home. Collected 'chippy' dinner en route. Followed by long sleep(s). Sometimes Mum doesn't even remember the hospital stay, even now @ 2-30pm; though both 'Fear' & 'Oh mi legs' have [re] appeared. Things to watch: -

1. The 'wearing down' of the patch.
2. The subduing (tranquilising) effects of the Morphine. [In the patch].
3. The right time to change the patch. (She may be in more pain towards the end of the 7 days).

T/c to T. He will collect 'overdue' medication [from hospital] about 6-30pm, & retain it 'til Thurs. [By way of early 'rehabilitation'], decided to try Mum in cemetery. Walked from 'circle' to Dad's grave & back. Nice to be out. [Despite 'patch'], plenty of 'Oh, mi

263

legs' with regard to (vascular) lower leg pain; but, and encouragingly, not much moan about Hip – morphine-based patch working on hip? Soup tea. 1st moans about walking frame. Mum not happy. Quickly insisted on it going in back bedroom – never to be used again! Opportunity to show her bed 'fitting'. Not happy. Told her it had to stay, 'cos fitted by social services. I think she might get used to that & it might be useful to lean on. Then she [got upset] 'cos clothes everywhere & neither she nor I knew where they properly went. 'You're no good to me', she said.

For L, some are in the bedding box & some are in bag in back [bed] room. I'm just too knackered to [think] where they go. She's still a bit disorientated. A tough & tiring 1st day for us both; but I'm hopeful she can get near to where she was with the help of the '3Rs' (Routine; Reassurance; Repetition). [Ready for bed. Saw her off to sleep]. Told her several times of tomorrow's visitors".

Looking back, I probably should've stayed over that first night, but I was 'out on my feet' myself by then, and in desperate need of a good night's sleep in my own bed. (It had been the 'longest day' in more ways than one!). So, once I'd seen her comfortably re-installed back in her home, and then safely tucked up in *her* own bed and off to sleep, I unthinkingly assumed she'd be fine until one of my siblings arrived early next morning; and, in the sense that nothing untoward happened to her, physically, she obviously did cope; but probably not so well in terms of her mental and emotional re-settlement and security.

22nd Jun. (Wed): [Mum] not happy. Cried all morning. Half undressed. Got her ready to go out. Wouldn't go. Made dinner. Peeped in house. Mum cleaning & straightening cushions. No problem. 2 paracetamol given. Turns out she doesn't want people looking at her". (L).

23rd Jun. (Thurs):

AM - "No tears on arrival, but plenty of moans. Mostly hip & legs. Had to take bathroom mats away. Full of sh-t. Could not be cleaned. Put down 2 sub mats until we can get another set. Had a short nap. Cannot remember being in hospital. [I] will not mention it again. Put all clothes in w/robe & drawers. Not a bad morning". (T).

PM – "Arr. 11-40 to support T. Not really needed. Useful update. T left. Stuck up some 'prompters' on kitchen [cupboard] doors. [To remind her of what went where]. Chit-chat. 'Oh, mi legs'. (Can't see point of using patches if they don't help). Relaxation – only able to practice slow, deep breathing; as leg pain (hip) too recurrent for exercises. Nap. 3pm – with lots of coaxing, I persuaded her to come to cemetery. However, she was back to normal on walk, and unable to take more than a few steps. 'Oh, it does hurt'. (Left her in car & walked dog).

Either (a) The existing 'patch' is 'spent' or (b) The 'patch' isn't providing the necessary relief. Big disappointment if latter. Let's struggle thro' to Monday & see if new patch provides some relief. It may provide stronger side-effects like sleepiness, dizziness, confusion. Have put up basic labels on kitchen cupboards. Beans on toast tea. Ps She never used the 'frame' all day. Hard to score today, because lots of moaning (with pain) offset by 'I keep trying', so 7/10".

As primary carers, we found it, by parts, both exasperating and annoying, (not to mention a little scary) to be facing the likelihood that Mum (and her Dementia) had spent 2 difficult and restrictive weeks in the foreign environment of a hospital medical ward, in order to supposedly undergo 'tests' to determine the most appropriate pain relief for her leg problems, only to find that the prescribed new pain relief seemed NOT TO BE WORKING! Indeed, Mum seemed to have, arguably, *less* mobility than *before* she underwent her disorientating hospital ordeal - perhaps due to muscle loss, following so much bed-bound inactivity. Moreover, (and despite her already limited recollection of ever having *been* in hospital), she also seemed to have been discharged from the place with both her 'fear' AND the Dementia further augmented!

What a well-intended, but totally unnecessary, disruptive, frustrating, and most-of-all unproductive, farce it all now seemed. We were not very amused! Yet we had no option but to go on. My sister's next day visiting did nothing to change that perspective, as Mum struggled both to walk far or to rid herself of the 'fear' that appeared to have 'upped its game' in her life. My sister had mentioned chasing up the physio, but, beyond that possibility, and now feeling totally impotent to affect the situation in any truly significant manner, we simply 'dug in', and struggled on.

25th Jun. (Sat): "Arr. 11-20. Door unlocked. Mum sat in chair. Soup on hob, but not lit. Mum cried on seeing me, & immediately began 'Oh, mi leg'. Asked where it hurt. She cited both hip AND lower leg. Gave her 2 paracetamol from new medication pack. (They're no stronger than Tesco). Also gave usual Sat. tablets, 'cos hadn't taken them. Soup & rice pudd. T rang for update. 10 mins later, L rang for update. No indication of Physio having been. Relaxation period. No exercises, due to leg pain. Nap. Dosette done. 3-15 – Took some motivating, but, with a couple of paracetamol, I persuaded Mum to come on *drive* to Tesco. Once there, she insisted on 'trying'. With my regular nod to the Tesco wheelchair [as an option] Mum struggled round; stopping, and whinging, a lot. But, to be fair, she struggled round. Well done, Mum.

At home, I set about making salmon butties, but she insisted on finishing them. [Psychologically], nearer to normal today. Good effort to deal with Tesco. We put out tomorrow's knickers & tights + her nightdress in bedroom [before I left]. 7/10".

26th Jun. (Sun): "Surprisingly, no phone calls & not too bad on arrival; apart from leg pain. I found Mum just that bit better in her mind. Good conversation this morning. She was asking questions. Seems to be using stick on occasions. Must be in a lot of pain from the leg. Brave woman. Reminded her I would [now] call [i.e. ring] between 4 -4-30pm. Made Mum 2 sarnies. At least she is having something. Never be 100%, but it's encouraging. Mum had same skirt on since she came home". (T).

Equally encouraging, and in spite of all the upheaval, and of the apparent ineffectiveness of the newly-prescribed morphine-based 'patches', and therefore of the ongoing 'double-barrelled' leg pain when mobile, was that all 3 of us had commented on the 'silver lining' of Mum tending towards a return to something near pre-hospital 'normality' in our latest couple of logs. Could it so? Could it continue? Moreover, the 'patch's' first week was now up, and a brand new Monday 'replacement' was due. Would the 'full-strength' effect of a 'fresh' one offer any better pain relief than the week-old one? Like the residents of the small Derbyshire village of that name, we could but live in *hope*.

27th Jun. (Mon): "Well, not a bad day. P/Office & hairdresser's. Yes, tears & pain, but had worse! Patch changed. Physio coming Tues. between 12 &-1-00pm – Don't interfere! P s Gas left on! (L).

My sister's 'don't interfere' note was intended specifically for me, wearing my 'social worker hat'; as, in that guise particularly, I did have a tendency to ask more searching questions.

28th Jun. (Tues): "Arr. 11-20. Door unlocked. Mum in chair. As usual, a little weepy on arrival, before responding to Reassurance. Soup. Noon - Nazir, the physio arrived. Commode coming to try... [Mum eventually] accepted the bed-pull & walking frame, so let's try commode. [Alas], Physio said he was unable to help with any physio for arthritic hip OR vascular lower leg pain. He only does physio on muscle/ joints. Offered other 'aids' (perching stool), but [Mum] only accepted commode [for bedroom]. Otherwise, as Mum said afterwards, 'waste of time'! He suggested we contact the GP about the ongoing pain. [He] did recommend exercise where possible. Not too many [noticeable] side-effects from patch. 1-00pm – Relaxation Exercises (not leg ones) & 45 mins nap with only the odd pain – so some relief whilst asleep.

Finally motivated her to do drive to Netto. Once there, she insisted on 'trying' – tho' it was a slog & took forever. Fish finger tea. But for the leg pain, it would have been a decent day. Still worth 7/10, 'cos a good day mood-wise. 5-30pm. Sarah arrived with commode. We unpacked it, and placed it in bedroom; & Mum 'tested' it. Will see how it goes".

Once again, our faint hopes of some really useful input from either the clinical medical, or the usual associated, professionals had been 'professionally' snuffed out; for once again (this time in terms of the 'physio'), we (Mum) had 'drawn a blank'. It just seemed to be one dead-end disappointment after another.

Not surprisingly then, the main theme of my sister's next day 'shift', and log, was the all-too-familiar, "Managed [Garden Centre] for dinner. Very limited mobility now".

As I said, besides the bed-pull, the walking frame, and the commode, another key element of the approved Discharge Plan had been the Social Services' offer to have one of their 'carers' visit Mum twice-weekly, (we had agreed on the Weds & Fri), for half an hour at 4-00pm (prompt, so that Mum could be told exactly what time to expect them), for a few weeks, to help with her 'rehabilitation'; that is, to help with practical tasks like making her something to eat or washing. Ever-desperate for *any* additional support by now, though, (practical or otherwise), we had persuaded Mum to accept those visits; not because Mum actually needed *too* much help with such basic tasks, but, rather more opportunistically, for the potential psychological benefit of having someone 'nursey' fill a little more of her 'lone' time, and provide a little 'extra' *social* company, by simply calling in to see her, and being there; and the first Wednesday was upon us; but, as in most of our involvements with the public 'services', in this increasingly desperate Dementia saga, we were not off to an ideal start.

30th Jun. (Thurs.): AM – "Not too bad on arrival. Usual moans. Pills for Fri. But none there for Sat. May have taken double. Also, note time of Carer last night (18-15). Not what was agreed. [Usual] leg pain. Lots of good chat. All-in-all, Mum seems to be getting better in her mind". (T).

2nd Jul. (Sat): AM - "Called for brew. Mum a mess, pain etc. Gave paracetamol. When the carers are here, she puts on an 'I'm OK' show". (L).

PM – "Arr. 11-20. Usual brief weep & 'Oh, I'm glad to see you'. Noted L been too. Interestingly, hip 'alright' on arrival, but lower leg 'jumping'.

Friday Carers ['log' shows they] arrived 5pm – including Carer Manager. Mum appears OK with them. It's when alone she gets most anxious/confused. Soup + rice pudd. Brief Relaxation Exercises, but Mum quickly fell asleep. 45 mins nap. Talked her into 'trying' Tesco. Hard work, 'cos of 'Oh, mi legs' & 'I'm frightened'; even when I was with her. Could it be side-effect as morphine enters her bloodstream? Feeling dizzy, sick, dry mouth & feeling confused being some that [are mentioned]. She deserves credit for handling them in her situation. Salmon sarnies for tea. 7/10".

4th Jul. (Mon): "Usual stuff. P.O. & Garden Centre. Little mobility & fear. Patch changed. Am speaking with GP for a ref. for wheelchair. We need it – if not now in near future. Bad day Sun. with phone calls". (L).

5th Jul. (Tues): "Arr. 11-30. by arrg't with T; to discuss 'suspending' carers. Mum keen for this to happen & one carer had been told not to come by her. T/c to Pat C [Carer manager]. Explained lack of Routine of Carers [was leading to] anxiety/ confusion. We agreed to 'suspend' the Carers from today; for 1 week in the 1st instance. Agreed to ring Pat same time next week; & perhaps have meeting on alternatives; if any.

[Due to attendance at a friend's wedding on Sat afternoon] hope to come up for 2 hours on Sat morning; and then on Sunday from 3 to 7.

1-00pm. – T/c from SW. Ran thro' the 'suspension plan' once more. Agreed to ring her next week. Relaxation Exercises (tho' not legs) & 40 min. nap. Netto. Hard slog again! Wheelchair definitely needed. Fish finger tea. 7/10".

The next few days were little different. Hard work, and underpinned by Mum's daily struggle with both her Dementia limitations and her physical leg pains when walking any distance; but now, at least, without the unsettling effects of the erratic visits and timings of the (clearly over -loaded, would-be 'Rehabilitation') Carers from the Local Authority.

And despite the prescribed use of the morphine-based 'patches', it was still hard to see any tangible benefit from *their* use to date; as the chronic double-barrelled leg pain, whenever Mum tried to get mobile for any length of time, just seemed to carry on regardless. It was also hard to know if Mum was being affected by any of the potential side-effects that the 'patch' *literature* made mention of; either solely or in combination with the already inconsistent imbibing of her long-established, and any supplementary, medication. For sure, since her discharge, (and despite her continued lack of mention or recall of the ordeal), being 'frightened' certainly seemed to have made its way back to the top of Mum's agenda; and to be exerting its influence on a daily basis.

Perhaps a little prematurely, though, (in his search for the most likely cause of so many of Mum's most recent, anxiety-induced, out-of-hours, telephone calls), my brother's log of the 7th included, "Mentioned w/chair. Mind working o/time. Will be interesting. No t/calls for 2 days. Missed them - NOT! Looks like it was the thought of the carers coming".

Meanwhile, 'behind the scenes', as it were, Mum's increasingly limited *outdoor* mobility had forced further discussion about *wheelchairs* to the top of *our* current domestic and management agenda. How to acquire a suitable 'rig', and, (far more tricky), how to introduce one to Mum without 'getting our heads bitten off', were now amongst our most pressing issues.

The obvious first 'port of call' here, of course, was the local social services. Having recently provided us with those other practical 'aids', (albeit as part of Mum's statutory hospital Discharge Plan), logic suggested that we make our initial enquiries there. So, my sister obtained the necessary form from the GP's surgery, and we made our application. Alas, it was an option that was doomed to fail and we met with a pretty 'short shrift' rebuttal. The very strict criteria for successful '*free*-wheeling' with the social services required that the applicant should be in more or less *permanent dependency* on the thing; both outside the home and IN it; and because Mum was still living, and moving, relatively independently in the *home* setting, her application for provision from the *public* purse was speedily dismissed.

If we wanted a wheelchair, WE would have to source, and pay for, one privately. So I was soon back searching the internet.

9th Jul. (Sat): "Arr. 9-55am. Mum not bad. Usual moans. [Despite 8 early-morning T/cs to T!]. Lower leg causing [most] pain. Hip 'not too bad'.

'Carers Plan' [already suspended] arrived. Shows no carer due 'til Weds. 13th. I'll ring [SW] to cancel altogether on Tues.

Do we want a meeting?

Do we want info on Volunteer Service?

Do we want anything else? Contact for Care UK, say, for future? I expect to be here Sunday, 3-15 to 7pm".

10th Jul. (Sun): AM – "Not in best of moods on arrival. 'Oh mi legs'. Mum only wants to see our 3 faces and no-one else. I wouldn't have anyone else coming. We have tried it in the past, to no avail. Mum agitated about w/chair. Does not want one. Said she would try and walk. Question after question about w/chair. May give us problems. Reminded her Keith was coming at 3pm. I may get phone calls. He is out of Routine.

Ps Changed sheet on bed – stained.

Pps Mum has been wearing the same 3 items of clothing since Tuesday". (T).

PM – "Extra, Extra. Arr. 3pm. Door unlocked. Mum in chair. 'Oh, Keith, please help me'. [Anxiety] Soon passed with firm Reassurance. Brought groceries. Put away together. Cuppa. Having read your notes – unless I hear differently: -

1. I'll ring [SW] @ Tues. @ noon & cancel 'carers' permanently.
2. I will not seek meeting unless U2 feel differently.
3. I will ask for info to be sent to us, re a. Volunteer Service; b. Care UK; c. Any other options. 4-30pm Corned beef & tomato butties".

12th Jul. (Tues): AM – "Mum sat in kitchen crying on arrival. 'Oh, mi legs'. Soon passed when someone here. First question: 'When's the w/chair coming'? It continued all morning. No phone calls since Sunday night. Mum got same clothes on for last few days. No washing done. Sh-t all over bathroom & banister rail. [Cleaned]. Brought clean sheet back. No pills for Sat." (T).

PM – "Arr. 12-05 with Kate. [My daughter; Mum's grand-daughter]. Mum recognised her straight away. Useful 'distraction'. 12-15 - T/c to [SW]. Message left cancelling carers. T/c to [Carer Manager]. Message left cancelling carers. Soup. Mentioned to Mum that she was wearing same clothes again. She said she changes her 'pants'; but other clothes are OK! Replaced Sat. pills in dosette. Relaxation + 40 mins nap (including Kate). Tesco – and wheeled Mum round in a Tesco WHEELCHAIR! Much easier. Further T/c to [Carer Manager]. Spoke to her directly. Carers cancelled. No reply from [SW]. Will e-mail tomorrow. Kate made cheese on toast for our tea. 7/10. If it wasn't for the perpetual 'Oh, mi legs' (except when asleep, sat, or being pushed round Tesco) I'd have given 8".

The latest (this time LA) carers were no more. Mum's case would once again be closed to social services; and once again we felt that we'd 'drawn a blank' from 'official channels'; and effectively been left to fend for ourselves. It was all rather dispiriting and depressing but Mum needed us more than ever, so it simply *had* to be 'business as usual' and on we went.

16th Jul. (Sat): "Arr. 11-45. Mum OK. Soup & cake. [Seen] 'wheelchair letter'. Not surprised. Only those wheelchair-*bound* likely to fulfil criteria in current financial climate. Appeal unlikely to win. I suggest we buy our own - AND Mum is willing to TRY one! Relaxation & 30 min. nap. Tesco. Mum in wheelchair again, but his time with special trolley attached. Better for Mum and pusher. Salmon butty tea. T/c from L. Explained T/c with T.

Plan - Keith will order [agreed] wheelchair tomorrow, from Amazon UK @ £99.99. Delivered to T's. Oi'll give [Mum] 8/10 - for coping with Tesco wheelchair set-up".

The wheelchair was duly ordered online.

19th Jul. (Tues): "Mum OK. Soup. Relaxation & 40 min. nap. Short cemetery walk. (1st time for ages; needed us to move 'in stages', between benches, to Dad's grave & back). Fish finger tea. 5pm – T/c from T. Wheelchair has arrived. (Only ordered Sat night). T will bring it up Thurs. I will try it round Tesco. 5-15pm Mum is currently out back, bent over & weeding. Leg pain?? 7/10".

21st Jul. (Thurs): AM- "Arrived to blood & shit everywhere (esp. B/room). Changed Mum's clothes, sheet; hands full of shit & blood. Looked like a slaughterhouse. Mum had cut on right hand. The shit must have come out in sympathy. Eventually got cleaned up. Mum not impressed with wheelchair. Got agitated. Eventually took [it] upstairs. Left near rad. Took sheet & her clothes for washing. Mum, unusually, had nap. Had better mornings". (T).

PM – "Arr. [without dog on a Thurs.] 11-45. Early, to check use of wheelchair before T left. Looks great. Got Mum to sit in it for wheel round kitchen but she said she wouldn't use it. T told me of cut to back of hand. (Now scabbed) & of blood & shit everywhere. T left. Cleaned kitchen floor with mop & floor cleaner. Cleaned stair banister and bathroom paintwork. Soup. Relaxation + 40 min. nap. [Have put] wheelchair Instruction Book & Spanner in letter rack. Tesco. Used new wheelchair!! I pronounce it a (relative) success. Easy to use & push - including with Tesco 'disabled' trolley. Final clean with Tesco's upholstery & carpet cleaner – relative success here too!

Ps Plus point – wheelchair does just fit in my boot with shelf removed.

Pps Caught Mum peeing in [and missing] bowl in kitchen and wiping it up with old cloth!! Spoke firmly to her about hygiene; then rang physios to request 2nd commode. [Coming tomorrow]. It's clear Mum [often] can't get, or can't be bothered getting, upstairs to loo! So 2nd commode can go [in kitchen] where frame was; frame in back bedroom, and wheelchair 'fits' in hall, by telephone table. T/c to L to update".

What a day that turned out to be! Mum had somehow managed to cut her hand, which must have been bleeding significantly, whilst she was in the bathroom attending to her 'ablutions'. In the process of trying to 'manage' two pressing matters at once, she had presumably decided to make her way downstairs for some reason and had thus managed to trail elements of both blood and shit onto anything she touched as she descended. Not that she could now recall, nor therefore confirm or deny, *anything* of what had *actually* gone on, so it was all something of a 'best guess'! That said, my brother's analogy with the 'slaughterhouse' was perhaps a bit OTT. The incident was still a 'relative rarity', (although a worrying one), and I felt sure that a second (*downstairs*) commode was the obvious way to avoid any repetition of such incidents. Moreover, an explanatory phone call to the physios had brought an empathetic response and a prompt, *next day*, delivery that meant things were soon back to something that passed for 'normality' these days.

23rd Jul. (Sat): "Arr. 11-35. Mum not bad. 2nd commode still in place. No sign of usage yet. Soup. Rice pudd. Dosette done. Relaxation Exercises +35 min. nap. Managed Mum, dog and wheelchair on inaugural cemetery tour! Hard work & military-style organisation required. Wheelchair pronounced 'success'. Salmon butty tea. Decent day. 8/10.Ps Mum used commode as chair, just to sit on, on 2 occasions".

My sister also found few problems with Mum on her following Monday 'gig', and had positively trialled Mum's new 'means of transport', logging, "Yippee for wheelchair, so much better".

26th Jul. (Tues): "Arr. 12-05. Mum OK. 1st job – change Mum's 'patch', (L forgot to do it yesterday), but there was no patch to change. [Either] it must have come off [or Mum *took* it off]. Soup. Relaxation + 35 min. nap. Then, a strange, short cemetery walk. Mum wanted to try & walk. Picture this: Mum on right handle, & pushing empty wheelchair, & me on left [one], with dog to my left & 'the invisible man' in the wheelchair! Mum walked to Dad's grave & back without ever getting in wheelchair. Weird. Fish finger tea. 7/10".

28th Jul. (Thurs): "Mum crying with hip & leg pain on arrival. Soon settled. Mum will not accept her age, and her body is knackered. Mum asking why she has got the patch on. 'To ease the pain in your back'. She said she sometimes takes it off". (T). My suspicions about her taking the patch off herself had been confirmed.

Next up, our Carer's Routine again came under threat, when my sister's log of Fri. the 29th included, "In future I will be working Fridays, so can't keep to the calendar, as I have to work to pay the bills. Will keep you posted". At least my usual Saturday visit was just that - usual; with (thankfully) nothing untoward to report or 'carry over', because my brother was away on the Sunday, and I was also providing *that* afternoon's cover.

31st Jul. (Sun): AM- "Crying with back pain. Seem to be going backwards. Patch changed [early] for pain relief. Managed trip to M&S. Couldn't walk. Came back. [She] went to wee in bowl. Little row. Asked her to use commode". (L).

PM – "Arr. 3-45. Usual weepy start, & 'legs', 'get frightened'. Reassurance worked. (Most pain in lower leg – patch mainly for hip). Soup for tea. Lots of moaning today. [Disrupted Routine?]. 7/10".

2nd Aug. (Tues): "Called out at 6-50am. Mum said house on fire. In fact, just burnt toast, so smoke detector gone off. Fireman Sam (me) got it all under control. Stayed 'til 7-30. Mum said, 'You can go now'. Back at 10am [for standard visit]. Mum never mentioned the incident all morning. Neither did I. No mention of hip or legs. Offered to take Mum out in wheelchair. WW3 broke out. Typical morning". (T).

As luck would have it, I'd bumped into my brother *en route* to Mum's, when our paths crossed as *he* headed home from his 'standard' morning shift. So, I'd already been party to a quick, cross-vehicle, update, and had arrived *expecting* the strong smell of burnt toast. Accordingly, I simply took the opportunity to release another discrete blast of air spray, when the moment presented itself, made no mention of the incident at all to Mum, and instead, just cracked on with our soup lunch and the Usual Routine; including a pretty successful 'roll' round Aldi in the new wheelchair.

My brother's *log*-of-the-day, however, had gone on to re-raise the dual matters of Mum not changing her clothes as often as he thought she should, and his perceived main-involvement with the laundering of her stained sheets; with the 'hard-done-to' implication that he alone had these matters in hand.

Of course, he did not; though he did seem to be arriving just in time to 'draw the short straw' on stained sheets on recent occasions; and, in consequence, he was *logging it more*. Living more locally than I, he was better placed for dealing with these necessarily 'quick-turn- around' laundry issues, anyway, and I had logged *that* point; and the fact that I had dealt with other issues; such as taking Mum shopping. That said, his logs did serve to remind me how easily perspectives could differ, and tensions and resentments still take hold and fester; and thus raise potential 'management 'issues'; and how open communication and a considerate sharing of views was ever vital between we carers. And the point took on a keen sense of good timing, (as if we didn't have enough to contend with already), when the need to cooperate in finding a quick solution to another pressing and practical household problem cropped up. Mum's cold water kitchen tap had suddenly, if intermittently, begun to lose pressure again. It was not, of course, something that we could 'sweep under the carpet' (to mix metaphors), as she drew on it umpteen times every single day. Indeed, *she* had expressed both her anxieties and her very understandable practical concerns about the situation on a number of occasions already. So a nagging sense of culpability and accountability, on this *and* the matters raised in my brother's log, bade me try to address and press my perspective once again in my *next* log.

6ᵗʰ Aug. (Sat): "Arr. 11-35 – early, 'cos L away, and [conscious of] tap problem. [Immediately] squeezed a little WD40 on tap. It began to work better. Needs replacing asap. It's unreliable. Can we identify someone. I'd have a go myself, but being 17 miles away, I need to be certain of completing it. Dosette done. Told Mum she [should be] changing her clothes more. (I would take stuff home, but I'm 17 miles away, and if I forget it, I can't just 'nip back'). Also, I'm here 22 hours per week [+travel time], & already working my sox off with Mum + shopping [for her] in my [days off]. All without a break so you'll understand if I don't seek extra tasks. Relaxation Exercises + 30 mins nap. 2-30 Tap problem again! Mum quite agitated. Managed to get her out to Tesco, where she soon forgot about tap. Also went to Wickes – bought similar taps to Mum's. Came home & tried to undo existing cold tap but couldn't get leverage. Professional urgently needed. Salmon baps for tea. Mum [still] agitated over tap [pressure]. Can only go 6/10 today, 'cos Mum had poor day (& therefore so did I for 7 hours)".

Of course, the dodgy tap *was* professionally replaced, (by one of the bright new shiny ones we'd obtained from the DIY store), within just a couple of days; but it served as another timely reminder of just how easily an everyday practical disruption to Mum's settled Routine could send a swift and significant 'ripple effect' through so many of the other problems inherent within her increasingly difficult, Dementia-damaged, predicament; and of how it might trigger, or add to, the existing and taxing tensions, pressures and anxieties that now pervaded so many days for both she and we - but on we had to go.

8th Aug. (Mon): "Usual moans. Patches are not staying on. [Could be her talc]. If we can keep checking it daily. May have to move to lower back. Mum weeing in bowl! I said to use commode. She said she hasn't got one – this is a chair". (L).

And on we went but, both mentally, (the Dementia), and physically, (the almost constant leg pain was now beginning to affect even *home* mobility), the signs were increasingly worrying.

For example, in my sister's 'clutching at straws' log of the 14th, she wondered, "Is it worth increasing the dose of morphine, 'cos she's having paracetamol as well", whilst elsewhere:

16th Aug. (Tues): AM – "Took an age to get in. Mum asleep in chair. Had to knock on window. Could hear her coming, saying, 'Oh, mi legs'. Had a joke, saying we'd have it put on her headstone. Old age has now taken over [what] any pills can do, no matter what strength. Offered to go [for walk] in the Merc. (w/chair), but she said no". (T).

PM – "Arr. 12-00. Mum moany. Not sure how to reduce pain if patch not helping – medical problem – see GP again? Soup & rice pudd. Relaxation & 30 min nap. Argument with Mum when I caught her peeing in bowl. Got a bit heated. Mum told me to 'Go', rather than accept that peeing in bowl was wrong. Calmed it down. Aldi & cemetery for 'roll round'. Cottage pie tea. 7/10".

Mum's 'standards' had definitely been slipping down the 'hygiene scale' in recent days/weeks; and more often. Her leg pain alone seemed to have dampened her enthusiasm for either changing her clothes *or* washing too regularly; and to have persuaded her that climbing the stairs too often should also be avoided whenever expedient; not just for washing, but, we suspected, even for sleeping, (as her bed had seemed remarkably pristine/undisturbed on a couple of recent occasions). Of course, the Dementia offered a handy source of collusion here, in helping her to quickly forget/ deny both the pristine standards of the past, (and thus accept/ignore the more unsophisticated, *slipping ones,* of recent days), *and* where she had perhaps chosen to spend the night sometimes, i.e. asleep in her downstairs armchair. Disappointingly, the recent arrival of the commode(s) hadn't particularly done much to alleviate either problem; with a *lack* of 'evidence of use' suggesting that *constipation* might once again be a force to be reckoned with. Potentially, we were heading into yet more 'unchartered waters', and to even *more* potentially dangerous 'depths'; but still we had no easy alternatives to just carrying on.

18th Aug. (Thurs.): "Usual moans on arrival, but not bad. Put piece of fluff in [downstairs] commode on Tues. Still there today, [so not been used]; also Mum still has same clothes on again. Brought back clean bedding & towel. Not a bad morning". (T).

To which I had added, in my otherwise 'Usual Routine', (dog-day Thurs.) *afternoon* 'shift', and log, of that day, "Not easy to have a fresh conversation these days – since [her] memory recalls so little [at least with any reliable accuracy]".

19th Aug. (Fri): "Usual fears. Tesco & cafe. She doesn't seem to be eating much. Maybe something to watch. Tired today". (L).

As it was turning out, the hygiene and sleep issues were far from the end of our problems; for not only were we having to accept that *they* had taken a 'turn for the worse', but Mum's appetite was also now threatening to lose what was left of its 'edge'. So now we feared that some sort of *eating disorder* might become the next significant issue to demand our urgent consideration and, of course, close supervision.

"What next?", I found myself wondering rhetorically, to myself, most days. As rhetoric, my 'wonderings' were destined to remain unanswered, of course; but had they *not* been, they would have told me that matters were about to 'come to a head'. That's what!... and, initially, *because of* that loss of eating 'edge' - and therefore weight. In fact, Mum's days in her own home were now 'numbered'. She was about to undergo another unplanned, initially déjà vu, but this time permanent, 'no-going -back', departure from her age-old domestic 'comfort-zone' - and from her beloved *home*. For the moment though, but only for a couple more days, she *remained* there, and on we (still) willingly went.

21st Aug. (Sun): "Not good on arrival. Mum seemed very down. Complaining of hip & back pain. Certainly going thinner. Piece of fluff still in commode. Proves she's not using it. Put heat on in living room. She said she was cold. Kept trying to be sick, but nothing happened. Slept on & off. Gave her some warm water. Seemed to settle the sickness" (T).

22ⁿᵈ Aug. (Mon): "Called out 8-40am. Mum seemed to have got up late, therefore mind all over the place. Phoned [siblings]. Left messages. L arrived 10-30am. Mum refused breakfast. Only [had] cup of tea. Calmed down, but kept feeling sick & leg hurting". (T).

Rightly concerned by Mum's *general* decline, the specific issues of recent days, and her particular worry about Mum's appetite (on the day in question, of late, and now taking into account the lack of evidence of any 'bowel movement'), my worried sister came to the view that Mum should again be seen by the GP as a matter of urgency; and, with the full backing of my brother, sought the earliest possible appointment. Indeed, after describing Mum's symptoms at length, and expressing her concerns over the phone, my sister actually managed to secure Mum an appointment at the end of *that* morning's surgery - and, from that came the decisive, *'same-day-return-to-hospital'* outcome that is detailed elsewhere. Ironically, and after 4 long-years-worth of scribblings that had become almost 'second nature' in our lives, our daily 'loggings', and the 'days of the diary' in general, were even more 'numbered' than my poor Mum's.

There would be but *one* final entry, following her latest hospital discharge - just 3 days later; and, as fate would have me collecting her from there for a second time, that would fall to me.

25ᵗʰ Aug. (Thurs): "Arr. Hospital 11-30am. Unable to find spare wheelchair. Reception sent me to other end of building. Arr. Bay 5 @ 11-45. Mum ready, but not medication! Complained to nurse. She sent for Dr. S; who had promised me medication would be there @ 11-30, so she went herself; [but returned *still* 1 item short]. (Clopidogrel 'cleared' for use).

[Finally] left hospital with Mum 12-20. Home @ 12-40. I made soup, which she ate slowly with slice of bread. T/c to T to advise we're home. T/c to L – message left. Relaxation time + nap. Checked Medication – seems to be a 4-week renewal of [existing] medication + Movicol [laxative for chronic constipation] + paracetamol + New Medication (Lansoprazole) – for inflammation of Oesophagus. [Ulcer]. Removed 'old' tablets from dosette - so just Fri & Sat left. Relaxation & long nap. Mum was 'well away', when L arrived. Mum proved difficult to wake. Indeed, we thought she might *not* at one stage! However, as L left, [some 40 mins later] Mum was awake, and agreed to go to [local mini-mart] for basics. We 'rolled round' OK. Back home L returned, and was here 'til 6-00pm. Mum slept a lot. Helped her get ready for bed".

All was far from perfect, though.

Firstly, and once again, on Mum's latest 'Fred Karno' discharge from the hospital, the prescribed medication had been promised 'on time', but then *hadn't* been so; resulting in the needless and unhelpful 'on-ward' hold-up that we encountered. (That, as I say, is detailed elsewhere). Of course, this had resulted in a significant degree of raised anxiety for Mum and frustration for us both.

Secondly, Mum still seemed really tired and lacking in energy, and certainly didn't seem to be in the *very best* of 'nick', but on the hospital 'say-so', I was more than happy to get her out of that dispiriting 'sickness' setting, and to try and get her resettled in her own home - and hopefully back to something that approached a 'normal Routine' as soon as possible.

Thirdly, despite Mum having been on her dose of Clopidogrel for what seemed like forever, Mum's long-standing hospital records apparently still noted that she had previously shown at least one allergic reaction to this drug! This imprecise, presumably out-of-date, information had obviously remained on her records, and been transferred, unchecked, willy-nilly, and as a matter of routine, to appear in the notes on her latest bed chart; where *I* had stumbled across it during a recent visit. I had, of course, raised this surprising inconsistency with the medical staff at the earliest opportunity, and after supposedly looking into the matter their learned physician had apparently pronounced it safe for her to continue to take.

Finally, I had received no advice at all on how I might best find support, or 'manage' Mum, after her discharge here; nor on how best to get her to take her latest supplementary medication (including the new Lansoprazole for a newly-forming stomach ulcer that was said to be the likely cause of Mum's recent bouts of 'retching' and loss of appetite), alongside her existing stuff; whilst any formal 'Discharge Plan' seemed to have been conveniently dispensed with altogether this time around.

I was worried. Of course I was. Who wouldn't be? But alas, my worries had no time to take root - for Mum was back as an in-patient in less than 24 hours! Once again, with hindsight, I probably should've stayed over with Mum on that first night back at home, (it may have been the difference between her remaining in her own home, or not, and, in that crucial sense, between life and death), but once she was 'well away' in her own bed, and with my sister having made her second 'flying visit', and then departed promising to be back there 'first thing', I had again taken the tired and poorly considered decision to head for my own much-needed good night's sleep, in *my* own bed.

Regardless, there would be no more 'loggings' after that of the 25th of August 2016. The diaries were effectively 'done and dusted'. History. They had served their purpose, and would, henceforth, be 'surplus to requirements', and confined to posterity, because...

Mum would never again live in her own home.

CHAPTER 6

(Care) Home From Home.

So, Mum would not be returning directly to her own home this time; indeed, it was considered by most of those involved, (including, as I say, hospital *medical and social worker* opinion, and that of both my siblings), that the Dementia had worsened significantly during the weeks that she'd been away from (the familiarity and Routine of) her own home, and that there was the real likelihood that, given her current level of functioning, she might *never again be* fit enough, either physically or mentally, to return there 'under her own steam'. I remained alone in not giving up hope entirely on that option for her, (not least because, throughout all the hospital visiting, she had *never* failed to recognise, or interact with, the three of us), but at least in the short term, I had been outvoted, and it had been decided that her immediate needs would be best met by her being 'looked after' in a care/residential setting. And in pursuit of that eventual 'ideal', it seemed that Mum was to be left, languishing unnecessarily, (not on a Dementia-friendly, but), on the (general medical) ward, and in the hospital, and without need or therefore plans for any further 'treatment', for some time yet, pending the pressing *identification* of a Care Home vacancy. (*Any* Care Home vacancy!). In the common parlance of the time, she was 'bed-blocking'.

It was still early September (2016), and just 2 days after the house-meeting of the 6th, with the hospital social worker, he had rung my sister to give her advance notice of just the "possibility" of an upcoming, luckily local, care-placement vacancy. Ironically, it was within just a few hundred yards of my sister's own home; and she was therefore quick to call round to make contact and view the set-up. It traded under the pleasant-enough name of Maple Mount. (For legal compliance, neither the home's name nor any subsequent use of the names of its residents and/or staff are *real* names).

She had been well received there, liked what she saw, and was then keen for my brother and I to see it as soon as possible, and to claim the available place, before it was lost. Geographically, it was just a mile and a half or so from Mum's *own* home, so in an area that she knew quite well, (and equally handy, of course, for 're-introductions', if a return home became a viable option at any point), and, as I say, barely 300 yards from my sister's home; and but a mile or so from my brother's. Logistically, it seemed as good as we could have possibly hoped for, or were likely to get; but could it provide the right type and quality of care that would suit Mum? My sister's first impressions had most certainly persuaded her so.

Both my siblings still tended towards 'wearing those rose-tinted spectacles', of course, and, as I say, remained hopeful that Mum could enjoy many more years of fruitful life, being lovingly 'looked after', by devoted carers, (with one of the 3 of us continuing to visit her daily, and, hopefully, able to take her out), whilst living amongst people with similar backgrounds and needs; and on my sister's ready recommendation, my brother arranged a separate viewing for he and I on the very next day, (on Friday, the 9th), and I drove the 17 miles to meet him, and to make the visit.

From the outside the signs were promising enough for a Care Home. It was a 'traditional-looking' home, positioned on its own, and within its own small 'grounds', top right, at the end of a short, gradually-rising, in theory tarmacked, but in truth pretty uneven, dead-end street, and was a robust-looking, but attractive, 2-storey, red-brick-built property of significant age and size; but not so big that it looked impersonal or 'industrial'; like most others we'd viewed from the outside. Conveniently, it was not only in a locality that Mum knew, but also directly opposite a small car park, and tightly adjacent to Mum's GP's surgery, which faced us squarely at the very top of the street; so we must have seen it often, without realising that it *was* a Care Home.

In plan, it was roughly the shape of a left-handed right-angle or 'L'; if that's not a contradiction in terms. Also conveniently, we were actually able to park right outside on the day, before climbing the three small steps, passing through the black wrought-iron gate, and small front garden, and approaching the solid, grass-green door, (with its single, upper, round and opaque window). We rang the bell, and waited beneath the apex of a small, slated, door canopy.

We were greeted by "Annie-May", the pleasant Head Nurse. She was attired in her requisite royal-blue nursing tunic, and invited us to step through into the Hall; where she took the time to explain that the large oak bookcase that sat behind two collapsed wheelchairs and an aluminium walking frame, and hugged most of the wall on the left, the sturdy oak dresser, with its fresh vase of flowers, and signing-in book, and single old oak dining chair, on the right, and the traditional-patterned, warm-red-themed, deep-piled carpet, (like most of their in-house furnishings), had been chosen to try and reflect styles that their mostly elderly residents might recognise, find an affinity with, and feel comfortable amongst. That was an encouraging early touch. We were then shown into the first room on the left, the "Front Sitting Room", which was one of the main rooms generally available for residents' use. In keeping with the 'age-appropriate' theme that Annie-May had just described, this too seemed to be quite 'traditionally' furnished - with a similarly-patterned deep-pile carpet, flower-print curtains, another well-stocked, hard-wood, bookcase, and a gas fire with 'matching' hard-wood fire-surround, a small TV, and a number of cloth-covered high back chairs in various pastel shades arranged around the walls, but not encroaching into the large bay window.

In there too, though, were a couple of mature male residents, each clearly with significant reduction of both physical, but particularly mental, capacity, and one of whom was being spoon-fed his dinner by a single carer in a *light* blue tunic. As a transitory and 'visiting' interloper, it felt rather intrusive to be in attendance at such intimacy, especially as they were both clearly unable to respond to my standard "Hello", so I quickly scanned the room, acknowledged them, respectfully but nominally, and suggested to Annie-May that we move on.

We then proceeded with our conversation in the very *next* room down on the left; which, handily, turned out to be the (suitably-appropriate, suitably-furnished, and suitably labelled, if somewhat untidy) 'Office'; and housed an array of predictable office furnishings; including 3 well-used wood desks, each with a phone and a number of wire 'in/out trays', 2 large filing cabinets, 3 shelves full of official-looking reference tomes, various wall-charts, etc. - and, currently, "Sally", smartly dressed in smart civvies.

It was here that we first 'got down to brass tacks', though, and where the actual practicalities, and especially the financial factors, and conditions of stay, were first raised and aired with both Annie-May, and particularly Sally, (who introduced herself as one of the 2 joint-owners of this "personal", one-off, business), with regard to the home and care set up.

Sally advised that she had both a relevant degree and a nursing qualification, that various members of her staff were also fully-qualified nurses, that she had a loyal group of trained, well-established, staff, and that Maple Mount had recently re-achieved the level of 'excellent' under its latest Care Quality Commission assessment; (simultaneously pointing to a collection of named photos of all members of her staff, all the relevant framed certificates and qualifications of both she and those members, plus that obviously-prized certificate from the CQC; all of which hung in a neat group on one of the walls). She added that Maple Mount had both an allocated GP from the adjacent practice, who visited regularly, plus a designated / link social worker from the local office who did likewise. She went on to tell us that Maple Mount was jointly owned with one other person, and (unlike some competitors), was their *only* Care Home; arguing that this allowed Maple Mount to cater more personally for the (maximum of) 18 residents that it could accommodate. So far so good. However, when I brought up the delicate matter of the actual *costs* involved in living at Maple Mount, I was unknowingly letting my brother and I in for a veritable 'snowstorm' of mind-boggling information.

Sally advised that residents here (as elsewhere) either qualified for 'Continuing Health Care', (CHC), and were fully funded by the NHS, or they did not; in which case those currently with total assets of less than £23,250 (including any property or savings), qualified to have their costs met by the Local Authority; whilst those with *more than* £23,250 (by far the majority), were termed "self-funders", and (effectively *subsidising* state-supported residents) were legally required to use all and any 'estate' assets above this threshold, including the value of any property, plus any welfare benefit entitlements, to contribute towards their 'private' care costs. (At the time of our visit, we had been buoyed up by the then Conservative government airing the possibility of actually raising this tiny threshold to £72,000; but their proposals had been quickly deemed too costly and withdrawn; and so, of course, never actually 'saw the light of day' in terms of legislation, though, as I write they are being aired yet again. Alas, of course, the moment has now passed for Mum).

Either way, in *this* Local Authority, like most, in times of austerity, there was an upper limit to the contribution that the LA would be able to pay and it fell more than £60 *short* of the (£554) weekly cost of even a shared room in Maple Mount. And it was a *shared* vacancy that might be in the offing. (This £60+ shortfall would later crop up under the guise of the County Council's "Top-up fee", and would be yet another cost and problem to be laid squarely at the *customer's* 'door').

Apparently, in the whole of the Local Authority, there was but one solitary, (it not only reeked of being the 'nominal', but also happened to be the only *council-run)*, Care Home where the weekly fees actually *matched* the maximum amount (of £489) that the LA was willing / able to pay; but it was way across the other side of the county, and would have been just logistically-impractical for us to consider; not that, surprise, surprise, there were vacancies there, anyway!

Despite her worsening Dementia, and the real and additional physical limitations being imposed by the combination of her 2 chronic, left-leg pains, and the certain agreement of all but myself that Mum had 'no chance' of currently managing 'home alone', our early and, as it turned out, naively-optimistic application, (via the hospital social worker), for Mum to be assessed as in need of *nursing* care, and thereby qualify for her all costs to be met by the NHS, (under the 'Continuing Health Care' system), had already failed miserably, even before she had left hospital; and with Mum's small, 2-up-2-down, house (and therefore 'estate' assets) being worth more than £23,250, it looked like we were going to be forced to *sell* Mum's home at short notice, and probably quite cheaply, and use the proceeds from that sale to 'privately' fund her Care Home placement. The only other alternative was to delay the sale, by arguing that it had not been proven, 'beyond reasonable doubt' as the lawyers have it, that Mum would not recover sufficiently to return there, (indeed, and in principle, Sally was quite happy to take Mum short-term on that basis, in the first instance, if she came), and, using her continuing benefit entitlements, make up the difference by taking out an interest-accruing loan from the LA, (under their Deferred Payment Scheme); with the latter then taking a legal 'charge' (first call) on the value of the 'estate', including her property, to an amount of debt loaned /accrued.

If Mum were to live for a further 4 years, we had estimated that ALL the value of her home, (she had very little in terms of savings), would be payable to the Local Authority. At least then, with her home sold, and all the proceeds (above the £23,250 threshold) gobbled up by the Local Authority, her assets *would* meet the criteria for her costs to become payable by the LA; but even then, *only* to the (£489) threshold set by the LA! Accordingly, if Mum *did* manage to live beyond a further 4 years, and her health still hadn't worsened sufficiently to meet the stringent 'death's door' criteria for *nursing* care under the CHC scheme, the weekly £60+ difference (and that likely to rise, if only in line with inflation), between what the LA would fund and what the (shared) room at Maple Mount cost for it to continue to be economically viable, would have to be made up (*'topped* up') 'privately' that is, by the 'self-funder'; that is, by the resident; that is, by Mum. In practice, that is by relatives, that is by US! If we refused to pay, or were unable to find, the difference, then her place at Maple Mount (or wherever), might be deemed 'at risk', and Mum (or any other resident in such similar circumstances), could, in theory, be uinceremoniously uprooted, and required to move - to a (cheaper) Home that *did* match the LA's threshold. (And of course they only had the 'full' one on the other side of the county!). My brother and I looked askance at each other as we tried to absorb the complexity, absurdity, and indeed enormity, of the financial undertakings involved. Even as a seasoned social worker, it took all my concentration to 'get some sort of handle' on it. If nothing else, financially, it was already looking a 'bit of a minefield', and it was abundantly clear that we still had much to ponder on here - *wherever* Mum was 're-housed'.

(Perhaps most worrying of all though, even if we accepted the next vacancy here, or elsewhere, for Mum, as I touched on earlier, it was equally clear that, with her house sold, and the entire proceeds spent on her care, leaving her with no 'fall-back' position whatsoever, there was still no *absolute* certainty of tenure - or even of the Home remaining profitable - or therefore, in business!).

Are you following me so far, dear reader?

No? I'm not surprised.

As a 'big-city' social worker of 20-odd years standing I was well used to dealing with umpteen levels of bureaucracy, but even *my* head was starting to 'spin' after almost an hour of trying to absorb the 'knotty' facts, figures and possibilities in play here, so I was more than happy to move on when Annie-May finally brought the 'sales-pitch' and cost considerations to a temporary end, with a timely suggestion that we continue with our 'tour' of the Mount.

Immediately outside the Office, Annie-May paused us briefly by the adjacent and fully open door of the long, thin, not exactly personal or cosy, indeed, essentially 'commercial', slightly 'industrial-looking', slightly old-fashioned, kitchen on our left. There, we were briefly introduced to "Jan", one of the two full-time cooks, and to a paper copy of a suitably-varied, perfectly acceptable, and apparently 'typical,' menu for the current week, whilst being advised that the Mount's "vulnerable" residents would not normally enter here unsupervised. (So, could not normally, for example, make themselves even a cup of tea). The kitchen appeared to be equipped with all the standard catering essentials you would expect, as well as a currently -closed serving hatch at the far end. Annie-May then escorted us along a dog-leg-left corridor, (past the solid kitchen wall, now on our left, and past the wide open door of a neat, single-bedded, currently-vacated, room of one of the luckier, 'downstairs' residents, and then that of a principal downstairs bathroom and toilet, that was also currently unoccupied, but quite clearly equipped with a full gamut of 'appliances' for all likely disabilities, on the right) - and on to *the* most depressing, disconcerting and affecting of unanticipated sights, as the end of the corridor opened up 'naturally' (through the also wide open door) into the "Main Sitting Room".

Given my years of social work experience, you might think that I would have been prepared for the sort of sight that confronted me; but, caught unawares, I just wasn't. On first viewing, and with no 'forewarning', it was a sight, and a moment, that I actually found quite traumatising, and a major shock to my system. So much so that I have never managed to fully erase it from my memory. (Although it was also a sight that I, like all visitors, would have to, and eventually did, learn to live with).

As I would come to realise, and for this type of Care institution, for the elderly, there was nothing unusual or amiss with the sight, the Home or any of the residents. Indeed, the experience might well have felt *more* traumatic, and a deal *less* personal in a bigger, more impersonal, unit.

Just seconds ago, in the 'Office', we had been told that Maple Mount catered for a maximum of 18 residents; of which my brother and I had met 2 in the 'Front Sitting Room'. However, we appeared to have arrived in the main sitting area just after the majority of the remainder of the residents, and the vast majority of them pretty elderly, (say 70 and upwards, and nearly all in various limiting stages of both physical and mental incapacity; much of the latter Dementia-based), had finished their lunch - and with every one of them, in a rather disarming state of inelegance, now at rest in one of the many high-back chairs positioned around the mainly off-white-striped and mint-green perimeter walls of what Annie-May formally reiterated *was* "The Main Sitting Room"; with just a couple more at their similar repose in wicker-type chairs in the small, but quite pleasant and airy, conservatory, just off to the left. No matter where they were, though, not a single resident seemed to be even close to what I would call consciousness, or therefore aware of, (let alone bothered by), the fact that we had entered their personal/living space; indeed, many seemed effectively comatose. The 'shock', I suppose, was in the simply unappealing *vision* of this accumulative *mass* of lifeless elderly residents all sat nominally upright, but either asleep, heading that way, or worse (!), at one and the same time. (My mind was mischievously moved to think that perhaps one of Dr. Who's more stealthy, but more malevolent, adversaries had been at work). It just wasn't an immediately uplifting or optimistic image to encounter at close quarters, as they sat in their various states of slouched inactivity in those high-backed chairs; some with heads and shoulders lolling forwards, others with their heads fallen backwards; quite a few with their mouths wide open, (a couple noticeably dribbling); and one or two actually emitting quite audible inharmonious variations on snoring, wheezing or similar breathing-based noises. Moreover, it was immediately obvious that very few, if any, were in a position to make rational conversation; or therefore to offer any views on what it was *like* to be a resident at Maple Mount. As Annie-May hurriedly restated, we had perhaps arrived at an inopportune time to catch the residents at their most active; but what concerned me most was that we had surely been introduced to the sort of scenario that was likely to become a 'normal' part of Mum's daily living if she came to live here; at least during this sleepy, 'after-lunch' period.

As Annie-May guided us quietly down the middle of this clapped-out collection of well-knackered 'sleeping beauties', deftly ensuring that we avoided clattering into a number of 'waiting' walking frames and adjustable, over-chair, tables, or randomly outstretched, often surgical-stockinged, and variously-slippered, feet, she again took the time to point out the consistent and careful choice of more 'traditional' furnishings, (including another 'old-looking' gas fire with 'teak' surround at the far end, but with a large-screen TV above it silently playing an old 'black and white' film to no-one in particular, and an upright mahogany piano, supporting a fresh vase of flowers, tucked into the near alcove on the right, that was apparently 'properly' played for the residents on a weekly basis by a local pianist brought in for the specific purpose of an 'old-time sing-around'), before escorting us through some white sliding doors just off at the far right, and into the pastel-green-and dark-wood-themed dining room. There, she briefly introduced us to "Donna", another member of staff, (also in a *light-blue* tunic), who was just putting the finishing touches to the room's half-dozen clothed tables, and to its return to 'ready' status again.

Our 'tour' then carried on with us back-tracking to where we had entered, and through an easily-missed, small-windowed, door in the corner of the Hall, (and directly adjacent to the rear of the *front* door), that lead upstairs. It was immediately obvious from the sturdy staircase 'rail' that it was fitted with a standard 'stairlift'; which was about to present we 'able-bodied tourists' with a narrowed gap to wriggle through at the top; because the *seat* was currently set at rest there. As we squeezed by, Annie-May confirmed that few (currently just 1 of the more able) residents with 'upstairs' rooms could 'come and go' without being fully supervised, and therefore have *free* use of their upstairs rooms. This, she continued, was due to their own very real limitations and disabilities, requisite health and safety issues, and the consequent, and impracticably disproportionate, *amount* of both assistance and supervision, by a finite number of staff, that would be needed if such free movement upstairs were to be liberally afforded. Consequently, the majority of 'upstairs' sleepers normally remained *down*stairs until bedtime once they had been helped to rise; even if they were ill; whereupon one of the quieter downstairs residents' bedrooms was usually commandeered for manageable supervisory and nursing purposes during the day. (Though Annie-May did concede that during visiting times, a resident's relatives would usually be allowed to take on any 'upstairs' supervisory role if/when they requested it).

Facing us, fractionally right, and across the upstairs corridor, at the top of the stairs, was the bland beige door to Room Number 9, which Annie-May advised was the shared bedroom where the next vacancy was most likely to arise. We all entered together. It was light and airy, with a high ceiling, a good-sized radiator, a free-standing brown-wicker room divider, currently collapsed and pushed into one corner, predominantly white and magnolia walls, a handful of framed floral prints on the walls, and a 'warm' good-piled, patterned carpet on the floor. My brother and I wandered slowly around, trying to get a 'feel' for what it would be like for Mum. It was immediately clear that the bed in the far corner was already occupied, and that the currently sheet-less one onto which the door opened was about to become the vacant one. Annie-May confirmed it as so. Each bed had its own adjacent, sturdy, matching, but, (out of keeping with the Mount's more 'traditional' downstairs theme and furnishings), fairly modern, white, nondescript, flat-pack-type wardrobe and chest of drawers, with its own small bedside armchair in pretty, chintzy-pink cloth, and a shared pedestal sink in the other far corner. The good-sized window that was also a central feature of the far wall looked down onto Maple Mounts' own small garden, its' patio and grounds, and, beyond the boundary fence, into the small back gardens of a sloping row of stone-terraced houses opposite.

Annie-May advised that Mum would be sharing with "Martha", another resident struggling with both advancing age and Dementia, if she came. (It would later turn out that Martha's Dementia was quite a bit more advanced than Mum's!) Annie-May was quick to point out how Martha's bed and environs had been personalised with her own 'bits and pieces' and mementos; including two photos from her past; one a slightly fading black and white print that, rather poignantly, showed off Martha as an attractive, dark-haired, young woman in her pomp, and happily dancing arm-in-arm with her (presumably) now long-gone husband. The implication was that Mum's bed-space could be similarly personalised.

At first glance, it was a perfectly acceptable room, but my abiding thought was of how Mum would respond to permanently *sharing* a bedroom again, let alone with someone other than Dad; for she had shared with no-one at all since *his* passing over 20 years ago, and this a bedroom that was *not* even the same, and, of course, very familiar, one that had been hers for over 60 years. For now, I kept my counsel, and my ambivalent thoughts to myself.

The 'tour' was completed by a nominal stroll along an *upstairs* dog-leg corridor that mirrored the downstairs one. It took us past several more residents' bedrooms, (all currently unoccupied and rightly unavailable for inspection; except for one that was receiving its daily dose of 'upstairs maid's attention, by "Penny", another *dark blue*-clad member of staff), and a mirror-image version of the well-equipped *downstairs* bathroom and toilet facilities. There was also the addition of a large broom / storage cupboard, and one small, extra, toilet and washbowl, (handily *opposite* Room 9), that was for the use of staff and visitors.

Finally, we were ushered back to the 'Office' again; where Sally was waiting to re-engage us, seek our views, and query whether we were likely to accept the place for Mum. She advised that the health of the current incumbent of the likely vacancy had deteriorated substantially, that she had been hospitalised for some time, and that, even as we undertook the 'tour', Maple Mount had been advised, by telephone, that she was unlikely to recover; and, regardless, would not be fit enough to return to there. Accordingly, Sally was advising that the vacancy was now effectively 'on offer' immediately, and could only be 'held' for 48 hours; because of the dual pressures to not 'carry' empty rooms, and those coming from the social services, due the general bed shortage county-wide. My first thought was not to rush in, and to take at least a couple of hours to 'mull it all over', and to check, for example, with the local social services if *other* placements might be in the offing. My brother, on the other hand, advised more urgency, and argued strongly for us to accept the place immediately. We asked for a few minutes to consider things, and were left alone in the 'Office'.

My brother was (rightly) keen to avoid Mum remaining on that hospital ward for a moment longer than was necessary, and, from that pressure alone, I was easily persuaded that we *should* accept the placement on offer at Maple Mount, at least by taking up the flexible offer of a '4-week initial placement', with the option of longer, that Sally had said could be the case. So, when she and Annie-May returned, we duly agreed, on that flexible basis, to accept the place that was on offer in Room 9.

The 'tour' was complete, the die was cast, and we were shown out, with the advice to contact the social worker 'as soon as possible' to advise that we had accepted the place. I was left with the nagging realisation that, for better or worse, we had committed Mum's limited future, at least for now, (and for what would turn out to be the penultimate chapter of her life), to being in residency at Maple Mount.

Just a few days later, on Thursday, the 15ᵗʰ of September, 2016, and after nearly 3 weeks of being defined by a particular hospital bed, and ward, and by the accumulating confusion, deterioration and lack of stimulation therein, (the bulk of that time just a 'holding' exercise in the absence of more appropriate living space), and with the fortunate identification of a suitable Care Home placement, Mum was finally released from her 'bed-bound' existence. As I fretted at home, my sister (and sister-in-law on behalf of my brother), duly kept my siblings' side of the bargain. The 2 women drove the 7 miles there, collecting Mum from the ward on the morning of the 15th, and similar back, and then spent several hours 'installing' her, with plenty of suitable reassurances, (and a few of her personal effects and 'essentials'), in residency at her new home - Maple Mount. The next, potentially final, phase of Mum's long life was under way.

Although it was a far from perfect 'initiation', (Mum often found her new environment predictably perplexing at the outset, 'though, thankfully, she didn't seem *overly* distressed), the early days seemed to go well enough, as far as we could determine.

In theory, visiting was unrestricted, but in practice we were asked to try and refrain from visiting at mealtimes and bedtimes, when staff time was at a premium. Bearing that in mind, we immediately implemented a daily visiting schedule that broadly tried to reflect the pattern and routine that had been in place when Mum was last in her *own* home. Accordingly, (and with the upcoming Saturday, the 17ᵗʰ as my inaugural visit to her in her new setting), I quickly settled back into a routine that re-established me in visiting Mum each Tuesday, Thursday and Saturday afternoon;

usually timing my arrival for around 1-45pm, and then departing around 4-15 pm. In between, and for both our sakes, and sanity I suspect, I was usually keen to get her out into the 'normality' of the local community for at least *some* part of that time. Not only for a change and a 'break', but also for the opportunity to drive past her house, (and to gauge her reaction to it), slowly through her 'old' neighbourhood, and on to a few other familiar haunts and shops; and, of course, to the local cemetery, to visit Dad's grave in particular; all of which, incidentally, she still continued to recognise, and to be able to name in situ. My *overarching* motive was to try and inject some semblance, and thus recognition, of her 'old' routine, life and past familiarity into her 'new' one. However, the unswerving, Dementia-lead, reality was that whilst she could usually tell me where she *was,* when currently *at* any of those familiar places, she could rarely tell me, nowadays, where she had just *been* - sometimes even just 5 minutes ago; including any unprompted recall of *any* details of where she was now living, once she was *outside* Maple Mount. (Indeed, on most occasions, once we were out, her active, but struggling, brain was usually quick to seek my confirmation that she had actually risen in her *own* home that morning, and that I had just collected her from there. Somehow, though, she still *knew* that her memory was letting her down, and would get extremely frustrated because that 'missing link' in her brain just couldn't, or wouldn't, confirm it as so itself; and the more so when I too had to disappoint her with a Maple Mount reality she barely recognised). Regardless, what remained clear, despite her drawn out hospital admission, and some further, consequent and predictable (irreversible?), loss of muscle mass, and thereby physical strength, mainly due to lack of any real use of her muscles whilst abed at the former, was that the damage being inflicted by Mum's Dementia was still mainly to her *short-term* memory. Albeit with some occasional prompting, her recall of the *familiar* present, and the outlying past, was still, surprisingly, and indeed quite hearteningly, pretty good. And as always, she *never* failed to recognise the 3 of us.

Of course, the return to a familiar visiting schedule (not that Mum, like the vast majority of her fellow residents, had, or now needed to have, any precise idea of just what day it was at the Mount, or who to expect, until someone actually appeared), still meant that we were not present with her for the bulk of each day's hours 'in residency', and were thus reliant on the busy (usually rotating) staff there to advise us on 'how things were going'; and they, in turn, entirely reliant on just the 2 night staff for 'out-of-hours' feedback.

Nevertheless, Mum's new, and of course unfamiliar, indeed much-transformed, 'home-life' was under way; Dementia, medication, 'Residential Care' setting and all. It would bring plenty of new issues to tackle, too. Not only were there those actual, if relatively minor, 'settling-in' problems, (as I'd predicted), around the lack of familiarity, ownership, routine, self-selection and independence in her Dementia-beset day-to-day, (and indeed night), life, at Maple Mount, for us to try and help her with, but, all too suddenly, there were also the parallel, ever- present and seemingly endless, always seemingly 'urgent', mass of unfamiliar administrative, fiscal, and 'agency' issues that were now 'bursting' around us, and needing our pressing and resilient attention on Mum's behalf. At their base, I suppose, most of these could be boiled down to being *financially-related* matters, but, regardless, they came 'thick and fast', and few ran smoothly.

During the 'Dementia years', and whilst Mum was still living in her own home, she had, of course, been throwing up plenty of worrying 'episodes' of 'forgetfulness', and, in consequence, very real, logistical, and practical, everyday care problems for us. Thankfully, though, her *financial* affairs hadn't really been amongst them. *They* had remained relatively straightforward to both organise and to manage for/with her.

Mum and Dad had always lived a very frugal, unsophisticated life, and especially so in retirement, barely having 'two ha'pennies to rub together', and apart from a basic Post Office Account, into which their only income, from their state-provided 'old-age-pensions' were paid, they had no other pensions, bank accounts or savings; and Dad had always taken the lead in *organising* the family finances. *His* (1996) passing had thus required us to help adjust them in favour of (a fully compos mentis) Mum; and the sheer simplicity of their finances had meant that we'd managed to do so relatively quickly; although enforced adjustments to all their provider's accounts, soon afterwards, did mean that Mum, (and of her own volition) ended up with the *very* simplest of all the Post Office's accounts, in the shape of a 'Post Office Card Account'.

At the time, that pretty active, fully compos mentis, physically very fit for her 70+ years, Mum of ours was well over a decade away from her 'Dementia days', and had insisted on having her state benefits paid into what would henceforth be her *sole* Post Office Card Account; not least because the Post Office was the only financial institution that Mum (and Dad) had *ever* used, was familiar with, and was most easily, and locally, able to access. At the time, of course, it made sound-enough sense. However, it was so simple that it only allowed for her benefits to be paid *in*, and for her to draw *out* any benefit monies that arrived thus. It paid no interest, received no other deposits, and offered no cheque-book, or any kind of facility to *transfer* money, or, say, set up a Direct Debit. Nothing beyond 'Pension paid IN, and pension drawn OUT'. However, once in place, and for well over a decade afterwards, Mum managed it very well on her own; using the same post office as a sort of one-stop shop, to both draw out enough cash for her everyday needs, and to pay her bills in situ. It was all that she really required and understood; and therefore felt comfortable with; or, indeed, was willing to try! But it would most certainly complicate matters the more during the 'Dementia years', and, perhaps most poignantly of all, when Mum had to leave her own home and established routine, and take up residency at Maple Mount.

To the largely inexperienced and uninitiated, just dealing with the related *finances* involved in moving an elderly relative, not to mention one suffering from Dementia, into a Care/ Residential Home can be painful and trying to the point of excruciating. Both the direct procedures and the 'peripheral', indirect, ones present as extremely complicated regardless, but can be even more so depending on what forward planning and foresight (or lack of!) has been deployed; and hence on what steps have been taken earlier, (or not), and before *the proverbial* 'hits the fan'! I would describe the situation as a bit like putting off making your own will because you think it might be prophetic, and somehow precipitate your demise, but thereby leaving the inescapable and equally-complex problems for those that survive you to sort out.

Whilst our generally healthy, compos mentis, Mum's life ticked merrily by then, we had certainly been happy to procrastinate thus regarding any planning for her likely decline, and demise; much preferring to believe, like the Queen, (who, I might remind you, was born in the same, 1926, *year* as Mum), she would just go on forever. Luckily, though, I had spent most of my working life as a front-line social worker in a major city in the north of England. It carried its own levels of complicated procedures and stress, and so I had become fairly used to finding the patience and stoicism necessary to deal with the in-built elements of 'checks and balances' paperwork and multi-level bureaucracy involved in working with any type and number of individual 'clients' and public agencies; but my perspective here, from the 'other side of the fence', as an under pressure *client/customer* trying to access the limited services available, still came as a real, and acutely frustrating, eye-opener!

So then, before I regale you further regarding the time Mum actually spent living and coping at Maple Mount, let me first set the *structural* scene and context for it, by shedding some (hopefully) useful light on the many, mind-boggling, and yet largely unavoidable, financial and administrative issues that our Mum's largely unanticipated, and therefore poorly-planned, admission to a Care Home threw up for *us* - *we*, her naive, trusting and unwary offspring.

I should again re-emphasise that Mum's admission into residential care triggered *several* financial/ administrative imperatives; very few, if any, of which ran either smoothly, singly, efficiently, or even in any neat sequential form, and many of which overlapped and needed managing *concurrently;* and in some cases over several weeks; indeed months. A few were particular, and indeed peculiar, to Mum, but most applied generally to all would-be 'Care' seekers. Anyway, since I have already mentioned the limitations of her Post Office Card Account, perhaps I should start from there.

Before I do though, I should confirm that, after urgent discussion, my siblings and I had at least reached one crucial decision. My brother and sister had been more readily persuaded that we should not *rush* to sell Mum's home, in order to see just how Mum *settled* in residential care; and from my point of view, to ensure that Mum had been given every chance to make the sort of miraculous recovery that might yet allow her to reconsider returning to that home. Our agreed decision, instead, had been that we would take up the 4-week initial 'trial' of residential care, offered my Sally, and very probably the 12-week period that we *thought* had been the minimum recommended by the social services, with an acceptance that a more comprehensive review after a year might well be more realistic; and that if she were still in residence at that point, such a review might well conclude that her stay should be redefined as officially long-term. In effect, and on behalf of Mum, we wanted to keep our options as flexible as possible, 'bide our time', reassess regularly along the way, and just see how it went. Eminently sensible, and not at all unreasonable, we thought. In the meantime, we would apply for the necessary Local Authority 'Deferred Payment' loan. We appeared to have a plan.

However, no sooner had we settled on that plan, and after a robust exchange of e-mails with the hospital social worker, (following our visit to view Maple Mount, and our decision to 'give the placement a go'), we were informed by that social worker that to apply, let alone qualify, for the LA's Deferred Payment Scheme, we had to accept that the placement was *permanent*, from the beginning; and that it was his recollection that we had done so. Otherwise the 'customer', as self-funder, would be responsible for paying any *short-term* Care costs themselves. It appeared that the 'rules' had been changed yet again. Indeed, the social worker, both verbally, and in his long-winded written report, (dated the 10th and received in the post on the 12th), was claiming that we had *definitively* agreed this 'permanency' at the house meeting of the 6th. That most certainly was *not* the case, and, whilst my position had been noted, it did not make any *practical* allowances for MY firmly stated hope of Mum returning home! Even so, with no obvious funding alternative, we were effectively, and belatedly, forced to change the basis on which Mum's planned move to Maple Mount would commence, and accept it as 'permanent' from the beginning. That may have *seemed* something of a technical change, (in that it did not actually *rule out* her return home if that 'miracle' came to pass), but it would prove to be an important one, whilst also adding to the growing sense of confusion and of feeling that we were being dictated to, hamstrung by, and fighting against, instead of with, a sort of 'Big Brother' *establishment* power at every turn. I, for one, most certainly wasn't happy that, at the last minute, our hand had been forced so but feeling impotent to affect the situation, in the face of the behemoth of 'the system' and the County Council, we felt obliged, to accept the latter's avowed conditions. Our plan had been strategically modified from without, but at least we still seemed to have one, going forward.

So, from that base, let me return now to the Post Office Card Account. Once she had entered Maple Mount, it became readily apparent that *we* would now need to manage Mum's affairs on her behalf, from thereon in, that the Post Office Card Account could no longer 'cut the mustard' for financial management purposes, and that we needed to do 3 things pretty rapidly. Firstly, we needed to gain flexible access to her Account, monies, and in-coming benefits; in order to be able to pay ongoing house bills, insurance and maintenance costs, any newly-arising care costs, and to buy everyday 'essentials' for her, etc. To do that, we needed, secondly, to open in her name, but to be able to operate ourselves, a more flexible bank account that would allow us to deposit monies from her Post Office Card Account, so that we had the option to pay for things more efficiently; say, by cheque, direct debit, or occasionally via our own credit cards, and eventually take reimbursement; and thirdly, in order to achieve the first 2, we were advised, from *several* quarters, that we needed to apply for something called Lasting Power Of Attorney, (LPA) and at the earliest opportunity.

Applying for LPA involved us in 'registering' our application with the 'Office of the Public Guardian', (OPG), and with Mum's ('the donor's) signed agreement, and supposed cognitive awareness, (and for if/when the donor loses the mental capacity to make the relevant decisions for themselves), for the legal right to manage and make decisions on the donor's, (Mum's) behalf; but always "in her best interests". It was available, and independently, on 2 'fronts' - LPA for 'property and financial affairs' and LPA for 'health and welfare'. (At a cost of £82 a 'pop'). And, once gained, these 'powers' were far from *trivial.* Having LPA for the 'donor's' *property and financial affairs,* for example, meant that, if/ when the donor became mentally incapacitated (say by Dementia), an attorney could make decisions about not only the donor's household bills and bank accounts, but even about selling their property and any investments; whilst having LPA for the donor's *health and welfare,* in that same circumstance, for example, meant that the attorney(s) could, theoretically, make decisions about both where the donor lives, (say, in a Care Home), and what medical (including any potential life-saving!) treatments the donor receives. (Or doesn't!). Potentially, pretty serious stuff.

So, just days after Mum's admission to Maple Mount, and with both financial and health matters already pressing, we began our 'parallel' application for LPA on both 'fronts' by downloading the long-winded forms from the internet. Consequent sibling discussions then concluded that my brother and I should *both* apply to be Mum's attorneys, (as the forms allowed), so that one of us could still act for her if the other was, say, away on holiday, ill, or otherwise indisposed. However, to complete the forms we needed to both identify an independent witness, (our initial request for the hospital social worker to undertake the role of independent witness was turned down by his line manager, on the grounds that it could compromise the social worker's own independence, so we eventually managed to enlist an old friend for that role), and get Mum to sign her part of each form; as the (supposedly) 'informed' *donor.* That latter, by itself, was arguably 'iffy', because Mum's lack of strength, dexterity, and general mental understanding in such matters, plus her already significant level of Dementia, rendered the whole affair potentially unachievable. (Had that been so, Mum's 'best interests' would have then been assessed, decided and sorted out, doubtless very slowly, and most certainly impersonally, via the so-called 'professionals' that were the mental health medics, social services and the Courts). Niftily, however, we got round that problem by arranging to take Mum to my brother's house on the afternoon of Tuesday, the 20th of September, and, after giving the simplest of explanations for her to sign, got her to practice until we felt she was 'ready' to keep her decidedly weak signature within each form's required 'box'. It took a while, but more by good luck than good management, we achieved 'success', had a literally laughable, (and in that respect very enjoyable), few hours together, and ensured that the forms were duly ready for dispatch to the OPG the next day.

Meanwhile, our relationship with the County Council, and with its Deferred Payment Scheme was still providing perhaps *the* most confusing and stressful cause for concern. From early on, we had come under further pressure to complete and submit our application to that Authority *for* one of their 'Deferred Payment' loans, if that was to be our chosen route; so that, if/when approved, Maple Mount might begin to receive the regular and necessary income from them, loaned on our behalf of course, for 'looking after' Mum. To this latter end, and in the course of the preparation of that requisite written Care Plan that actually contained several significant inaccuracies, the (over-?) industrious hospital social worker had already given us some appropriate leaflets and information, and had even arranged for some number-juggling superwoman from the County Council HQ, (and going under the grandiose title of 'Financial Assessment Benefits Officer'), to meet us at my brother's house.

This latter event eventually took place in early October 2016; ostensibly to thrash out some 'final' figures; her subsequent, and supposedly definitive, *written* offerings carrying the date of the 10th of the month; but they turned out to be something *less* than definitive, and rather susceptible to changes; and thus *far* from final; not least because of the potential for changes to the *government's own* interest rates; and therefore to those being added to the loan offered by the County Council at its different stages. As if that wasn't woolly enough, there were a couple of other really annoying reasons for a lack of clarity from, and therefore for dispute with, her and her County Council crew.

Firstly, the written information we'd been given about the Deferred Loan, (as well as an additional leaflet we'd obtained, independently, from the Alzheimer's Society) had stated, (we thought clearly), that, "For the first 12 weeks" of (Mum's) placement (at Maple Mount), the property known as [her home], "is disregarded for assessment purposes". Naively, we siblings had cheered with relief as we each 'read' this as meaning that, (even) under the 'Deferred Loan' system, the *full* cost of the first 12 weeks of her residential placement were effectively 'free of charge', and would be picked up by the Local Authority, since that 'disregard' put Mum under the £23,250 threshold. Not so! (*That* applied only to eligible *temporary* residents). We really should have known better, but under pressure we'd clearly been clutching at straws! Anyway, superwoman had barely got through the door, on said date, before we had been fully divested of our version of the relevant phraseology, and left in a state of unreserved disappointment. For, despite vigorously disputing *her* officious interpretation of the County Council's own wording of the 'disregard' information, and quoting the Alzheimer Society's leaflet, we had been made fully aware that there was no room for negotiation, and that the version that would prevail would be hers; and that Mum would *still* have to contribute her full welfare rights income from the start, (less £23.50 for 'personal' needs), plus that 'Top-up' fee mentioned earlier, (though this latter could be added to her loan). In this way, the County Council could, and would, ultimately, absolve itself from picking up *any* of Mum's care costs, both in the first 12 weeks, and for *any* of her ('private') weeks in residence thereafter. I guess we really *should* have known, (especially in a time of austerity and cut-backs), that nothing comes free - from the Council or elsewhere!

Secondly, the Council Superwoman had failed to reckon with an equivalent level of doggedness from the equally bureaucratic people from 'Pension Credit', who, in generally re-assessing

303

Mum's welfare benefit entitlements, (after we had been required to inform them, by telephone, of Mum's move and change of circumstances), disputed those (lovingly laid out in a letter) 'final' figures that the woman from the County Council had sent to us, by stating that, in her Maple Mount (residential) setting, Mum was only entitled, at the outset, to state Retirement Pension, plus the re-start of her Attendance Allowance after 12 weeks, and indeed no longer *qualified* for Pension Credit at all! The County Council's superwoman initially begged to differ, and initially retained the Pension Credit in her calculation, and an impasse appeared to have been reached! (I ask you!).

After trying to unravel the dispute myself, in a futile and frustrating search for any kind of personal understanding and final clarity, of just what we had signed up to borrow, with futile and frustrating go-between phone calls to both parties, I eventually 'gave up the ghost' on this aspect, advised both that it was beyond me, and insisted, as so-called 'professionals', that *they* 'get their fingers out', 'sort it out between themselves', and 'let us know' when it had been resolved. (See what I mean about having to deal with so much clanking inefficiency and clearly uncoordinated bureaucracy and red tape!). In the end the Pension Credit people had it, and superwoman was forced to issue revised figures to us; and then again when first government interest rates changed, and then Attendance Allowance eventually kicked in again. Regardless, in principle, all Mum's (regularly) re-assessed weekly welfare benefit entitlements, in her new setting, (eventually less the new and increased rate of £24.90 for her 'personal expenses' allowance), would henceforth be paid (direct by the State) to Maple Mount as her individual contribution to her fees there. And still the various bills for the upkeep of Mum's empty house continued to roll in. Financially and administratively, it all seemed to be 'kicking off'.

So you can see why the limited and rigid offerings of the Post Office Card Account would no longer be suitable for servicing Mum's changing financial affairs. Even here though, nothing was straight-forward. In order to gain the financial flexibility that we needed, we had to first book an urgent appointment with my brother's (local) high street bank, with a view to opening a new bank account to accommodate Mum's latest monetary requirements. So, on the 29th of November, my brother and I gathered all the necessary paperwork together, in a folder, and attended an hour-long meeting at his bank, with their 'specialist'; and the new account was officially opened in Mum's name, but with each attorney having access; although we would have to wait for well over a week for the official paperwork and Bank Cards (one for each attorney), to arrive via our respective postmen. Even then, alas, as the 'specialist' had made clear, it would be of little use to us until and unless we managed to transfer in relevant funds i.e. from the Post Office Card Account! For that, she advised us to ring a number for the Post Office Card Account's *customer service* people in Preston. I'd duly done that the very next day, and a man who's 'ethnic English' I found so difficult to understand embarrassed me by continually and patiently repeating his advice for me to "wait on", until I finally *got it*. Ultimately, his message was that I had to *write in* with my request to transfer the required amount from Mum's Post Office Card Account to the new High St. Bank Account; making sure that I included copies of the LPA, the respective account numbers, and all other relevant information as long-sufferingly listed by him. He further advised that the matter might take up to '10 working days' to complete. I followed his advice to the, and with an appropriate, letter; that I prepared and posted the very next day; and then we waited; during which time the Post Office Card Account should still have only been *officially* operated by the named account holder i.e. Mum. Unofficially, we got round this quite easily; by formally asking Mum's permission to take the actual card from her purse, in the cupboard where she kept it 'at home' (down the years, we'd often been in attendance when her *compos mentis* self had requested our help with the "fancy" ATM 'technology', anyway, and we already knew the password), and just simply continuing to operate the account ourselves, (on the odd occasion with Mum still actually present, but more often than not in her absence), and withdrawing monies from the Post Office ATM, up to her (£600) daily limit, as proved necessary and expedient.

Earlier, on the 2nd of November, and some 6 weeks after submitting our applications, we'd been able to welcome our *one* relatively *trouble-free,* and vital, break. Thankfully, our manoeuvrings to get Mum's signature on her LPA applications had brought their crucial reward. The applications had been approved without any real hitches, and we'd received our official letters from the OPG, confirming that they had indeed been successful; and that we had been duly 'registered', and now had LPA on both 'fronts'; so at least we could *operate* as Mum's official attorneys thereafter. That was, of course, critical on a number of counts. Firstly, for example, we had then been able to authoritatively book that appointment with the 'specialist' at my brother's bank, and to render the necessary bank account open and ready for use. Secondly, we were *officially* able to accept and sign the County Council's 'Deferred Loan' proposal on Mum's behalf. Thirdly, we'd been able to use our LPA to authoritatively contact the Post Office's Customer Service people in Preston and apply for a transfer of significant funds. And last but most certainly not least, I had been tactically able to invoke it on Mum's behalf, in the New Year, and for what I judged to be 'in her best interests', for what I believed to be potentially quite serious care and *medical* grounds.

Quite by accident, it came to my notice, in the January of 2017, after I unassumingly enquired about one of the pills that a member of staff was blithely asking Mum to swallow on one occasion, that the GP servicing Maple Mount had been prescribing a particular medication, for Mum, (Sodium Valproate), without informing us, (even as attorneys). Moreover, according to the staff source, the original prescription apparently dated back several weeks, to mid-November. (Clearly, the 'medicalisation' of Mum was still ongoing, even in the supposed 'safety' of the Care Home).

Mum was already 'rattling' with so many prescribed pills and medications, so back at home I ran an exploratory internet check. This revealed that Sodium Valproate was a particularly potent drug, used primarily for the management of epilepsy and bipolar disorder; but also, apparently, in severe cases of mania ('abnormally elevated mental states'). Worryingly though, that same check also revealed that the drug had potentially significant

306

side effects. (The latter included, and under "common" ones, potential risks of liver toxicity, and even that of *memory loss,* for goodness sake!). However, my enquiries revealed that it had apparently, and regularly, been prescribed for *several* of the patients at Maple Mount, (now including Mum) for anxiety-based issues judged to come under the banner of 'mania'.

Although Mum had exhibited occasional bouts of both raised anxiety and low mood, (who wouldn't in such a communal but relatively foreign, claustrophobic, ill-health-affected setting!), there had been no noticeable evidence of such 'mania' in Mum whenever I, or any other of my siblings, had been in situ. Indeed, none of us had witnessed *anything* that even remotely approached either hyper or unmanageable behaviour problems from a largely acquiescent Mum, let alone 'abnormally -elevated' ones that evidenced mania. Moreover, none had been reported to us by Maple Mount. So I was most definitely in something less than a generous mood myself when I found out about the unilateral prescribing of this Sodium Valproate, and immediately made my concerns known to both the Home's senior staff and the GP; and in consequence, and wearing my relatively new 'attorney hat', straightway requested the relevant forms, and applied for the right to access Mum's medical records online at my personal convenience; whilst advising all relevant parties that I would hence- forth expect, (as Mum's attorney) to be consulted and kept 'up to speed' *before* any further non-urgent medications were proposed or prescribed.

The (bitterly ironic) upshot of my complaint was that Maple Mount referred Mum to their linked Dementia doctor/ advisor/'specialist', who was based at a hospice near to, (and serviced), the hospital, and he duly dispatched his specialist nurse to Maple Mount to make an assessment.

This nurse made just one official visit to Mum, (albeit, and taking into account my own strong views, by making it on a day when I was actually visiting), before submitting her report to the specialist. The outcome was that this specialist doctor (and here comes the bitter irony) actually recommended *increasing* the dose of Sodium Valproate a little, and instead, proportionately reducing her dose of the antidepressant called Mirtazapine. Given this nominally *independent* assessment (the specialist doctor never actually saw Mum), and the recommendation for its continued, if sparing, use in reducing Mum's anxiety and 'fear', and that, as my siblings pointed out, Mum was already well- established on her apparently "minor" dose of the drug, I allowed myself to be persuaded, though more than a little reluctantly, to heed the supposed 'independent' medical advice *not* to press further for her to be taken off it.

Eventually, as April dawned, and yet another needlessly long-winded bureaucratic process ground to its ever-coming end, my application to access Mum's medical records, as her attorney, was (finally and officially) approved. Henceforth, so long as Mum shall live, and at my leisure, I would be able to check online precisely what Mum was 'taking', and whatever else was on her records, etc. And I did.

Administratively though, the potentially biggest, (and quite freakish), 'stumbling block' of all, occurred as we'd entered December (2016). The initial problem cropped up at the Land Registry, and with regard to Mum's (empty) house. Yet it threatened to undermine the already erratic progress that we were making elsewhere, and, potentially, to derail the whole 'kit and caboodle'. This latest, and entirely unforeseen, not to mention quite worrisome, problem had reared its very peculiar head when the County Council had sought to formalise their legal 'charge' against the house, with regard to the 'Deferred Loan', and found a significant incongruity on the house deeds. In fact, the 'problem' was that the 2 purchasers' signatures on the deeds of the house were not actually 'Frank and *Nellie*' Brocklehurst, as per the respective birth and the marriage certificate names of my parents, but for some unknown reason, 'Frank and *Helen*'. This potentially serious anomaly not only threatened to derail our nominally 'agreed' application for the Deferred Loan, but also brought into question whether Mum (Nellie) was even the rightful *owner* of the property that she had lived in for over 60 years! Accordingly, the County Council required us to consult, and then appoint, (on the 15th of Dec. 2016), a local solicitor to *officially* act as go-between for us with the County Council and the Land Registry on this quite bizarre legal matter; and it took 4 *long bureaucratic months,* to finally untangle and resolve the problem to the ultimate satisfaction of all interested parties; and that, in the end, largely boiling down to my *own* amateur, and wholly flukish, 'gumshoe' efforts.

With the matter long unresolved, and little movement apparent at any official level, and by a stroke of sheer good fortune, whilst browsing nostalgically, but not expectantly, through a couple of old biscuit tins of fading old paperwork that I found tucked away in the bottom drawer of the dressing table in Mum's (and Dad's) bedroom, back at the family home, *I* was finally able to bring the matter to an acceptable closure, by identifying a particular solicitor's receipt, dated "Nov. 1953", and clearly for their initial mortgage deposit on the property that was about to become our family home; along with a couple of further receipts for the first two payments to the original, now long-gone, building society. Each of these receipts had been signed in the two names of Frank and *Nellie.* Armed with those, along with their marriage certificate in the same two names, and dated 1949, I was able to convince the Land Registry 'beyond reasonable doubt', that 'Helen' was an aberration, (of whom there was no other traceable record), and that Nellie and Helen were indeed one and the same person. That was still not quite the end of the matter, though, for, legally, the Land Registry could only accept a written 'Statutory Declaration', agreed, drawn up, and signed, by our *solicitor,* to that end. That required a *further* meeting with our 'legal eagle', our supplying of the relevant paperwork to 'prove' the case, and the solicitor's definitive acceptance of that evidence, and his subsequent Declaration letter being accepted at the Land Registry. Eventually, finally, and fully 4 months later, on the 17th of April, (2017), to be exact, the land on which the house stood (and therefore the property itself), was *confirmed* (in a phone call from said solicitor), as being officially 'registered' in the name of Nellie; and all the administrative paraphernalia that had effectively been 'put on hold' during the questioning of the validity of Mum's claim to be the owner of the property that she had lived in all her married life was 'returned to active service'; including the Deferred Loan that was finally and officially 'rubber stamped'!

So yes dear reader, and to repeat, as well as one of us visiting Mum each day at Maple Mount, and fretting about her on our *non-visiting* days, whilst keeping both a 'maintenance eye' on her still-empty property, and in daily touch with each other into the bargain, and whilst each of us were respectively trying to keep the merry-go-rounds of our own domestic lives going, we soon found ourselves being engulfed in a right royal administrative and financial 'snowstorm' of seemingly unavoidable *processes, procedures and legalities* too; some of them, as I say, peculiar to Mum and some common to all those going through such similar moves and changes. And, in order to just 'keep up' we had, of course, in the end, to instigate, and maintain, our own records. At times, it was like we had acquired a joint, but full-time and unpaid, secretarial job, and were taking on the whole of the relevant care, financial and legal establishment as well - the very agencies that we thought were supposed to be of help to us!

Luckily, my sister only worked part-time, whilst I'd been retired for a few years, and my brother just recently so, and between us we could, ultimately, free up the very considerable amounts of time required; whilst my siblings and I were also able to work well and discuss things together, and act either solely or in tandem as agreed and expedient, on Mum's behalf ; but for someone acting as a *sole* relative, and whilst in full-time work, not residing locally, or perhaps in serious *dispute* with other siblings or relatives, it could quite easily have become utterly overwhelming.

Meanwhile, back at the 'ranch' and with all that going on in the background...

Despite the staff's generally effusive early reports, it was soon clear to me that Mum was taking time to settle, and, (hardly surprising), appeared to be searching for some sort of reference point within her new setting to call her own; for a Routine and a sort of in-house base and mini-sanctuary within the 'Main Sitting Room', (where she was spending most of her day), where she could feel 'at home' and perhaps keep a few personal items to hand. To that end, Mum had soon laid claim to the same, slightly worn, pale-green-cloth-upholstered high-back chair, in the same corner of that 'Main Sitting Room'; to where she would consistently return, and appeared to feel a degree of familiarity and safety. She often claimed the adjacent small shelf to boot, for those personal items, (glasses, sweets, tissues, own cup, etc), and quickly came to guard both the chair and the shelf quite protectively; as that place to call her own amid the 'madding crowd' of so many knackered old brains and bodies; quite a few of whom, (usually with the help of their walking frames), were able to shuffle themselves slowly about the ground floor, but often without obvious or cognitive purpose, and apparently on 'autopilot', in the random search for somewhere else to alight for a while. With a half-indignant air of suspicion, Mum often said that she felt 'her' chair might be their destination and, if vacant, her prophecy often came to be fulfilled. Perhaps predictably then, she came to vacate it less and less. But it gave *me* a vital insight into how Mum was perceiving, and dealing with, the challenges of her new, shared, unprecedented, and much-changed 'home' environment.

So, in no time at all, that was where I was pretty much guaranteed to find her, (usually half-asleep, in the supposedly age-appropriate, necessarily warm, breezeless, and, with the exception of the small conservatory, light-limited, ambience that prevailed), whenever I visited.

In the early stages, she would usually respond enthusiastically and appreciatively to the recognition and stimulation that my arrival, and gentle touches and intonations, evoked. If I then managed to persuade her to come out with me, for example, (as I usually did), and she found someone else in 'her' chair on our return, she would initially insist that I remove them personally. When I tried to explain why I couldn't do so, she would become noticeably anxious and even indignant, and, on occasion, would crossly suggest that I 'didn't care' about her. So, despite her degree of Dementia, (and unlike most of the other *lost* 'inmates'), she still 'knew' that *her* 'space' had been invaded. I would then feel obliged to stay there longer and comfort her. On those occasions, I usually tried to usher her into the conservatory where a lighter and airier tone, and a more refreshing view of Maple Mount's small garden, might provide my best chance of briefly 'distracting' her with the sights and sounds of the flora and fauna beyond the glass panes; but only so long as 'her' chair remained within sight, and only until it was eventually vacated (say by the discomfited occupant needing to be taken to the loo); whereupon Mum would immediately struggle to her feet and insist on re-taking what she saw as her 'rightful' place back in 'her' chair, and in 'her' corner. Only then would she settle sufficiently to let me finally leave.

Over time, the more aware staff would attempt to save us this 'returning' agony by trying to free up her chair just before we were due back from any outing, and I was certainly most grateful to them for that!

Almost from the 'off', I noticed that, though the 'inmate' membership did occasionally change, the vast majority continued to have two things in common. They were both physically elderly (say 70+ to a tad over 90), with an associated degree of infirmity, and almost without exception, functioning, mentally, with a readily notable degree of Dementia, as a minimum. It also seemed pretty obvious, from the pills that I observed being served, that most, if not all, were on prescribed medication, (including, I suspected, the 'sedating' likes of the sodium valproate, for example), so rarely fully awake or aware, and not therefore approachable for *any* rational, or reliable, let alone lengthy, conversation. Indeed, Mum was probably among the top 3 or 4 for still showing any degree of real awareness and I quickly learned that even one of those 3 or 4 was already 'on notice' to quit. Like Mum, he too seemed beset by mainly *short-term* memory loss, and, (according to his committed, and regularly-visiting, wife), he had been deemed to have shown an unacceptable level of aggression to at least one member of staff. Accordingly, some four weeks after Mum's arrival, I arrived to find this elderly man was no longer in residence; my discreet enquiries revealing that the guy had indeed been 'relocated' elsewhere in the town. (In fairness, this appeared to be a 'one-off' during Mum's time there, but it hinted at what was possible for those that threatened trouble; and whilst other 'departures' did occur, and at quite regular intervals, all those that followed thereafter directly reflected ill-health or 'end-of-life' issues. (i.e. either periods of ill-health requiring an 'inmate's hospitalisation, or, sadly, reflecting their passing).

To be honest, I'd always suspected that Care Homes for the elderly in particular, and most 'closed' communities in general, (and there was no obvious reason to exclude Maple Mount), with their ever-ready potential for hygiene issues for their oft-dependent and essentially 'incarcerated' residents, were classically ripe breeding and collecting areas for bugs and viruses, and therefore further ill-health developments, and it wasn't long before my theory was put personally to the test, as *Mum* was inaugurated into the 'bug club'.

I arrived one Saturday in mid-November, at my usual early afternoon time, to find that Mum was not in her chair, and, indeed, was nowhere to be seen. On this occasion, as fate would have it, I'd actually been let in by another visitor who just happened to be leaving as I arrived, rather than by a member of the busy 'other-wise-engaged' staff, and had also chosen to by-pass the closed door of the office, rather than knock and seek an advance update, and instead made my way directly along the corridor to the 'Main Sitting Room', and to 'Mum's chair'. As usual, I'd sneaked a peek from the door jamb, to see if she was anything other than 'nodding'; because the staff insisted that she was *often* more active than I (or my siblings) always seemed to find her. However, on this occasion Mum's chair was actually filled by another resident, and her absence there, or elsewhere, had quickly fuelled my anxiety; and it wasn't long before Annie-May had sought me out to confirm my suspicions. Mum was actually in that downstairs bedroom reserved for supervising any 'poorly' residents, and I was advised by Annie-May that she had a chest infection, and that, being a Saturday, the on-duty '*locum*' doctor had been summoned from afar, and was en route. Annie-May escorted me through to where Mum was abed, and propped up on 3 pillows. She immediately recognised me, and managed to raise a weary, rather resigned, smile. She did look tired, (when *didn't* she, these days?), but didn't seem unduly poorly, though she was indeed harbouring a spasmodic, audibly-raspy, and clearly discomforting chesty cough. She was happy to sip water, but, according to Annie-May, had no appetite, and had eaten little; and no amount of persuasion from me made Mum any keener to eat now. Then, just as I started to worry that a worsening of an 'old' diagnosis (of 2014), of 'diffuse pulmonary fibrosis', might be at the root of her latest infection, and might be putting her at increased 'risk', the door-bell rang. Annie-May departed, and was soon ushering in the locum doctor.

Once again, I wasn't overly impressed with how things looked to be going with this latest, and apparently 'nomadic', medic. For, after taking a few standard 'readings', with his stethoscope, and with his blood-pressure gear, etc. and despite my advising him of her significant Dementia from the 'off', he naively began to ask Mum questions to which the answers were almost certainly going to be unreliable, (not just by way of an 'inclusive' bed-side manner, but actually appearing to expect fully-remembered, fully-accurate answers - about when she'd last eaten, and what, or been to the loo, for example) - before proposing that, (once again 'to be on the safe side'), she be taken to hospital 'for tests'.

It was at this point that I felt obliged to remind him once more that Mum's answers were almost certainly unreliable, and, on Mum's behalf, to point out how previous hospital admissions to purely 'medical' wards had further confused and worsened her cognition, and I argued strongly for the chest infection to be given the chance to respond to the familiarity and lack of disruption that in-house treatment at Maple Mount might offer. Luckily, Annie-May took pity on me, and concurred, saying that she felt her staff could manage such an option, and between us we persuaded the locum that Mum was not 'at death's door', and to go down that in-house route. Thankfully, he prescribed a course of antibiotics, (predictably) advised Annie-May to contact the GP on the Monday if the condition persisted, and left. I breathed the heaviest sigh of relief, and consoled myself that I had managed to save Mum from another desperately disruptive and almost certainly unnecessary hospital admission. (It was a 'one-off', and I would never manage to do so again!).

Thankfully, I was proved right though, and she recovered within a day or so, and then remained (relatively) healthy through Christmas, the New Year's onset, and even beyond her 91st birthday at the end of January. Indeed, we were able to share in her apparent, if limited, sing-song enjoyment of the talents of a hired guitarist-singer of old 60's songs at Maple Mount's Christmas 'party', and, just over a month later, had even agreed to share the costs with Maple Mount for the hiring of another karaoke-type singer, this time of 'old' music-hall songs, for Mum's 91st birthday 'party', and for the inclusive benefit of *all* the residents; and, on both occasions, a pleasant, (if limited) amount of a 'slow, slow, never quick, slow' supported shuffle that passed for dancing, and of the imbibing of sherry and cake, took place; and good times appeared to be had by quite a few!

During that relatively (and the *most*) settled period at Maple Mount, 'routine' was essentially back at the forefront of my thinking. So, once again, Mum was being visited every day by at least one of her offspring, and for a minimum of 2 hours. My siblings covered the visiting on the Sunday, Monday, Wednesday and Friday, between them, whilst, as I say, I had attempted to reinstate *my* Tuesday, Thursday, and Saturday afternoons to as near parity as possible; invariably spent, to reiterate, with a general drive round familiar local places, (including past a house in which she had lived for over 60 years, but to which she had somehow become 'frightened' of entering), before finally alighting at the local branch of Aldi, one of 2 parks or a cafe, (depending on the weather), and the local Tesco supermarket, respectively; and invariably capping each off with that brief 'wheeled' visit to Dad's grave, (and, if time and weather allowed, those of her own much-loved mother, and other once-valued relatives and friends) - so as varied, yet as familiar and as stimulating, as I could possibly make it, given Mum's real and creeping physical and mental limitations.

In the beginning, and for some time hence, Mum seemed to enjoy all of our outings. She took little motivating, and seemed to relax quickly in my familiar company, and freed from the perceived boundaries and 'expectations' of her shared new 'home'. There were still definite glimpses of the fun Mum and playful personality

I used to know; still hiding *in*, yet still hidebound *by*, the cranial confusion. She just seemed to enjoy the 'open', restriction-free, chance to converse with me, the personal and trusted reassurance, the steady stimulation of her senses by the places we (re)visited at leisure, the simple partaking of a shared cuppa or ice-cream, and the familiarity of places that triggered 'old' memories; but, over time, and certainly towards Spring, fighting her tiredness, (and, I suspect, the sedation), meant the motivation for getting her out began to take just that little bit longer; whilst, once out, her concentration and stamina would increasingly begin to waver and wane the more, and her sense of frustration would nearly always kick-in towards the end; usually, when faced with her continued inability to resolve her mental battles, and to successfully confront, and 'fill in', the 'gaps' in her recent (short-term) memory. By the end of Spring, and post-Easter, then, this, in combination with her chronic and ongoing *physical* pain and limitations, could be almost guaranteed to wear her down to the point where eventually, and wherever we went, she would usually end up lamenting, stoically, and with evident awareness, (especially as I loaded her into the wheelchair that she hated being both dependent *on*, and being seen out in public *in*), something along the lines of "Eeee - I never thought I'd end up like this".

To lighten the mood, my response was invariably a gentle tease that asked what she *did* think she'd be doing at 91 - "Climbing Everest?", "Playing centre-forward for Manchester United?", and "Running the London marathon?", were among my stalwarts here. And any of these were likely to bring a brief smile to her face, but it rarely displaced her underlying lament, for her lost years, and especially her lost health and mobility, and would often cue her to add, rather pathetically, "I never did now't t' nobody"; as if simply trying to be a good person all her life should somehow qualify her for an entirely pain-free end and exit from her 'Maker'. It was as if she couldn't quite understand why the (Catholic) God she had believed in (and feared) all her life would, in the end, let her suffer so - but she always accepted that He had a reason, and I never once heard her question her own faith in Him.

On irregular occasions, just for a change, or a treat, we'd venture to the other side of town, and for tea and a scone or something at the cafe of the newish M&S food-store, or even further out to take similar at a local Garden Centre. In both those less-familiar settings, it was as if she felt we'd gone a little more 'off-piste' and 'upmarket', and would absolutely insist on struggling in on my arm, and on her "own two feet", regardless of the real pain and discomfort being generated, rather than be seen entering such establishments in her wheelchair. Once again, despite the ('short-term') nature of her Dementia, a significant element of her ingrained self-respect, and indeed some degree of cognition, seemed to be still at work and in attendance. Alas, none of this ever seemed to help in returning Mum to Maple Mount.

Wherever we were, and whenever I suggested it was time to 'take her home', the conversation, and her immediate reaction, was pretty predictable. Firstly, she would ask if I was taking her to her *own* home. Then, when I explained for the umpteenth time that she was now living at Maple Mount, and that was where we were heading, she would ask me if anyone *knew* her there, and whether she would "be alright" there, as if going for the very first time, and would start to get anxious that she would not "fit in there"; even though, with the onset of Spring, say, she had been in residence for around 6 months. Of course, she would always receive my most carefully-worded reassurances as necessary.

To more poignantly illustrate this cognitive deficiency, let me recall the February occasion, whilst rolling Mum round Tesco's, in her wheelchair, when we bumped into an off-duty member of the Maple Mount staff whom Mum should have known well. The woman was shopping with her small daughter, and began to chat to Mum as if she knew her well, (which of course she did), but Mum completely failed to recognise, let alone make any meaningful connection with, the woman, and apart from the odd polite and accommodating smile and nod here and there, she just looked on vacantly throughout; and as soon as we set off down our separate aisles, she insisted on asking me who it was.

So, her raised anxiety at the thought of returning to Maple Mount was unlikely to be because she feared something in particular there, but more likely because of the complete lack of recollection of anything specific associated with it - until we got there.

Just to try and understand even a tad, I used to compare it loosely to the anxiety we all get when confronting the 'unknown' for the first time; say, when starting a new job on the very first day, or arriving on day 1 at our new house or foreign holiday destination.

One potentially and particularly awkward response in such anxiety-raising situations, was to cause Mum to need the loo, and after a couple of early, and *very* awkward, encounters, (through which, by the way, I came to realise that the Maple Mount management unilaterally took it upon themselves to fit the bulk of their residents, including Mum, with incontinence pads as standard; this, my enquiries revealed, was to 'safeguard' the hygiene of the residents, their home environment, and it's furnishings, as a priority), I was required to become passably skilled at escorting her in this dreaded, inelegant, unenviable, yet very basic and personal need whilst out in the community! (In her more independent, 'compos mentis', days of but a handful of years ago, like most of us, her sheer embarrassment at such a prospect would have consigned the notion to 'unimaginable'!)

Back in the 'early days', when the issue first cropped up, I had given it not an iota of pre-thought; and when it first presented, ("Keith, I need the toilet", I remember her whispering anxiously, as she sat beside me in her local Tesco's cafe, and started tapping fretfully at my arm), it still did so as so *very* awkward (for both mother and son), for the latter to be required to help toilet the former; especially in an untested public place. So much so that it subsequently crossed my mind to 'play safe' in future, to *not* take the risk, and to *not* take her out at all, (an option I knew my siblings' anxieties had often persuaded them to follow here); but, deep down, I knew that, for *me*, the answer was not to deny us either the stimulus, the familiarity or the pleasure, (and what I therefore saw as the obvious benefits), of our outings, but instead to find acceptable solutions to *managing* the problem. And so, by thinking it through, by a sort of trial and error, and, of course, by talking to the Maple Mount staff, it quickly dawned on me that I needed to be absolutely sure that Mum had been taken to the toilet by a member of staff, fully 'emptied', and fitted with a fresh 'pad', and that I'd packed appropriate 'spares', before I ever left Maple Mount with her; though even that ground- work never guaranteed anything, of course. So, I also researched our likely venues and destinations more thoroughly, (Tesco's, M&S, the local cafe, and Garden Centre), to ensure that we were never going to be far from sites that had loos suitable for the disabled should I have urgent need of them!

These simple 'solutions' may seem obvious to those 'in the know', but when you start out on this 'road', as a hopeful, enthusiastic, well-meaning, fresh-faced, naive, 'newbie', (just like you might do in your new job, or at your new house or foreign holiday destination), you don't really 'know the ropes' properly, and end up learning many of them 'on the job', don't you? And so it was here.

Soon though, and with the aforementioned pre-planning, I was able to manage both our invariably pleasant outings and the usually anxious 'returns' relatively competently, until the Spring and beyond; the 'returns' always better facilitated once I'd made arrangements for a reassuring member of staff to meet us at the front door, and re-welcome her, warmly and personally, by name. From there, we would all enter together, and in no time at all it was as if she'd somehow re-entered a previous 'present moment' - cue the customary 'chair dance'!

By the time she was safely ensconced back in 'her chair', though, the accompanying experiences and sensations of our outings, (including any lingering feelings of awkwardness regarding toileting and the likes), often appeared to have largely dissipated; and sometimes to no longer carry any recallable effect or clout of significance. For a while, Mum might still seem vaguely aware that something had just taken place, but, often, the detail had simply disappeared; almost as if those specific sensations had never been experienced; as if she'd never been to Tesco's or the like. Obviously, these outings had taken place. I was there. For Mum though, the experience somehow seemed to have been locked away somewhere in that part of her brain that no longer *released* the detail of such short-term stuff to her; and whatever had gone on 'out there', be it for good or ill, that detail appeared to have only occurred at the time - in *that* present moment - for Mum.

Once back at Maple Mount, and once back in 'her chair', she was back in the twilight, labyrinthine world of both her Dementia and the shared physical setting, and, encumbered by an increasingly dependent body, was back struggling to make sense of the still relatively recent, still relatively unfamiliar, and always subtly changing, comings and goings of the 'world' of the Care Home.

Of course, and especially on later occasions, especially when Mum seemed truly tired (perhaps fighting sedation) or 'under the weather', and couldn't or wouldn't be persuaded out, when the outside weather was against us anyway, or perhaps when 'eye-catching' in-house 'entertainment' was to hand, we might opt/'be forced' to 'stay home'. Those were the devious occasions when, despite my reservations about Care Homes in general, 2-hour confinements, and the subsequent shared experiences and enforced interactions with both the staff and the inescapable residents, meant that certain 'bonds' and relationships were unknowingly forming regardless; and the increasingly-familiar personalities of both were slowly having their formative effect on *me*.

To be fair, Maple Mount usually had some sort of pre-planned 'entertainment' on offer on each weekday afternoon for the 'inmates'; plus tea and biscuits *every* mid-afternoon. (The former tended to be on the weekdays because more staff tended to be on duty then). And of course the TV was an easy and ever-present fallback 'entertainer'.

Again, to be fair, the 'entertainment' could be quite varied, and included those occasional, bought-in, singers, (mainly on 'special' days, say when it was someone's birthday, or at Christmas), a regular (usually weekly) piano-playing local woman, another woman that came fortnightly to offer the residents gentle arm, leg, foot and shoulder massages with various oils, and a variety of musical, simple quiz, drawing 'themed',(usually with crayons or coloured pencils, like you did at early primary school), and other ad hoc offerings conjured up, in-house, by the whims and varying abilities of the loyal staff.

Alas, and despite these gallant efforts, only a handful of 'inmates' tended to have the ability or motivation to take part for long, if at all. Apart from a valiant few 'triers', (which, with a little coaxing and support, usually included Mum), most tended to remain only minimally responsive to, or completely ignore, the gentle cajoling of the staff, and continued to slip in and out of their various, often involuntary, stages of 'rest'. So, staying in was still usually something of a rather disheartening, rather downbeat, 'last resort' for me.

Amongst other, and more specific, in-house *drawbacks* for me, I should add, was the apparent ease with which Mum's (and presumably other 'inmates') personal *belongings* went missing; in particular her false teeth, prescription glasses and personal laundry; triggering the eventual need for us to 'room-check' and 'stocktake' regularly regarding the latter. (In the end, and from around late November, my brother and his wife agreed to actually take much of Mum's washing home with them to try and improve, if not resolve, the latter). Then there was the barely-changing, 'zombie-like', status and moanings of a handful of the saddest, most incapacitated 'inmates', the inevitable and literally demented ramblings of so many of the rest, and the short length of time before a personal leakage nearby could be guaranteed to fill my nostrils with the unmistakable whiff of urine etc, and trigger the (not always instant) arrival and involvement of the necessary 'tools', 'machinery' and personnel to take the (often unaware) culprit for a bout of appropriate 'cleansing'.

Whilst it might often be quaintly amusing to see another 'inmate' shuffle by in an item of Mum's clothing, (say her cardigan, blouse or skirt), losing Mum's teeth and/or glasses had potentially immediate effects, and was a particularly irksome issue. I can recall at least half a dozen occasions when one or the other, and usually both items, had gone missing, leaving either myself or one of my siblings to find a toothless, gummy, mummy at various stages of awareness, or not, of the missing 'basics'. Of course,

Mum never knew why she had been left so, or where the said items might be, so urgent enquiries of the *staff* had to be made. *Their* first response was always that they had looked "high and low" around the Mount, but had hitherto failed to unearth the missing item(s), that the search was ongoing, and that they were "sure" they would "turn up sooner or later". The slightly blasé way in which they appeared to handle the matter always suggested that it was a regular occurrence amongst the 'inmates' in general; but to members of an 'inmate's' family, it was often of singular, personal, and therefore more than minor, concern. In Mum's case, for example, it could have major implications for her levels of anxiety, and therefore management, for her practical ability to eat and drink, (anything other than 'thin', soup-like, stuff), to see anything close up, and, in my case, for whether she would be willing, or *I* would think it practical, to go out to eat; or go out at all; and if so, where. Sometimes the items were missing for a couple of days but eventually, as the staff knew, the said item(s) would be located. For example, her glasses were once found deep down the side of her own, and once when she'd been temporarily re-located at some point, another, chair; (along with old tissues, sweet-wrappers and similar, potentially-lurking sources of infection!). Her teeth on the other hand often turned up in the *most* unexpected places. For example, there was the occasion where they'd somehow managed to slip into the lining of one of her skirts, before it had been packed for washing, and the occasion when they were eventually found in the dressing-gown pocket of *another* 'inmate', in another bedroom, and who had presumably purloined them, either intentionally, or otherwise.

Yet further potentially embarrassing downsides to staying in were that it was almost impossible to avoid those more irrational, eccentric, compromising and unsolicited contacts and interactions with the more mobile 'inmates'. For example, they were prone to shuffle up close to you, and, even if you were *seated* in their vicinity, would touch your face or arm, sometimes try to hold or stroke your hand, and might well, in their confusion, tell you, a little disarmingly, that they 'loved' you. Sometimes, however, they were trying to get the (equally-compromising) attention of the rational, kind-hearted, but unsuspecting, visitor in the expectation of gaining their more practical, unofficial, and nearly always inappropriate, "help". For instance, 2 or 3 of the 'inmates' would regularly ask me (and I presume others), to take them "home". (Mostly they meant to a previous address that they had lived at, but sometimes they were actually requesting to come home with *me*). On the other hand, many, (perhaps mistaking visitors like me for staff, but more likely just not too fussy), asked me to take them to the toilet, (obviously inappropriate), or to take them to the front door and let them out of Maple Mount altogether, (equally inappropriate); or might just look dolefully into my eyes and utter what amounted to some kind of incomprehensible gibberish akin to 'talking in tongues', just to give some sort of focus and vent to their jumbled thoughts, or simply to have someone's extended personal attention for a while.

Only Mum and one other 'inmate' appeared to have *daily* visitors, just a very few 'inmates' appeared to have regular visitors, (say more than twice a week), quite a few appeared to have only limited ones, (say weekly), and some sad souls, alas, appeared to get no noticeable visitors at all.

In the face of all that, Mum barely moved from the 'defence' and 'safety' of her chair whenever I was indoors with her, presented her quiet, unassuming and biddable self, with a ready, if sometimes 'vacant', smile, and was invariably among the more easily managed; just a bit slow, and confused, and on occasion depressed and noticeably frustrated, about why she couldn't break through those barriers to her missing short-term memory!

Amongst the few *positives* to 'staying in' was that free 'entertainment', the decent, good-humoured, well-meaning staff, those free tea and biscuits, the chance to meet and 'compare notes' with other 'inmates' visitors, and if lucky, and in the cook's 'good books', the occasional offer of a tasty but 'surplus to requirements' portion of the (always attractive) dinner that the residents had enjoyed earlier!

So, on the whole, I *was* generally keen for both Mum and myself to 'break free', and visit 'the real world' for a while, whenever possible.

As for the nights, apart from a couple of early 'settling-in' issues, whatever was happening up there still tended to remain largely unspoken/unknown, and rarely came into our conversation, via either Mum or staff; and when I did occasionally enquire of the latter, I tended to elicit the same, safe, second-hand, (the day staff were only able to report anything that the 2 night staff had logged), and catch-all "she slept well" response. That couple of reported 'exceptions'(?) were one very early occasion when they advised that Mum had been found propping open the bedroom door, and then occasionally wandering on the landing, (perhaps looking for the loo or the like in her strange new surroundings?), and another when they reported that 'Martha', her 'room-mate', had actually got into bed with Mum for a cuddle, in an apparent search for close 'comfort' and 'company'. The night staff were deemed to have dealt sensitively, supportively and appropriately with each situation, and on each occasion had reported no significant distress shown by Mum; and no further episodes of either. Otherwise, and in the absence of any evidence to the contrary, and, of course, feedback from Mum, who would most certainly have forgotten any concerns well before we arrived, we had no option but to presume that such incidents *were* 'one-offs', and to accept that she probably had 'slept well' enough most nights.

Anyway, Mum too was soon very much an 'inmate' here, and, sadly, becoming ever-more dependent, in a necessarily warm, soft-lit, slow-moving, sleep-inducing, (probably sedated) environment where time sometimes seemed to have almost ground to a halt; but where a sort of visiting 'routine' had nevertheless been pretty well established for her by her committed offspring; and for the latter to manage; and so it went on, until:

CHAPTER 7

"Am I Going To Be Alright?" (Hospitalisation)

The 'writing was on the wall' when Mum was initially admitted to hospital, from the Care Home, some weeks *earlier*; in fact, in *June* of that year. (2017). On that occasion a *chest* infection, and a noted deterioration in her breathing, had been the focus of the Care Home's, and then the GP's, concern. On the day in question, the home had contacted my older brother, by telephone, as per agreement, to update him, and advise that an ambulance had been duly summoned to take Mum to hospital.

Once made aware that Mum had been so 'dispatched', we 3 siblings dropped what we were doing, and hastened there, individually; and were soon gathered round a hospital trolley, in the corridor at A & E, to offer our confused Mum full support. (Not just by our still *recognisable* physical presence, and our familiar voices, but also psychologically, via our oft- repeated explanations and reassurances in response to her all too predictable but nonetheless regular, "Where am I?", "What's wrong with me?", and "Am I going to be alright?" questions).

A&E was predictably busy, with patients aplenty, and hospital staff scurrying hither and thither, and Mum was initially held for quite some time on that trolley in the corridor; with triage prioritisation and processing predictably deeming her non-urgent; but, thanks to the Dementia, and ironically, Mum wasn't really aware of just how long the wait would be. Eventually though, with the wait approaching an hour, she was allocated one of the single-bedded cubicles, and after being installed there for perhaps twenty minutes, (with nurses coming and going, and setting up pillows, drips etc.; and re-asking basic questions that we thought we'd answered umpteen times already), Mum began to settle in her bed. Then, just when she'd got comfortable, and her anxiety and breathing was lowering slightly, a porter arrived, and she (in her bed) was trundled off for an X-ray (my sister accompanying her for continued reassurance); and duly returned perhaps twenty minutes later, to said cubicle; and efforts to resettle her were soon in progress again. Eventually, the young Indian doctor dealing with her case came to offer his prognosis. He'd presumably had sight of the X-rays, and he suggested that her pre-existing, but non-urgent, diagnosis of Pulmonary Fibrosis (a condition first diagnosed in 2014, but not considered serious enough for, or likely to be improved by, major and/or intrusive surgery/ treatment at my Mum's then late-80s age), was being subjected to added pressures and complications from an assault by a *new* viral lung infection. She was to be admitted, and was started (with an injection) on a course of antibiotic treatment; and with Mum getting irritable, we were all left to wait a further hour or so whilst a bed was identified on the MAU ward (Medical Assessment 1 Unit).

Once identified, and made ready, Mum, in her A&E bed, was trundled off down further corridors, with her entourage of loyal offspring in tight, reassuring, bedside attendance. Then, barely seconds after her arrival there, and during her initial installation, she suddenly launched into a severe coughing bout, and brought up an inordinate amount of thick yellow phlegm, just as she was being tucked up in bed. Luckily the deluge was caught in a spare sheet destined for the laundry, by the attendant nurse, and the bed did not have to be remade.

During a brief, (3-night), stay on the MAU, (and despite her Dementia limitations, for which little allowance seemed to be made on this, or any other, essentially 'medical' unit), Mum had managed to respond well to the antibiotics, and this latest infection was actually deemed 'treated'. We were informed accordingly by the medical staff, and she was summarily discharged, again by ambulance, back to the Care Home and all seemed (relatively, and *medically)* settled again.

Then, less than a month later, on Friday, the 14th of July to be precise, Mum was again deemed 'poorly', by the Care Home staff, and after they had again consulted the GP, much the same reaction and protocol ensued. That is, Mum was re-referred to the same hospital's A&E ward, (again being ferried there by summoned ambulance); this time with a suspected *urine* infection. Again we siblings were soon by her side.

This time, alas, and though we had not the slightest inkling at the time of re-referral, there would be no early discharge, and, indeed, no recovery. This time, she would not leave alive.

Again, a similar procedure to her last (June)admission followed, and after another lengthy wait on a trolley in the corridor of A&E, she was allocated another cubicle, and 'tests' and x-rays followed. This time, the GP's early suspicion of a *urine* infection was further reinforced when that was relayed to us as the likely cause of Mum's problems by the young junior doctor on duty here; and once again she was admitted onto the MAU ward for 'treatment' with antibiotics; where, tired and drained by all the 'toing and froing' of the long day, she finally gave in and nodded off. It was after 9pm by now, and equally tired and drained, we all headed wearily to our respective homes, just relieved that Mum was now asleep, and safely tucked up in a hospital bed, where she would, hopefully, be receiving the very best care and attention.

The next day, (Saturday) I returned to the MAU, at the official 2-00pm visiting time, to begin what would become my standard, daily, two-hour, (minimum), afternoon visiting stint.

Apart from a general confusion about her situation, and from her ongoing Dementia issues, (and ensuing and repeated questions about where she was, and why, and for which, once again, NO obvious extra allowance seemed to be made, on this essentially 'medical' ward), Mum was clearly in some significant additional *physical* discomfort. She was clearly anxious, and was moaning, and occasionally writhing in significant rectal distress, with what appeared to be acute constipation. Mum managed to *confirm* this as the source of her discomfort.

As became my equally standard practice whenever I arrived on a ward to see Mum, I looked round that ward for appropriate professional help and advice, and to seek out information/ updates from the busy and sparse ward staff - usually one of the nursing *auxiliaries* (the least qualified, and usually identifiable, I came to realise, by the *lightest* of the parade of blue nursing uniforms), in the first instance. (This small number of generally willing workers appeared to be the frontline 'dogsbodies' of the ward, and to not only dish out the food, and some non-prescriptive medication, but also to attend to most of the personal, routine, 'bog-standard', and often messy, nursing and hygiene tasks for their respective ward's patients).

Eventually, I managed to attract the attention of one of these very busy souls, as she was scurrying by in her clear-plastic apron. She confirmed that Mum was indeed struggling with a bout of acute constipation, adding that she had recently been given an enema, (an injection of liquid into the rectum, to try to free up and expel its reluctant contents); which, time duly elapsing, would hopefully bring about the required relief. Without me yet being aware of, or therefore raising, the issue, this same nursing auxiliary advised that this same problem was also likely to be the cause of Mum's limited intake of food so far that day. Then off she shot, and I was again left alone with Mum, (and with her still obvious discomfort), to try and both occupy and distract her, whilst the enema did its work; and the auxiliary spent some of her precious time attending to patients with equally pressing needs elsewhere on the ward.

It was during my (largely fruitless) efforts to reassure Mum, and to keep her calm, amidst her ongoing constipational pain, repeated worry that she was in impending danger of embarrassing herself by soiling the bed, now standard, Dementia-lead, confusion about where she was, and why, and her regular vocal requests for a nurse, and for "help", that Mum made the first of a pair of sudden, and quite startling, claims that, "I'm going to die today"!

Her death was not (yet) being even remotely *contemplated*, (at any level), let alone imminent, and, as on her previous admission, I was still (naively?) expecting her to return to the Care Home after her 'brief' period of in-patient treatment; so I had genuinely (and yes, naively) been able to offer her further Reassurance to that end, and to implore her not to worry. (Perhaps, however, she'd had some sort of premonition, as her death would turn out to be but a couple more weeks away!). Regardless, her utterance had come completely out of the blue. What on earth had invaded her mind, to make her blurt out *that* heart-rending assertion, and at that particular moment - and then again a few minutes later, despite my attempted ministrations?

As the enema eventually got round to working its dragged-out magic, and after our auxiliary had returned for a third time to check on its progress, I was eventually asked to vacate the bedside, and wander aimlessly elsewhere on the ward, as an additional auxiliary was enlisted, and the bedside curtains were slowly drawn around Mum's bed, to exclude me. Clearly, there was further medical/ rectal 'jiggling' going on in the now curtained bed-space, as more of Mum's discomforted moans and groans emanated from behind; but, (like Mafeking) Mum's constipation was eventually relieved!

As I waited and wandered outside on the main body of the ward, alternately casting a, probably intrusive, but essentially idle, and neutral, eye over the rest of the ward, and the other patients there, and looking equally idly through one of the rear windows nearby, to some far hills beyond, the clues were suddenly there; not just in Mum's audibly expressed relief, but particularly through the ginormous *stink* that leaked out through the drawn curtains. As I was taught to write at the end of so many of my school chemistry experiments, all those years ago, 'a pungent odour was given off'; and this time, it was retchingly caught by my usually poor nasal detectors! Poooey! (Phew, these 'dogsbody' auxiliaries don't half earn their pittance).

Then, suitably relieved, re-dressed and yet barely resettled, and just half an hour later, Mum, and her bed, were on the move again. She was being moved elsewhere; and with me scurrying along, and holding her hand for succour and reassurance, amid Mum's further disruption and confusion, and with one of the auxiliaries and a sole porter to hand, she was trundled away by the latter - off the MAU ward, down corridors, round corners, over a link bridge, and finally up in a long, thin, lift, apparently *designed* for such a trollied purpose, to arrive at the doors of a locked Ward 31, level 5, of another 'medical' block.

Our auxiliary appeared to have a pass to gain entrance, and on we went. The main corridor on Ward 31 was quite wide, and designed with a line of (about 8) 4-bed units/ mini-wards immediately down the right as you entered, with a similar space half-way down for the quiet/ rest room, (we wouldn't realise that there were just a few *single* rooms still further down on the right until quite some time later; when it would become all too obvious why!), and with offices, patients' toilets, small kitchen for basics, a nurses' station, and other service rooms down the left.

Mum and her mobile bed were carefully trundled down the main corridor, before being installed in the vacant, right-sided, space labelled for 'bed 14', in the 4th mini-ward down; where it became the first bed on the left as one entered. The other 3 patients there seemed to be elderly and female too, and each and all seemed to be well into varying states of slumber.

At the other (the far) end of this small, 5th-floor, mini-ward, and facing at eye-level, were large, ward-long windows, which gave rise to a rather pleasant bucolic scene outside on the far horizon, and a light airy feeling *inside*. Rolling green hills dotted with odd bits, lines and clumps of darker, *leafed* greenery and the occasional serene-looking, stone-farm-house-like property, afforded a rather relaxing and easy-on-the-eye sight to new arrivals, and thus encouraged a sort of 'continued-contact-with-the outside-world' feel for both patients and visitors alike. So far so good.

With Mum and her bed duly installed, and the porter released to take up duties elsewhere, the auxiliary from the MAU and her counterpart on Ward 31, began to chat openly about the work and running of their respective wards. It was clear from both that they were hard-pressed and relatively new to the work; the latter openly, and rather indiscreetly, disclosing to all within earshot, that she had been previously running a local pub, and had only been working here as a nursing auxiliary for just 5 weeks.

The longer Mum remained in the hospital, the more it became clear to me, (from talking directly to the auxiliaries, watching them go busily about their work, and overhearing their various work-a-day conversations with other 'professionals' in my vicinity), that staff turnover and retention was a major problem (at least at this level), and that the one's that remained were often called on to do long, 12-hour, shifts - and then even some extra ones on their days off, at times of severe shortage. Indeed, throughout all of this essentially *medical* input and 'treatment', on this first and foremost *medical* ward, the staff, and indeed the doctors, when they appeared, seemed to change often; which hardly suggested an ideal recipe for *consistency* of care; and getting to speak to one of the latter at short notice *certainly* wasn't easy. Moreover, Mum's Dementia needs, (like others with similar mental limitations), appeared, once again, to remain largely tolerated, but to go, frankly, unadministered to, on any regular basis; and most certainly not by anyone claiming any particular Dementia training, understanding or specialism. Of course, there was no definitive medical *treatment* to offer, since Dementia remained essentially untreat*able,* in the sense of 'making it better', but simply tolerating it meant that my Mum remained less than fully aware of what was happening to her whilst on the ward and often, sometimes just *minutes* later, of what *had* happened to her. Ironically, yet again, her limited short-term memory probably helped her through here. (Thankfully, and consolingly, though, her longer-term memory ensured that she still continued to recognise and to know who we 3 siblings were on all of our visits - right up until and including the very end).

As I've suggested, and for my own convenience, I elected to take responsibility for visiting Mum each and every afternoon, whilst my siblings tended to cover all the evening shifts; unless one of us had truly pressing engagements elsewhere; in which case we organised a 'swap'. In theory, this gave ME the most likely chance of accessing the relevant medical staff during 'normal working hours'.

On the following day, the Saturday, I arrived to find some 'notes', with charts, attached to a blood-red plastic clipboard, and hung at the bottom of Mum's bed; but they gave little away to the average punter. An auxiliary told me that Mum had eaten only 'a few bran flakes' for breakfast, and sipped some water from a drinking cup during the day. She suggested that Mum might be constipated, and seemed completely unaware that her constipation had supposedly been tackled and relieved on the previous day. I asked to speak with the ward sister, (dark blue tunic), who arrived towards the end of my visit to advise that she too was unaware of the actions of the previous day's enema on the MAU. My request for the truth of it to be properly established, so that all the current ward's carers were 'singing from the same hymn- sheet', was noted.

On the Sunday, I arrived to find Mum asleep, still on an arm drip (of antibiotics?), and now fitted with a catheter (a see-through plastic bag, and a tube that apparently connected with her 'nether regions', in order to collect, and monitor, the rate, and state, of her passage of urine). Yet another different (dark blue tunic) ward sister confirmed that this *was* for 'monitoring' purposes; whilst a familiar auxiliary raised my hopes by claiming that Mum had eaten a little cottage pie and rice pudding for lunch; though there was no food chart amongst her notes to confirm this. My later enquiries to a 'staff nurse' (also dark blue, but slightly different shade and different design), drew her agreed need to attend to this, and to provide both a food and a 'stool' sheet. When I asked about the clarification of the enema's outcome on the MAU, I was again met with a rather blank look. Slightly frustrated, I asked if I might speak with a doctor to get some idea of how Mum's treatment was going in general, (no nursing staff, not even those in the darkest blue tunics, can make judgement on *clinical* matters; they can only pass on relevant points and requests made, to the busy doctor, whose job it *is* to advise on clinical matters). Again frustratingly, I was told that, as it was Sunday, there was NO doctor *available* to speak to me, anywhere in the hospital(!), and I made the nurse politely but firmly aware of my incredulity, disappointment and continued frustration here. Then, towards the end of my visit, and despite this claim of there being no doctor available onsite, one arrived unexpectedly at Mum's bedside. So there obviously WAS at least *one* on the premises, and he had been duly summoned because the nurse had couched my 'firm politeness' in terms of *a complaint*. He was another young Indian junior doctor, and though he wasn't normally attached to Mum's ward, or case, he did have access to her notes, and agreed to try to update me on Mum's current position. He took me off to a side room/office across the corridor, and a little further down, and there, having accessed a computer terminal, he officiously ran through the likely scenarios - and he was the first to even mention the possibility that Mum might NOT survive!

For a significant, and of course disturbing, part of his news and advice was that, clinically, *the urine infection* that Mum had been initially diagnosed with *may* now have been complicated further by the possible presence of the potentially life-threatening Sepsis bacteria. ("Also known as blood-poisoning", according to the Sepsis Trust, "it is the reaction to an infection in which the body attacks its own organs and tissues"; and according to the NHS Choices website "the most common sites of infection leading to Sepsis are the lungs, *urinary tract!*, abdomen and pelvis"). Hospital tests were ongoing for this, he insisted. He further advised that, at this stage, there was every hope that the one (and apparently only) form of treatment for this combo, a variety of courses of antibiotics, would be successful; but still made the point that if these failed there was no other viable treatment, and in consequence, that there was the risk that someone of Mum's age, with Dementia, might not have the necessary strength of immune system to fight these attacks, and to survive. He further advised, honestly, that the course of antibiotics that Mum was currently on was a 'bit of a best guess', and something of a 'holding' option, at this stage, whilst blood tests, for which blood had already been taken, had been sent to the microbiologist in the 'lab', to try and establish the *optimum* antibiotic to *best* fight her particular type of infections. Each of these courses of antibiotics, he further added, would require several days to do their work, before any conclusions could be properly drawn.

Not only was all this very relevant and starkly to the point, and truly shocking, in inviting us to now contemplate even the possibility of this finality, but it was also pretty obvious that Mum was not going to be 'sorted' quickly on this occasion, and her hospital stay would be significantly longer, and therefore more risky, than we had hoped. Of course, I hastily relayed this new and vital information to my siblings.

333

By the next day, Mum's breathing seemed a little more laboured, but she was certainly, if a little sleepily, aware of my presence. Gladdeningly, at the very outset of my visit, Mum had even been sufficiently alert to see me coming down the corridor, and the wide and lovely smile that had filled her face as I arrived bedside suggested that she was clearly pleased to see me. Alas, it was soon very obvious that she was no less Dementially confused about where she was, and why she was there, and during the usual round of reassurances, she quickly lost focus and tended towards sleepy again. Moreover, her breathing continued to be laboured, and she started to actually 'nod off'.

On the practical upside, the bedside charts now looked more comprehensive. The food chart had arrived, and now showed that she'd taken a little porridge for breakfast, and was drinking OK, but that she'd refused lunch, apart from a few spoonfuls of her favourite rice pudding. Today's auxiliary confirmed this. I was eventually able to discern from Mum's other 'notes' that she was now on a cocktail of drugs to compliment the course of antibiotics, too; including some to proffer appropriate pain relief. It would never be entirely clear to me, from here on in, if/whether/when/ how much, this 'cocktail' was affecting Mum's general moods or consciousness; as opposed to the effects of her infections and Dementia.

However, the pattern of my visits was already beginning to take on a frustratingly familiar look. On the next day, I was able to speak with a young female junior doctor, who had arrived, quite unsolicited, at Mum's bedside. She may just have been on her routine 'rounds', but up she popped. This junior doctor was of an Asian background, and a similar conversation to that already undertaken with her previous day's male colleague followed. This time though she spoke about our need to be prepared to consider palliative care versus tube feeding IF/when the various antibiotics had all been fully tried, and been found *not* to have worked. Once again, the possibility of my Mum not surviving was being ominously raised; and that broadly in proportion with my anxieties. This doctor confirmed that the 'lab' was still looking for the *optimum* antibiotic, gave Mum the 'once-over', and left to continue her 'rounds' on pastures new. Then 2 auxiliaries arrived to fit Mum's bed with an air-mattress. This, they advised, would help to prevent bed sores forming, as Mum was now spending nearly all her time in bed. (The slight downside being that Mum, and her visitors, would never again be entirely free from the quiet occasional 'hummm' of its' tiny motor starting up, unannounced, for short whiles, whenever the bed-pressure dropped).

A few days earlier, my adult daughter (Mum's granddaughter) had arrived home for the summer, from her primary school teaching post abroad. Of course, she was keen to be updated on her Gran, and then keen to visit her at some point. Despite my cautionary advice that 'Grandma' might not recognise her, and that my daughter might be upset by 'Grandma's' deterioration over recent weeks, my daughter continued to press her request to visit. So, on the Wednesday, (the 19th), I took my daughter along on my afternoon visit, but continued to advise her not to expect much by way of interaction. Coincidentally, my sister had also arranged to visit that afternoon, and having 'beaten us to it', Mum was awake, and quite alert. Amazingly, and even though she hadn't seen her for over 3 months, and despite the Dementia, Mum seemed to recognise my daughter straight away, and she greeted her with a lovely beaming smile before hugging her warmly. Even more encouraging, Mum's chart showed she had eaten some porridge for breakfast, and some cottage pie for lunch, and had been drinking 'under her own steam'. Still further, Mum's breathing seemed a little more even, and less laboured. Yet, and despite all this positivity, Mum kept asking, disconcertingly, and at regular intervals, "Am I going to be alright?", which rather took the edge of an otherwise lovely and very encouraging visit. Her repeated enquiries here suggested that while Mum appeared to be doing surprisingly well that day, the Dementia was still at large, and ensuring that she remained unsure and anxious.

She was right to be; even though the next day's visit was also quite encouraging. Mum was again awake to receive me that Thursday; though no less confused about where she was; and why. Her food chart also showed that she'd eaten most of her breakfast porridge and her rice pudding dessert at lunch, and was drinking water and tea fairly frequently, and still doing so 'under her own steam'. She even ate a digestive biscuit during my visit. Moreover, the catheter had been removed, and a new bag of antibiotic was infusing its contents into her left arm. The only real downside seemed to be that her ongoing confusion, due to her Dementia, continued to hold selective sway; but we had had two extremely encouraging days in a row now, and I was very hopeful that she was 'on the mend'. I may have been right at the time, but not for long - because it was slowly, unexpectedly, upsettingly, and almost entirely, downhill after that 2-day 'high'.

Friday, the 21st of July; not too bad a day either; except that Mum had apparently eaten very little that day, and seemed back to her more sleepy mode; though she surprised me by actually asking, "Can I go home?" on one occasion. I fielded this, and the usual questions about where she was, and why, with my usual patient explanations and calm reassurances, before she eventually nodded off.

So far, though, the early days on Ward 31 had given grounds for a reasonable degree of hopefulness and optimism. Mum was now eating a little; and then 'little and often'; admittedly with the help of the auxiliaries encouraging, and even spoon-feeding, her on a few of those occasions; and after that polite but firm 'enquiry' to the staff nurse (dark blue uniform), from us, details of her daily food and drink intake had begun making their way onto her 'end-of-bed' records sheets. However, with hindsight, these would turn out to be her last few days of genuine positivity, and to have actually been nothing more than a very, very, 'false dawn'.

Over the next few days she continued to show a slow deterioration; eating less and less, (and on one occasion, according to the auxiliary, violently vomiting up the little that she *had* ingested), and, alas, sleeping more and more, too. Then on the following Tuesday visit, I noted that Mum was having some difficulty in coordinating the simple holding and lifting movements necessary to drink 'under her own steam', and after discussion with the ward sister, it was agreed that her standard ceramic cup with a handle should be replaced for a while, by one of the hospital's blue plastic drinking cups with a 'spouted' plastic top, and *two* handles, similar to that used by babies. Mum immediately found this easier, and, henceforth, she would come to rely on it. Later on in that visit, I spoke to Dr. Anca, (her first name, and hereafter referred to as Dr. A), yet another new doctor; and from the badge hanging round her neck, this one was clearly a *locum* doctor. Her speech and her accent persuaded me that she was from an Eastern European country, and I had to ask her to repeat herself on several occasions, when I couldn't fully pick up what she was saying. I did manage to pick up, however, that she too agreed that there had been some deterioration in Mum's condition in recent days. Moreover, and both worryingly, and surprisingly, this doctor advised that Mum was now on yet *another* antibiotic. (Not first and foremost because it was necessarily better or more effective, but because the hospital had apparently *run out* of Tazocin, the optimum antibiotic supposedly recommended by the lab's microbiologist, after the blood test!). Nevertheless, Dr. A remained upbeat and reassuring, and was "very hopeful" that this latest antibiotic would perform just as well, if not better than the last, and would 'come to the rescue' for Mum. (Whilst the reason given for the change of antibiotic was a little disquieting, I could only take her word for it that the latest one *would* perform just as well).

On the following day's (afternoon) visit Mum was already asleep when I arrived. However, not deeply so, as I was able to wake her by simply whispering "Hello Mum" gently into her left ear to let her know that I was there. Her eyes flickered, and cracked open in response, and just the hint of a smile crossed her lips, but I wouldn't exactly say that she was fully awake; and certainly far from fully alert; whilst her speech seemed somewhat difficult and slurred. But she was eventually able tell me that her mouth was sore. I asked her to open her mouth, to show me, and with my gentle index-finger support she had a brave try.

My cursory inspection revealed that she was minus her false teeth, for starters, (that sallow-cheeked look always made her look worse than she might be), and that her tongue was generally very red, and not only looked sore, but suggested, in a couple of *darker* red, and coarser, spots, that it was beginning to sort of *scab* in a couple of forward places.

I was, of course, alarmed, and discreetly 'collared' the first of that day's available auxiliaries as a matter of urgency. She did not seem as alarmed as I was, and advised that though Mum was apparently sleepy just now, she had actually been awake and talking that morning; before blithely adding that Mum had also refused all food, and only drunk a small amount of water; mainly because of the sore mouth. I asked what was causing it, and the auxiliary, unable, or perhaps (and rightly given her relatively lowly status) unwilling to say, went off to fetch the ward sister. The latter's best advice was that it was likely to be due to a lack of oxygen to the tongue, which Mum's own body seemed unable / unwilling to supply to it at present. By now though Mum had more or less nodded off again, after muttering that she wanted to go back to sleep because she could breathe more easily thus. Unable to properly establish how the tongue condition was being treated, I asked (again firmly but politely), to see the doctor. The ward sister seemed slightly irked, but strode off with purpose, and returned about half an hour later with Dr. A in tow. Dr. A advised that Mum's lung functioning seemed to have become a little less smooth; this 'probably' caused by both the existing pulmonary fibrosis and the new (Sepsis?) infection, which was still active. She advised that Mum was now likely to need more frequent access to a supply of oxygen than hitherto, both to support her general breathing and because of the lack of oxygen to the tongue; and by way of some sort of back-handed encouragement, added that Mum was also likely to need ongoing access to a supply of oxygen "when she leaves".

So, at that stage, there was still some sort of implicit expectation that Mum *would* actually be able to leave the hospital, and return to her Care Home at some point soon; even though, depressingly, she might function less well than before in the setting, and require regular access to that supply of oxygen, henceforth.

Dr. A also prescribed a mouth spray to help with the soreness, and took her leave, (though the fact that it took my persistence to get this, whilst none of the hospital staff had felt it appropriate to initiate its earlier acquisition and implementation, disappointed me somewhat). However, the ward sister remained to fit Mum with the latest antibiotic drip bag.

Whilst I had the ward sister's ear, I took the opportunity to suggest that Mum be tried with liquid 'Build-up', milk-shake-style, drinks whilst her mouth remained sore, as they had been effective in getting Mum to eat on a previous hospital admission, and the ward sister agreed to try this, and departed. (Again, I was left wondering why *I* was having to initiate the idea).

Mum then woke up and tried to make it known to me that she wanted to go to the toilet. At first, I struggled to make out what she was saying, and could see that she was getting frustrated with my failure to understand her, (which of course raised my own sense of frustration at being unable to respond promptly to her request), but, luckily, at the third attempt, I did make out the word 'toy... et', and was handily able to 'book' that service with an auxiliary just arriving with another pillow for a patient in the next bed.

Toileting was obviously a two-nurse job, though, and off she went; returning just a few minutes later with a colleague. They started the entirely orthodox, but to me never entirely dignified, in-situ, bed-pan, process by pulling the curtains round the bed, and asking me to step outside that now private space. It was approaching the end of visiting time, anyway, so I took that as my cue to leave altogether, kissed Mum fondly on the cheek, spoke reassuringly about 'seeing her tomorrow', and strolled, exhaustedly, off down the long corridor, before nipping conveniently through the open coded door just as another nurse was entering the ward, and over to the lift - and, 5 minutes later, unlike Mum, (but not unlike Elvis), I had left the building.

Thursday was another generally 'sleepy' visit, with Mum only waking in 'fits and starts'. On the plus side, that day's auxiliary advised that Mum had taken some sips of the (strawberry) 'Build-up' shake they'd provided, as well as being spoon-fed a few spoonfuls of rice pudding, and sipping water. On the down side, however, Mum's tongue still looked very red and sore, and was clearly causing her quite a bit of continued discomfort, despite the auxiliary's claim that the spray had been regularly employed. Also on the downside, oxygen was now being tube-fed up Mum's nose almost as standard, via a small plastic nose-clip that Mum would regularly find irritating, and try to remove, as she felt the need to scratch in the area; and the catheter was back; the latter apparently redeployed because Mum had passed so little fluid, and monitoring was once again required; and she was on a fluid drip into her left arm to help here, too. Yet further, and perhaps most worrying of all, was that, according to the bedside notes, she was *still* being treated for Sepsis - with which the latest (Augmentin) antibiotic was struggling to keep control. This was confirmed in a very brief, unexpected, and late-in-my- visit appearance from Dr. A; and all this, according to the latter, almost certainly taking place against a background of no help from Mum's own immune system, because the unrelenting Dementia was preventing this being appropriately triggered.

Friday the 28th of July; I was just a few minutes into my visit when I was taken aside by the ward sister. She had critical news for me. She informed me that the latest, and last available, antibiotic course would be coming to its end in the next few days, that none appeared to have worked so far, that no other was practicable, and that progress seemed to have, at best, stalled. At worst, she thought, it was likely that the antibiotics had not even halted the spread of infection, after all, and Mum's condition now gave grave cause for concern. Accordingly, I was also informed that the specialist, end-of-life, doctor, from the nearby hospice, had been called in earlier that day, as per standard practice in such cases, and asked to give his assessment of the situation. His verdict, apparently, was not good. In the absence of a 'miracle', he had apparently advised the relevant in-house doctor, and ward sister, that Mum's condition was now likely to continue to deteriorate further, and it was unlikely that she could be saved!

With Mum's *clinical/medical* care (treatment) deemed to be effectively failing, following this latest, critical, and supposedly specialist, prognosis, and her need now deemed to be primarily for *nursing* (palliative) care, the *ward sister* (rather than a doctor) was apparently deemed to be the appropriate 'professional' to deliver this 'specialist' doctor's devastating blow, prognosis and views, to *us*, and to make the case for we offspring giving our most urgent consideration to the only 2 viable options likely to be still 'on the table' when the current, and last, course of antibiotics came to its imminent end.

Firstly, of Mum being 'tube-fed' in the very near future, in order to just keep her alive; or secondly, for Mum to be placed on palliative care, that is 'end of life' care, in acceptance of, and preparation for, her actually dying and leaving both us, and the world!

Oh, my God!

Having had her in our daily lives since birth, (65 years in my case), it was, of course, incredibly hard to hear this. Incredibly hard indeed, and even harder to have to now contemplate the reality. Despite the evidence having, arguably, been before me for some days, my initial reaction was one of complete shock; like I'd been hit with a heavy weight of some sort, and was currently hearing the words, but not really taking them in. It just felt so unreal, indeed so *sur*real, so very *weird*, and just so (literally) unbelievable, to be suddenly faced right now with these 2 equally traumatic, no-win, no-hope, and truly terrible options. Barring that miracle, it was slowly dawning on me that there was to be no happy ending after all, to what was quickly becoming a stressful, prolonged, and now rapidly worsening nightmare for us all.

If we opted for the former, it sounded like Mum would effectively be put on a permanent, bed-bound, probably hospital-based, life-support system, and almost certainly tube-fed for the rest of what would, equally probably, be a very poor quality, (and very probably short) existence; and all this just to keep her going physically; whilst mentally, she would still continue to be imprisoned and confused by the unrelenting Dementia. Yet, if we opted to let her go, and for the latter, palliative, *end-of-life* care, it seemed to me that we'd be opting for something just short of euthanasia, and ensuring that she would soon be gone from our lives altogether. Forever.

At least with the latter choice, however, there were *palliative options*, according to the ward sister; but only options about *where*, not *whether*, her dying would take place. In fact, *three* palliative options were being made available. Firstly, for Mum to remain in the hospital, and on the same ward as at present, but to be moved to one of those 'single-cubicle' wards further down the corridor, for her own privacy, peace and quiet, and comfort. Secondly, for her to return to her place at the Care Home to die; with whatever conditions the home might be able to make available. (Mum had been *sharing* a room with another Dementia resident prior to entering the hospital and we were still financially responsible for its cost). Thirdly, we could take up an offer of a bed and single room at the nearby (hitherto unseen) hospice.

I nodded appropriately in places, as the ward sister spoke, but to be honest, I was still struggling to take it all in. As a matter of course, I agreed to have urgent discussions with my siblings regarding the developing situation; which I initially did by telephone on that same (Friday) night; but before they were due to visit. For most of the rest of *my* visit Mum had thankfully taken to sleep, because my mind was now predominantly engaged in computing and absorbing the shocking new prognosis and (literally) *deadly* information recently related by the ward sister.

In truth, the tube-fed option seemed both harsh and impractical to us all, from the off, as a long-term 'solution' to Mum's predicament, and to be simply putting off the inevitable. Moreover, we were agreed that Mum would not, herself, have wanted such a wholly dependent, and an utterly undignified, drawn out, final existence and end. (Objectively, my own crude view and benchmark was that when you have no chance of ever wiping your own backside again, it's surely time to call it a day, and head for the exit). From that perspective, of course, there was but a *single* option left to us!

It felt like *we* were being given power over her life and death. Like we'*d* been thrust into the role of deciding how/if /when Mum's life should end; and given the unenviable task of watching our choice borne out. What a task! What a responsibility! But better us than anyone else, and after only a few relatively short exchanges and considerations by telephone, it emerged that, in principle, we had broad agreement. Our foremost thoughts were that Mum had suffered enough, should suffer no longer, and given the prognosis of further deterioration, should be allowed to go on palliative care. We agreed to reflect further overnight.

Saturday, the 29th of July. I received an early morning telephone call from my older brother. Mum's lack of either communication or activity at his Friday evening visit had convinced him that she had already deteriorated the more. He was suggesting an urgent sibling meeting at the hospital that afternoon, in order to come to a final decision about our 'options'.

When we arrived on Ward 31, Mum was no longer in bed 14. She had already been trundled further down the corridor, and to the slot reserved for bed 22. In fact, she had now been installed in one of those single-bedded, 'dying' wards, as I, somewhat cynically, labelled them. This, the ward sister advised, would allow Mum to have peace and quiet, and more personal nursing attention, and allow us to visit as and when we wished, until we had finally made up our minds about the options still available to us (her).

The new, single, ward was shaped like an inverted 'L'; in golfing terms, like a sharp dog-leg left on entry. Once again, the eye was immediately drawn straight on, (over the projecting foot of Mum's bed and past the small roof-mounted TV directly above it), to the full 'wall' of window that filled the top half of the far end of the room, and thence to the same pleasant rolling green panorama as for bed 14; but now we were just a little further along to the left, allowing a tall pylon to just edge into view *hard-left* on the horizon. A few yards in, and Mum's head, and that of her bed-head, came into view, round the corner to the left.

The single-bedded ward was minimally, but adequately furnished. As Mum lay in Bed 22, the left-hand edge was positioned about 3 feet from the 'bank' of windows, with the bed-head tight against the wall behind her, and its foot about 3 feet from the 'footer' wall. Only the iron, black-and-white painted, oxygen bottle, its metal cradle, and delivery tubes, and some trollied hospital monitoring equipment, both near the bed-head, intruded permanently into the gap between bed and window. To the immediate *right* of Mum's bed-head was yet another monitor, then a thinner metal stand holding the clear plastic bag that was delivering the last remnants of antibiotic, and finally a standard sort of hospital locker, which was holding her minimal belongings, and providing a handy top surface on which to keep various personal and medicinal items. The room was also furnished with a single turquoise, faux-leather, high-backed chair, with wooden arms, a matching broad-seated stool, a couple of grey standard 'stacker' chairs, (more available from outside), and one of those wheeled, over-the-bed, tables; all free-standing and able to be moved around to suit; but in essence we had 3-sided access around Mum's bed. Yet further to Mum's right, and tucked discreetly into the corner, was a small stainless-steel sink.

With Mum asleep again, we withdrew to a vacant side/ meeting room to discuss those options one more time. Amid predictably difficult emotions, we did reluctantly, but alas unanimously, come to the inevitable conclusion that for both Mum's sake and ours we had to 'let her go'; that is, we had to allow Mum to go on palliative care, and progress as comfortably and peacefully as possible to the end of her long, well-lived, life. However, there was less immediate agreement on the options pertaining to *where* that should be allowed to progress.

The hospice, with its apparently cultivated lawns and gardens, personalised room, and peace and quiet, certainly sounded nice, and it *specialised* in end-of-life care, but it was unknown and untried by either Mum or us. We were also aware that back at the Care Home staffing vacancies meant current staff were doing long shifts, and had up to 18 other full-time and needy (mostly Dementia) 'inmates' to care for; whilst the current hospital ward was a busy one outside of the single-bedded side ward that Mum had now been given exclusive occupancy of.

What would Mum have gone for?

Initially, we felt that a return to the familiarity of the Care Home might be her chosen option, but then quickly realised that Mum *shared* her upstairs accommodation there. It also had only a limited view from the window. Moreover, we concluded that Mum's Dementia meant that her memory of the Care Home, now 2 weeks back 'down the line', was probably nil, anyway. (She'd certainly never mentioned it since *arriving* in hospital). We also thought that the lovely-sounding conditions and gardens at the 'specialist' hospice would be nice for her, before surmising that she would probably be bed-ridden, predominantly asleep, and might never be fit enough to appreciate, or even see, them, let alone get *used* to them.

In the end, we concluded that Mum would not now fancy being moved about, to effectively start again, in either of these other settings, and unanimously came down on the side of not adding any further or unnecessary discomfort to her final days. So we were persuaded that, if Mum were more compos mentis than she was, regarding her current sad state, she would almost certainly opt for no further disruption, and to stay put.

Here at least, we concluded, Mum had the quiet single-bed cubicle ward to herself, and, directly from her bed, a very pleasant green view over the middle-distance hills, through her extensive 5th floor windows - not that, unmoved, she seemed any more likely to wake sufficiently to take full advantage of things here, either! Additionally though, doctors were (theoretically) available on site if she had further urgent need of them, and we were being promised full palliative care from the hospital and nursing staff, (many of whom we had got to 'know' a little by now), and the freedom for we siblings, and any other potential visitors, to come and go as necessary.

The decision was made.

With heavy hearts, welling emotions, and a final acceptance that any miraculous recovery was now beyond our much-loved Mum, we sought out the ward sister and informed her accordingly. Mum would go on palliative care, and spend the final days of her life where she was currently and (relatively) comfortably ensconced.

On the Sunday there was little change in Mum; though there certainly was in *me.* Any previous mood of hope and openness that *I'd* brought to these visits was now clinging on by its fingertips. Thankfully, Mum opted to sleep through most of my afternoon visit, today, only offering a weak, "Uh" in response to my closely-whispered "Hello" on arrival, (but at least it signalled that she was still aware of my presence), and then half-waking at a couple of other points to accept a sip of water from me. Her new 'status', on 'death row', however, meant that my already much-frazzled emotions had been immediately heightened the more as soon as I'd clapped eyes on her again. To have had to look her straight in the eye today, and offer her *any* sort of *reassuring* answer to the, "Am I going to be all right, Keith?" question she'd so regularly posed on more interactive occasions, would surely have upped my sense of deceit and disingenuity to 'gibbering idiot' levels. Of course, I was pretty confident that she was in no fit state to ask anything like that just now, but even the *thought* of her doing so was enough to make me grateful for having to just sit in quiet, supportive, vigilance and reflection for the most part today.

The one physical change that I did note on arrival though, was that she was no longer on any form of 'treatment' medicine. The last droppings of the final course of antibiotics had presumably been completed, and the drip, stand and monitor involved in supplying it, had been removed from the room, never to be seen again. Henceforth she would only receive oxygen by nose-clip, as required, to help with her breathing, and appropriate pain relief. Equally depressing, was the fact that her food chart appeared to have remained untouched by human hand; suggesting that Mum had presumably eaten nothing at all so far that day. Nor did she do so whilst I was there. For more than *one* split second, waiting for the inevitable seemed just a little more tangible today.

By the Monday, I'd 'steadied my own ship', emotionally, and on my afternoon visit to Mum I met with a glimmer of alertness from her, too; and, at her *most* alert, her eyes would briefly, if blearily, open, and she might manage the suggestion of a smile. Regardless, I just wanted to cherish her continued presence now; the chance to enjoy her company still, and those precious few moments where she *was* susceptible to any meaningful communication between us. At intervals, I managed to persuade her to try a few extra sips of water and warm tea, and even a couple of feeble licks of the cool vanilla ice cream dessert that I'd ordered as part of her still-allocated teatime meal. In the back of my mind, I was probably trying to convince myself that all was not lost if she was still taking in even tiny amounts of potential sustenance. With hindsight, alas, I was probably just fighting another desperate battle with denial.

Who was I kidding? Only myself of course.

By the Tuesday, (the first day of the new month of August), my denial was officially, and starkly, if only administratively, exposed from the 'off'. Mum's file had acquired the dreaded, and official, black and white, 'end of life' papers in a new, but still appropriately coloured, *red* (for danger) file, that uncompromisingly signalled a change of status and a 'warning' to all. It was a denial exposed the more by the fact that, though Mum's bed-head, and therefore head, was raised up today, (encouragingly, at an optimum angle for eating or speaking), it was not because she had actually built on our token efforts of yesterday. Her chart showed that she had taken in nothing at all today. Nor was it because she had *said* anything of note, either.

Once again, she only woke spasmodically during my 4-hour vigil. She wasn't exactly *fast* asleep for much of the time, but when she did crack open her eyes and try to speak, it was now even more of a struggle for her, and, once I had again established that her need was not for the toilet, (by the slowest and slightest negative turn of her head), I was increasingly unable to hazard even an educated guess at what she was trying to tell me; both because of the ongoing sore tongue and mouth, and because, as the ward sister later pointed out, her vocal chords were now being affected by her condition, too.

Sadly, and exasperatingly for all, this probably meant that she was feeling both very frustrated and further discomforted herself; and on one sole occasion, going off her slowly gurned facial contortions, she seemed quite agitated, before quickly running out of energy, becoming discouraged by, and finally giving up on, my chronic inability to understand, and therefore to 'come to her rescue', and fulfil, her request.

Whether she wanted it or not, by way of my tendency to 'best guess' her, I'd take the opportunity to both whisper more reassuring words, and to just help her take a few more sips of water, whilst then inviting her to try again to make her request clearer. (Talk about feeling a sense of impotence through a shared language!). She did try, poor soul. At least I think she was addressing *me*, but, in the end, there may have been a level of frustration and confusion developing that was bordering on delirium; this latter being suggested to me by the couple of particularly brief, but arresting, attempts to speak when I could have sworn that I heard her utter, in her croaky, semi-comatose desperation, "Help me, Frank", and "Help me, Mam", of both my 21 years-deceased, father, (Frank), and her own, even longer-gone, mother, (Mam). It was incredibly distressing to witness her struggling so, and doubly distressing to struggle, so impotently, myself, to find any way to alleviate her plight. What it did do, though, was to afford me a latest potential insight into her pitiful, still demented, and presumably still deteriorating, state of both mind and body. Of course, I was just choked with emotion, but somehow I managed to keep a 'poker' face and carry on.

When the auxiliary of the day popped in later in the visit, she *confirmed* that Mum had already been toileted, so I'd asked if I could speak with the ward sister again, to see if *she* could make head or tail of what Mum was saying/asking. The ward sister duly arrived towards the end of the visit, but she couldn't understand what Mum was trying to say either; nor did she appear to have any further palliative ideas as to what might be done to improve the situation.

So, fearing the worst, I steeled myself, and asked the ward sister if she could say how long 'the waiting' might be, now that Mum could be barely understood, and might be dipping into delirium; and now that she was receiving no *treatment* for her condition(s), and only oxygen, pain relief, and personal hygiene comfort, as required, from nursing staff. Alas, the ward sister remained either unable or unwilling to proffer anything precise regarding the amount of time that Mum might have left; nor, therefore, about the degree of continued agony that both she and we would have to endure. All she would repeat was that Mum could go "any day", now that she was taking in neither food of note, nor any medication; but was equally, and non-commitally, keen to make it known that some patients had been known to "hang on" for several weeks.

WHERE DID YOU GO TO, MY LOVELY? DEMENTIA DAYS

I had been in situ there for so long now that I was still in attendance when my brother and his wife arrived (early) for their evening shift. They too expressed their alarm that Mum had been getting so frustrated, may have experienced delirium, and was still currently unable to make her needs known, either verbally or alternately.

Feeling unable to improve the situation any further myself, and reluctantly, I gave Mum an extra big hug, (just in case it might turn out to be my last), left them to take over the vigil, and headed home for some desperately needed rest and recuperation.

Later that night I received a reassuring telephone call from my brother to tell me that Mum had actually been calm towards the end of his 'shift' (largely because the ward sister had thought it appropriate to give Mum some sort of sedative), and that she had been sleeping comfortably again by the late-night time he departed - helping *me* sleep a little better that night.

Weds. The 2nd of August. Yet another lengthy, and generally lifeless, afternoon visit where Mum didn't really wake up properly at all. When she did stir, she once again seemed semi-comatose, (in part due to the painkillers?), and though she did seem to know me, and that I was there, she again seemed to be moaning and rambling to herself quite a bit, too. She also seemed to be breathing a little harder today; despite the oxygen; whilst both our auxiliary and the day's ward sister suggested that the previous evening's sedative might still be affecting her. At various points throughout the 5-hour stay, I dabbed cooling water onto her lips via a pink-sponged 'swab-on-a-stick' provided by the nursing staff, and a cup of water freshly run from the in-room tap. At one mid-visit point, when she was at her most awake and aware, I also managed to gently prise open her 'gummy' mouth a little, and dab some water onto the front of her now more badly-scabbed, scarlet-red, tongue. (She either couldn't or wouldn't now open up sufficiently to allow use of the largely ineffective spray, so I chose not to force that matter). For the rest of the time I whispered 'sweet nothings' to her, and even had a go at quietly singing some of her favourite 'old-time' songs, (such as 'Daisy, Daisy', 'We'll meet again', and 'Que Sera Sera'), by way of time-filling comfort and reassurance.

(Amazingly, the calm look on her face suggested she wasn't actually opposed to my offerings!).

When I wasn't either dabbing or crooning I remained predictably subdued, and just sat around, ministering where I could, and quietly reminiscing to myself where I couldn't. Mostly I sat on the stool, presently placed in the gap between the bed and our 'window on the outside world'. Sometimes I sat in the high-backed chair that gave both a close-up, bed-level, view of Mum, and one *across* her bed to the far horizon of that 'outside world'; and occasionally I even perched on the window sill, just for a change; as she alternatively slept and then came round sufficiently to wheeze and moan a little more loudly, (yet just as helplessly), for a few moments. And as the sheer sense of sadness, of utter powerlessness and of unending guilt at being unable to even help with, let alone 'solve', her problems, and just the raw emotion of it all, got to me, I wept quietly from time to time, too, and wished into the ether for a pain*less* end to such a pain*ful*, and pointless, dragged-out, no-win, no-hope, situation.

And all the while Mum 's (supposedly suspect) heart kept pumping away, and refused to 'call it a day'; even as her other organs continued to offer so little back-up, and her ever-weakening chest muscles continued to struggle so noticeably, with the slow wheezy breathing, and the lungs' ultra-laborious rise and fall, as they fought for air; and sometimes even seemed to stop, (and yet start again a few seconds later), as she puffed and strained to hold on to life - apparently in spite of its now pitiful quality.

Not surprisingly, my own thoughts and emotions remained all over the place. "What on earth is she (that is, what's *left* of her brain and body) putting herself through this slow lingering agony for?" I remember thinking, for instance, on more than one occasion, as she just refused to give in. Surely there couldn't be long left now. Then a strange mood would unexpectedly sweep over me, and I would suddenly realise that I was totally unprepared for that finality, and pray (again into the 'ether') that there *was*; and that she wouldn't go *today*.

The ward sister looked in to see if there was anything Mum, or I, needed. I took the opportunity to ask this different practitioner for *her* advice regarding the likely 'time left', and, remaining as non-committal as the rest of her colleagues had previously been, she suggested, from her own years of experience, that Mum looked to be a 'fighter', and may still have a few days left. (When my dog was this bad we had called the vet to ask for our pet to be put out of his misery, and the vet was able to oblige!) The ward sister left. I returned to my more melancholy musings, and to thinking how cruel it all was, and that, if there was a God, how cruel he must be too, to have my lovely mother, (who, to my knowledge, had never harmed anyone in her whole life), put through such end-of-life purgatory. And yet, somehow, as I say, I still couldn't shake off that parallel thought that I didn't really *want* to savour the finality of her breathing her last *today*, and to actually *have* her leave us altogether. Once more, the theory and the practice were somehow at odds. My mind continued its own inconclusive ramblings.

Outside, ironically, (and in stark contrast to the inner gloom), it was a lovely, bright, clear, early-August afternoon. Through the closed windows, and on that far horizon, a few pure white, wispy clouds clung lightly to the roof of the sky, to break up the dominant blue, and to suggest there was little breeze today. For a moment I felt the sheer sense of freedom being painted by the increasingly-familiar and gently-rolling green hills, dotted with their frequent splashes of hedgerow and trees; each dressed fittingly in their complementary-vibrant summer-green coats; and interrupted hither and thither by the contrasting greys and blacks of the 'odds and sods' of broken stone wall that, I guessed, once mark the boundaries of a farmer's fields; and by the solitary stone farmhouse whose occupant may yet still 'own' them; and by that lone, strangely attention-grabbing grey pylon: until it dawned on me that it was *just* the sort of lovely summer sight that Mum might never again have the chance to see and appreciate - and again the tears just trickled slowly and involuntarily down my cheeks.

"Damn you, Dementia", I hear myself mutter out loud, to no-one in particular, once more, as I look back forlornly at my once 'full-of-life', but now totally helpless, clapped-out Mum, lying there barely conscious, *on* such a lovely summer's day.

Again her breathing seems to have stopped. Is this it, I wonder? My anxiety levels shoot up, my own breathing 'holds' instinctively, for a moment, and my own heart almost seems to stop in sympathy at the thought of that possibility; but after a few seconds' pause, Mum's thin, blue and white, flower -print nightie begins to rise again in the chest area, and the strained, still distinctly wheezy, breathing pattern resumes. Again, I struggle to make up my mind whether I'm relieved or not.

Either way, I take a deep breath of my own, and stand up tall to face the window again, to stretch my legs, and to re-seek that fresh, broader and more sweeping panorama that might lift my spirits for a moment. Leaning slightly further forward than usual, and for no obvious reason, and then tight to my left, at eye-level, I can now just make out a few distant, red brick, buildings and the matching red-tiled rooftops of what seems like a small housing estate. A single-decker bus, of predominantly grass-green (and cream) livery, and a couple of following cars, of various hues, roll silently up a broad winding road that appears to run through the middle of the estate. I wonder, momentarily, how many people are on the bus, and where everyone is going, and note that nothing appears to be actually coming down the road, before my attention is diverted once more.

Back inside, and behind me now, and on the corridor beyond the open door of the ward, there's a noisy distraction, as another trollied hospital vehicle rattles past with its 'driver' in tow. Reactively, I turn towards the sound, but its' Doppler-like effect is fading already, and is soon gone. I look back at Mum, and she's effectively 'gone' too, as she's been neither moved by, nor taken a jot of notice of, either the serene summer sight outside the closed window, nor the passing castored clatter. Yet still she continues to hold on to this sleepy and now very minimal form of existence. I turn on the TV, and turn the sound right down, in a vain attempt to alleviate both my boredom and my sadness. I can't concentrate on it, and it doesn't seem right, anyway, so I turn it off again. I sit elsewhere; firstly back in the big high-backed chair for a few minutes, and then even on the wide window-sill again, before finally reverting back to the stool. I rise up spasmodically, and stroll over to the sink, to reload my sponge swab, and thence to re-dab my sleeping Mum's lips with cooling water, to kiss her fondly on the forehead, and sometimes to quietly sing 'Daisy, Daisy' yet again, and to whisper more sweet nothings about her being 'the best Mum in the world'. It all appears to be to no avail, as there's no sign that she actually hears any of this at present and yet she continues still with her scratchy, laboured, stop-start, uneven breathing; and so hangs on doggedly to the dregs of her life.

I hear another trolley trundling somewhere nearby. It's getting louder as it gets nearer. It stops outside the ward door. *Two* auxiliaries are in control of this one. A glance at my watch shows that it's 4-45pm, and they are clearly dishing up tea-time meals to the ward's patients. Wow, is it that time already? It might have seemed a long-winded and wearisome afternoon, and often like time had slowed to a crawl, whilst it had certainly been downright upsetting, but, like all time, *it's* kept trundling on, regardless - and now its teatime.

One of the auxiliaries approaches with Mum's teatime entitlement on a tray, (including a covered hot meal and a dessert), and places it on my Mum's over-the-bed table. She asks if we need anything else. I shake my head, with a polite "No thanks", and she turns to leave. I lift the largest metal lid. It's clearly a chicken casserole. Despite being barely aware of what's going on around her, and officially being on palliative care, struggling to digest or even swallow anything beyond water right now, and, indeed, having not eaten anything significant, (let alone solid), for well over 24 hours, and it being obvious that Mum is in no fit state to eat today, the hospital has to provide the option. (In case of legal action, or perhaps of that modern miracle, I guess). I thank the departing auxiliary again, and jokingly say I'll eat it myself. She says that's OK if Mum can't eat it. I'm provided with a proper (not spouted) mug of tea, too; and as the auxiliary returns to her task, and the meals trolley trundles onward and away, I pull the bed-table towards *me*, and (not entirely guiltily), tuck into Mum's casserole. It's not bad for hospital food. Suddenly, I recall that it was I who filled in a form for this food option yesterday. Even though I knew Mum was unlikely to eat it, I'd been asked to fill in the form anyway, to fulfil the hospital's obligations and procedures; and also ensure that tomorrow's bed 22 patient has a meal booked, regardless of who actually occupies the bed. I also remember that I requested the chocolate sponge and custard option for dessert. I check under the other metal cover, and there it is. Again I tuck in. Hmm. (No need to eat when I get home now - just catch up on rest and sleep, I tell myself to justify my tuck). By the time I've finished dessert, the tea has cooled, and, gently tapping her shoulder, I try to persuade Mum to wake, and, for a change, try to wet Mum's lips with the taste of tea. (Mum loved her tea, and used to drink several cups a day). My persuasions make little impact, though, and Mum has soon resumed her eyes-closed, laboured breathing, but otherwise non-interactive repose.

I push the wheeled over-the-bed table towards the corridor, ready for collection of the meal's non-edible remnants, and, casting yet another sad eye on Mum, slowly wander back 'towards the light'. This time my gaze is somehow drawn by a *lower* landscape. Beyond the closed windows, and five floors down below, and in a noiseless, Marcel Marceau/Laurel & Hardy, silent movie sort of way, life just seemed to be continuing as normal - continuing *with* Mum, for the moment, (or anyone else for that matter who was still able to join in), or *without* her (or anyone else who was unable to take 'normal' part). Yes, out there, life, like time, was just dispassionately reminding me that it was 'carrying on regardless', with no necessity for any of the apparently 'healthy' souls scurrying along down there, (or anywhere else), and with their own worries, needing to be aware of, let alone overly bothered by, the life ebbing away up here - and indeed, despite this being a hospital, those probably doing so elsewhere on the site, or wherever.

Fielding such thoughts as best I could, I stood there for a while, gazing idly upon this soundless, but subtly-shifting, scene. On the busy hospital site in particular there seemed to be a steady, but never-ending, trickle of activity. Some people were arriving by car, and driving round and round the large but packed public car-parks looking for a space; and some were leaving, perhaps at the end of their latest working day, shift, or visit, to vacate such a prized space. Watching the 'arrivers' silent battle for those scarce spaces was a bit like watching worker ants going quietly but unceasingly about their business 'on the hill'. Other people were on foot about *their* business. Some, not surprisingly, were in hospital liveries, and quietly going about their hospital business. Others were in their 'civies', and shirtsleeves, and less easily identified by their cause or position; but all *seemed* to be progressing in a sort of smooth 'gliding' manner towards their chosen destination, along the various tarmacked surfaces that criss-crossed and dissected the neatly trimmed lawns, assortment of buildings, and crammed car-parks, of this eerily noiseless summer setting. Then a double-decker bus, in post-office red, wriggled silently onto the site, and across my vision, to take my attention. I just assumed that it was bringing in the latest batch of foot-soldier visitors, and collecting those car-less others who relied on such essential public transport, and were done for now. After wriggling along for perhaps a couple of hundred yards, it veered slightly left, and then left my sight as quickly as it had arrived, so I know not if or where its potential passengers alighted or embarked.

All this outside activity only served to trigger yet more reflective, and more surreal, thoughts in me. Once again, they were broader, more neutral, less personal, almost philosophical in kind; and they offered another brief but most welcome, if limited, distraction to my otherwise unavoidably sad, and now predominantly upsetting, and very 'here and now', mindset that came with my in-ward Mum-minding.

It dawned on me, for instance, in those more objective-cum-philosophical moments that, at every minute of every day, around the world, *loads* of the 7 billion people that inhabited this incredible planet were probably busy dying; (whilst loads of others were probably just as busy being born); and yet, life, like the ever-rolling seas, barely broke stride in its incessant progression to goodness knows where. For those who *had* life, and were *not* yet ready to 'check out', and who still had need of an ongoing purpose and goal, and were busily taking their turn at 'time', and at keeping the wheels of their society turning, both down below, and around the world, by doing whatever was necessary to achieve that goal, and to keep the world functioning as it did, life still provided the fundamental 'stage' on which each individual might act it out. For whatever reason, it also crossed my mind with wonderment that in less than, say, 120 years, absolutely everyone who had been alive that long ago, and had also strived to pursue *their* goals, purposes and lives with appropriate vigour and belief, had sooner or later been replaced, and indeed added to, in profusion, by today. 'Ah, well, that's life', was my resigned conclusion.

Meanwhile, back in the land of the dying, there had been no discernible change whilst I'd been 'away'. Then, in truth, relief. The evening shift arrived, in the form of, first, my sister, and then half an hour later, my brother and his wife. After bringing each of them 'up to speed' in their turn, regarding my visit, and any relevant issues concerning Mum, my latest (Wednesday) vigil was over. It had seemed a particularly long, depressing and upsetting 'shift', and by far the worst to date, so despite knowing that Mum could die any time now, (though probably not *right* now, if the ward sister's experience was to be believed), I knew that I had to take my leave for a while, and to seek yet more vital rest and recuperation, and, hopefully, a more positive mind-set beyond the hospital; and thence to prepare for another day.

Thursday, the 3rd of August. I'm back again for another afternoon shift, and Mum is still alive; though once again there is only the minimum of response during my 4 hour vigil. For the most part, she's breathing slowly, but hard again, despite the oxygen, and yet her facial muscle movements, and the occasional flicker of her rarely, and barely, open eyes, suggest she *is* still hearing me whisper my 'sweet nothings', and now clearly false reassurances. (I could hardly whisper the truth, could I?). Once again I try some soft strains of those favourite old songs of hers, but despite just the hint of a mouth movement, (was she *really* trying to sing along?), that too makes no lasting or discernible difference, as she barely breaks the forced rhythm of hard breathing all afternoon, and never *really* wakes up. Sleep seems to be her preferred state just now.

When I'm not whispering or singing, I fill my time much like I did yesterday - and the day before - dabbing Mum's lips with cooling water, and then her brow with another dampened sponge, looking to both the hills and the lower 'campus' for outside distraction, and listening to the enforced and regular trundle of hospital trolleys, giving that decent impression of the Doppler Effect, going past her ward door. After a couple of hours of this though, my sister arrives unexpectedly to help break the monotony. She had been finding it all too much hitherto, and my brother and I had encouraged her to take a day off and to go out somewhere with her husband, to take her mind off things here. She had tried, but couldn't get past the guilt; so here she was to *share* the boredom, the whispering, the singing, and, most of all, the unending upset, at the saddest of sad, 'catch 22', sights (literally) laid before us.

With my sister in situ at the hospital, and my brother due soon, I eventually took my leave a little earlier than I'd planned; and headed off home to try once more to find some evening rest and recuperation of my own. After a bite to eat, I took a refreshing shower, and settled down with my wife to watch a little early-evening TV for a while. Neither of us was really taking any of it in, and I was pretty poor company anyway, so my much-neglected wife decided to pop round to see her friend and neighbour for a cuppa, and I found myself trying to relax alone.

I found it almost impossible. I sat watching some more TV trivia for a while, (it's amazing how so much seems trivia really, at a time like this), but my concentration was pretty limited, and constantly interrupted by the thought of Mum still puffing and blowing, on her airbed, some 7 miles away, and fearing, (as I had for several days now) that the next time the phone rang it would be a call to tell me Mum was gone. But I needed the rest, and whilst that phone call remained outstanding, and she presumably kept chugging on, I took myself off to bed earlier than usual, despite being permanently 'on pins'. Remarkably, my tiredness did eventually win out, and it's the following morning (Friday), at breakfast-time, when I next encounter consciousness.

Friday the 4th. I arrived early afternoon; about 1-00pm. My sister was already there, and into her second hour as it turned out, and quietly singing to Mum as I walked in. Remarkably, Mum was technically awake, and with her bed-head set for Mum to be at a comfortable elevated angle again, she did seem, occasionally, to be in a little less breathing *dis*comfort, and even trying to speak. However, her swollen and 'scaled' tongue was still greatly restricting her efforts to be understood, and, once again, it was almost impossible to decipher her words; and therefore her needs. She was actually quite weak now though, and she either couldn't, or couldn't be bothered to, put her limited energies into getting overly frustrated, or angry, and just sort of gave up, and returned 'to rest'. Yet again, it felt both deeply frustrating and incredibly upsetting to be so impotent as to be unable to offer her any really useful help, and both my sister and I were really struggling to hold back the tears at this ever-saddest of sad sights. I took hold of Mum's plastic spouted drinking cup, and, more in hope than anything else, asked her if she would like to try some water. I could just about make out her pathetic, babyish, half-utterance of the two words "Ye... plea...", (which I interpreted as "Yes please"), as they struggled out and, still barely holding back my tears, gently put the spout to her lips. With difficulty, she did take a drop or two, but I'd no real idea if that had actually sated her needs.

Just then, the ward sister made her timely showing, and, as usual, asked if we needed anything. From nowhere, I found myself requesting another 'Build-up' drink for Mum to try, 'by way of a change' as if that was going to sort her and save her! The ward sister set off for the small kitchen to fulfil my request; and was back within minutes with another strawberry version of the shake; and I was even able to get Mum to take a taste of it too. (Somewhere, in the back of my befuddled mind, I suppose that I *was* still clinging to the last vestiges of the possibility that a miracle might actually happen, and Mum would begin to take more of the shake, and start to recover).

The ward sister remained non-committal about how much time Mum might have left, but tactfully reminded me that Mum was now only on palliative care, (essentially only oxygen, water and painkillers; plus anything specific that might make Mum more comfortable in her final days. I guess she was telling me that the shake fell into the latter category), and was not receiving any kind of medication that would give hope of improvement, let alone help make her 'better'. So, essentially she was reminding me not to get my (false) hopes up, that the milk shake wouldn't make any difference to the ultimate outcome, and that Mum was just waiting to die. (We had not seen a doctor for several days; not that we had any real need, given that we had already received the *medics'* final, and of course fatal, prognosis).

By this time in the visit, and still struggling with her pulmonary fibrosis, (and presumably with her Sepsis, though that was never definitively clarified), Mum had returned to hard-breathing and sleep mode. My sister and I returned to chatting quietly, about our memories, and about Mum's life, and alternated between pottering over to kiss her fondly on the forehead, gently caressing her hand, by way of signalling our continued presence and support, and discreetly leaking our tears of sheer grief when the latter just got too much. Dabbing more water onto Mum's lips, sitting around dolefully, and taking up the option to look out of the still-closed, and therefore sound-proof, window, at the 'silent' life still going on beyond, also played their now regular part in the desperate search for some sort of relief, purpose and in-ward coping strategy; and then the silence might be interrupted again by another low-key start-up of the haphazardly audible 'drone and moan' of the airbed motor as it regulated the pressure in Mum's mattress. Eventually, my sister brought her own long vigil to a reluctant end for that day. *I* then continued with my lone efforts for a little while longer - I wandered over to the window, etc. etc.

After a run of similarly unproductive days attending Mum on this single-bed ward, the outside view was now pretty familiar to me. Essentially, there was the peaceful-looking 'far hills' perspective in the distance, to contrast with the more immediate busy-body scene taking part 5 floors below on the hospital 'campus'. The latter, with all its *silent* activity, increasingly tended to remind me of the sort of model 'toy town', 'garage', or 'hospital' play boards from my childhood, where you were able to pick up the characters and cars etc and physically move them around; and where you were able to provide your own story, and imagined conversations and sounds.

At regular intervals, too, the castored trundle of another, in-house, trolley-based, hospital vehicle could be heard passing the always open door, to reaffirm that supporting lives that were not yet coming to an end was still ongoing elsewhere on this busy ward. I sank into the King Canute-like chair, looked solemnly on Mum again, and thought about how I was soon to be deprived of even *this* simple, saddening, but nonetheless still *real*, living view of her; and wept again. As I dried my eyes, I remembered that I'd had the presence of mind to bring a small pair of scissors, and some manila envelopes, with the intention of cutting off 3 locks of her hair; one for each for her 3 privileged offspring, as a treasured personal memento for later.

So, whilst she slept, and whilst the 'coast was clear', I snipped away, top-back, and out of obvious sight, at her grey hair, put the snippings into 3 separate manila envelopes, and stuffed those into my coat pocket for my later attention at home. Then it was back to the silent vigil for another half hour or so, and until by brother and his wife took over for the 'night-shift' again. Off I went home, as on previous nights, to seek rest and recuperation, as best I could.

Saturday the 5th of August. In a perverse and ironic sort of way, the pattern of my afternoons on the ward was beginning to fall into something of a predictable routine now. Most times, Mum just lay there slowly drawing breath, and extra oxygen, with the sight(s) and sound(s) around her largely unchanging, and my hopes and expectations getting just as routinely predictable and limited, too. Most times Mum was barely awake. For great chunks of time she was *fast* asleep. Most times she moaned softly, with a hint of wheeze, and just short of an active snore; apparently to herself. (But not in noticeably *significant* discomfort; in part thanks to the painkillers, I presume). Most times the ward sister or auxiliary looked in at some point, but had nothing new to say. Most times I dabbed Mum's lips with water at regular intervals. Most times I sat impotently and just watched Mum's helpless puffing and blowing in her quiet repose. Most times I thought back, to happier, healthier, younger, times, and to more pleasurable aspects of Mum's otherwise well-lived life of 91 years, and then forward to its' imminent end; and to my own (our) subsequent loss, predicament and bereavement. Most times I surveyed the surrounding scene, both inside the 'leased' little ward, and out beyond the window, in my now routine manner. Most times I shed a few pained tears at the continuing sense of the fragility of life, and at the accompanying sense of impotence that had beset both she and me, in our respective attempts to find any effective solution to Mum's predicament. Most times I returned, yet again, to reluctantly having to contemplate the potential loss that was soon about to engulf me. Today appeared to be of little exception to that pattern...but little did I know, at this point, that today *would* turn out to be the exception. Today would be different!

Unbeknown to me, *this* time, *this* afternoon, *this* day, this *Satur*day, this *August* Saturday, this once-in-a-lifetime, this unique and forever unforgettable, August Saturday, *would* be different. Oh, yes! So very different. After 65 years of seeing my Mum at will, since my birth, *this* day, this August Saturday, would be the *last* that I would see my lovely, 91-year-old Mum alive so long as I might live myself.

I suppose the signs were there. (But they'd been there for days, so how was I to know; while *she* clung on, I guess *I* clung on, still in the vain hope of that modern-day miracle and cure). This day, for example, though, Mum had seemed even less awake or aware than usual, and had seemed to be moaning/snoring even more quietly/deeply than previously; but still the ward sister couldn't say if the end was nigh, or just *when* Mum might shed her 'mortal coil'.

So, as usual, if a little guiltily, I kissed her fondly, and left around 6-30pm, after another long, tiring, and no less upsetting afternoon vigil, and at the handover to an evening shift made up of my other two siblings. *Their* early observations had also been that there appeared to have been still further reductions in Mum's lack of activity. *They* too had wondered if the end might be a little nearer; and agreed to stay even later, just in case. They did. When they left though, according to my brother's pre-midnight text,

Mum had apparently been 'sleeping comfortably' so there was every reason to assume that the pointless purgatory would be continuing into yet another routine visiting session on the Sunday; and perhaps beyond.

Sunday the 6th of August 2017. *This* was to be Mum's day of 'departure'. *This* was to be her dying day.

It didn't so much dawn, as *burst* into being. In fact, it was night, and the 6th was barely under way, when the dreaded call finally came. It was just after 2-00am when my home phone rang, to 'jump-start' me awake from my already unsettled rest. I scurried down the stairs expecting the worst, but praying that it were not so; but it *was*.

It was my brother on the phone. As the eldest, it was to him that the hospital had turned once more, to inform us of changes in Mum's condition. And there *had* been a change! The *ultimate* change. The hospital *had* rung to say that Mum had finally, (though apparently peacefully), breathed her last, and given up on life. She had died. She had finally been released from her misery, mental and bodily 'imprisonment', and purgatory, by the Dementia. Bless her. I was immediately bereft, and broke down.

Ironically, though, and despite ample opportunity to expire whilst her loving offspring were at her side, over so many recent, yet barely waking, hours and days, (including up to almost midnight of the day barely ended), Mum (or more likely her knackered and demented old body, and its cruel infections and afflictions) had 'chosen' to pass up that opportunity and 'check out' alone.

Yes, and sadly, Mum had departed this life, alone, in bed 22, on ward 31, of the hospital, and in the very early hours (1-31am it would eventually say on the death certificate) of that Sunday, the 6th of August. Goodbye my lovely.

The call from the hospital had come with 2 options: To visit or not to visit? That was the question. Did we want to visit her one more time to see her at rest, or not, before her tenancy of bed 22 was brought to an end, and she was removed to the morgue? My brother was opting for not. He'd barely been home half an hour, and felt there was nothing further to be gained by returning now. Having not seen her for over 7 hours *I* didn't feel I could just leave it at that, so I 'pulled myself together', as best I could, and rang the hospital to say I was 'on my way'. I also rang my sister to see if she wanted to make a final visit. She did. I arranged to meet her on the ground floor, by the lift to ward 31 at 3-00am.

On the 7 mile night-drive there, on empty, middle-of-the-night roads, I was overcome by the sheer emotion of what had just happened, and suddenly burst into an in-car shouting, crying, sobbing, swearing, tirade, as the rivers of tears flowed fulsomely down my face. In truth, I was probably a potential danger, and probably shouldn't have been on the road, being both incredibly upset, and (perhaps selfishly), very, *very* angry - at a God that I didn't believe in, at both the medical services and myself for not being able to save her, at life itself, and, illogically, at Mum *her*self for 'deserting' me after all this time; but I arrived safely.

I met my sister on time and as arranged, and we hugged and consoled each other, and cried buckets, on the way up in the lift. We rang the ward bell, and were met by the night nurse. The general ward was almost *eerily* quiet at this time, compared to my usual *afternoon* visiting sessions, and we were escorted calmly down the hushed central corridor, and for the last time, past the sleeping, but still sentient inpatients, all tucked up in their respective 4-bedded wards, to Mum's now lifeless single-bedded unit. We were shown in, and left alone.

Mum was now *laid out* in her bed; bed 22 in that one-bedded cubicle that had been exclusively hers for over a week. But now there were no ongoing signs of life there at all. No movement. No noise. (Even the airbed had been switched off). No moaning. No groaning. No heavy, fraught, wheezy, breathing. No sighing. No blinking. No twitching. No laboured lungs rising and falling. No muscle movement. No struggling to speak. Nothing. Just complete silence and a strange stillness, and Mum's lovely, familiar, but now lifeless, expressionless, and entirely unresponsive, countenance and neatly tucked-in body lying there. Her false teeth were back in place, though, and a rolled, white, towel had been placed under her chin to prevent her jaw from dropping open.

When our tears finally cleared, we could see that Mum had also been de-cluttered of all the medical paraphernalia, (monitors, tubes, oxygen bottle, etc), and she looked so, so, serene, and so peaceful now. Like she was finally at rest. The pain and struggle (of the life that had been inflicted upon her in recent months, by the cruel Dementia and the body it had so teasingly drained of its faculties) was gone - but so was any active semblance of the life and lovely personality that had been hers for the past 91 years. Yet she looked younger, somehow. Her skin was somehow smoother, and a little less wrinkled now. (Had the night staff 'prepared' her, cosmetically, for our 'viewing')? We brushed her grey hair, and kissed her still slightly warm cheeks, and hugged her, and each other, in a desperate hope that it was all a bad dream. Mum, of course, remained unresponsive, literally unfeeling now, and stubbornly static in every way.

The room's blinds had not been drawn, and the dimmed lights of the room contrasted starkly against the twinkling stars, set in a clear, dark, August night, and the many artificial (street, car and house) lights of the urban night sky outside. "Oh, Mum... Eh, Mum", I remember uttering, repeatedly, resignedly, and of course rhetorically, as she lay there entirely stock still. Of course, I expected no response to my utterances. I got none. She was dead.

Then, after a while, we noticed that her skin was starting to become slightly colder to the touch, and just beginning to look a little more sallow. We had been there perhaps half an hour, and my sister and I agreed that this was probably the right time to leave; with the 'warm' memory still intact, and before the calm, serenity and peacefulness turned to something less pleasing, and perhaps even more distressing and pallid than anything seen so far. We each held and caressed Mum's hands, hugged her dead body in turn, kissed her one last time, on both her forehead and cheeks, spoke soft 'sweet nothings' to her about having been 'the perfect Mum', and about how much she'd been loved, and would be missed, and left, weepily, with a final, "Bye, Mum", to find the night nurse. We advised her that our visit was at an end, and that we were ready to leave.

The night nurse's final act was to hand us a small bag of Mum's personal belongings that had been made ready for us to take with us, and with due sympathy and courteousness, to escort us from the ward. We would not return. There was no longer a reason. The ordeal was over.

Mum was gone. She was no more. Let the grieving commence.

CHAPTER 8

Wish You Were Here (Letting Go).

So, my lovely - Now I *know* where you've gone to. Goodbye.

Mum's battle (with general aging, after 91 years of life, and with the Dementia that essentially 'did for her' in the end) was now lost. But at least, for her, it was a battle that was finally over. We would no longer have to watch helplessly as she struggled and suffered so. For she no longer had, or knew, consciousness; and unless you believe in some form of never-ending, happy-ever-after, heavenly, after-life, (which I sometimes wished, for her sake as well as mine, that I *could*, but, sadly, could not, and thus couldn't, rationally, take consolation there), the depressing reality for me was that Mum would henceforth exist only in my memories, supplemented by an assortment of lovely old photos, and (thanks to the advances of modern technology), a couple of treasured video clips, (one with a precious voiceover), and would now be confined to just 'pushing up daisies', probably making her contribution to the 'cycle of life' from 'down under', and no longer entitled to know or feel anything about anything.

(Though as a lifelong, God-fearing, Roman Catholic 'believer' herself, I can only hope that *she* passed away with the continued and consoling expectation that she *was* bound for 'a better place'; and if she *is* now cosily ensconced there with Dad, her own Mum and Dad etc. I'm more than happy to have been proved wrong. I await any confirmation!).

As in all bereavements in *this* (earthly) life, though, it's those loved ones left behind who have to bear the loss, find a way to cope, and battle on. For me, of course, the time to battle with *my* own grief was afoot. And it would certainly involve time, *plenty* of *time*, (as the 'great healer'), and a battle with my *own* consciousness. As such, it would be a predominantly *mental* battle; a battle between *objectivity* and *subjectivity*; between *theory* and *practice*; between *rationality and ir*rationality; between *logic and emotion*.

My lovely Mum had finally breathed her last. Like everyone else who has ever been, and like the 'Norwegian Blue' in the infamous Monty Python sketch, she too was 'no more'. She'd ceased to be. *Finally…Unbelievably…Quite, quite surreally, and so very, very, sadly, and after such a long and very sorry saga,* she was gone from this life - and from us and ours - forever.

Yet, despite her long, drawn-out, death, my supposedly 'helpful' social work background, and the oodles of time I had to prepare, her actual passing, and the sheer finality of her going, (in the form of her dead body, and, thereafter, her actual and permanent physical removal from our sight, access and reach), still came as a complete and utter shock to my system.

Whilst I'd occasionally given reluctant consideration to her *theoretical* passing, that is *objectively*, (not just during her desperate hospital demise, but over the past 2 or 3 *years*, as the creeping Dementia had dragged her slowly but unceasingly down to a level of more and more decrepit and *dependent* functioning), her actual, *practical*, death, (as I suppose I knew, at heart, would be so), proved to be a far, far, more, traumatic, overwhelming, 'here and now', *subjective* experience; and one that would need to be addressed, confronted, absorbed, negotiated, mitigated, and slowly, but ultimately, accepted, over many months.

In consequence, in the stark immediacy, and on into the shorter term, following her passing, I found myself to be pretty much *un*prepared, *sub*jectively; and forced to actually peer into the void, and feel the pain and anguish that was hiding there. To *feel* the 'loss'; and it was very real; and incredibly hard to bear; especially over the early weeks. And whenever I dared to think that I had it under some sort of control, it would flare up, without any warning; and might still feel just as hard to bear even months later.

So, not only did I have to find ways to cope with a mega serving of 'loss', and with my daily bouts of private grief and upset, (which, thankfully, I managed to keep under stoical control, and limit to quiet moments alone for the most part), and my constant sense of lethargy and acute tiredness, and an odd *physical* aching, in my muscles, but my *general* thoughts and emotions also seemed to be decidedly 'out of kilter'. It may have *looked* as though I was coping OK, but that was nearly all veneer in the beginning. In truth, I just felt like being on my own, and alone with my thoughts, much of the time. I felt like avoiding people and hibernating until it had all gone away; or, more preferably, had proved to be nothing more than a very bad dream from which I would soon awake. My motivation to do anything vaguely social, let alone pitch in with all the funeral arrangements and the inevitable post-death bureaucracy, (and *its* cold and immediate 'stripping' away of Mum's being and identity - beyond a closely-regulated memorial headstone at the local cemetery), was rock-bottom; but I knew that had to carry on; for her and others.

In the very early days, I rarely felt like getting out of bed, to be honest, and just wanted to sleep away every minute of every day. My usual, and normally 'half-decent', coping skills were being stretched to breaking point, as cherished thoughts, familiar feelings, and precious 'images' of Mum just kept popping up in my head, intervening everywhere, and *blocking* rational thought. I certainly wasn't thinking straight on many of *those* occasions. I suspect that I wasn't fully in control at times, either, but no-one seemed to notice - or tactfully chose not to say so if they did. At one early point in my mourning and propensity to self-pity, the idea that I was now an *orphan* suddenly popped into my mind, for example. Yes, an *adult* orphan, but no less an orphan.

On the same theme, (of surreal AWOL 'abandonment'), I also found myself thinking that, (albeit as an official OAP myself, at 65), I no longer filled the role of *son* to anyone, (at least not to anyone living), and felt more than a little unsettled by the notion that I had also been detached from my (literally) oldest, most trustworthy 'always there', life-long, stabilising, *anchor*. If I lived to be 100, I kept thinking, time spent having Mum IN my life would always be near *double* that spent *without* her there; and then tormenting myself by reflecting on how that was all 'in the past now'.

Perhaps most chastening (and selfish) of all such confusing and destabilising thoughts, though, was the periodic, (and not entirely irrational), thought that the awful arrival of *Mum's* time to 'fall off the conveyor belt of life' somehow highlighted and hastened my own mortality, by seeming to push *me* a little further along on that same 'belt'!

So yes, early on, I was often overcome by heavy-duty melancholic thoughts, and remained both recurrently heart-broken and generally distraught as they continued to hold sway; and yet they were spasmodically balanced by moments when I also found myself strangely *consoled* by such thoughts; ironically, as the fondest of fond *memories*. She *had* been that loving, unconditional, stabilising, and life-long anchor for me for well over six decades, and we *had* shared so many close and special times, both in my childhood and throughout my adulthood, (not least through the special closeness fostered in the 20+ 'post-Dad' years), so I was determined that such times should not be shut out or erased here, (just to try and deny or assuage the pain), and that no-one was going to take away all the wonderful positivity embedded in all those fond memories.

Moreover, on the random occasions when I did find myself 'logged in' to a degree of objectivity, I was able to both acknowledge and concede that her passing probably *was* now for the best. That she had surely endured enough, in those desperate and drawn out, and, in the end, vain, battles to defy the dreaded Dementia, and to cling on to even a *poor*, 91-year-old, quality of life. Well, 'Bravo' for that, my lovely Mum. Alas, she had become totally knackered in the process, and by the sheer, draining, remorselessness of those battles; not *just* by the final, futile, depressing, hospital-based fight, (where Sepsis also took its cruel chance and toll), but also, as I've said, by those many others that she had struggled with, in a slowly declining quality of life, (both in her own home, and for the latter 10 months in the Care Home), for perhaps 4 years or more.

Had she *managed* to survive this latest battle, I knew, in my heart, that it would only have been to delay the inevitable. For I knew that the Dementia would not have left her alone or relented, and would have simply set about her again in some way; and that she would have been both extremely vulnerable to a repeat appearance at the hospital, and only surviving (in the Care Home), to bear more of the same, and perhaps even worse (physical and mental) pain, purgatory, indignity, anxiety, and near total dependency to that she had just fought through. It had certainly become increasingly clear to me during her final days that the Dementia was always going to win. For there was still no known cure; and therefore no hope. It could be neither prevented, restrained, nor undone, and it was a near certainty that it would have continued to shut down more and more of her broken body's already diminished and limited faculties. Yes, objectively, I knew that both the battle, *and* the war, had already been lost, that the Dementia would have had its way (probably sooner rather than later), and that her passing was now the only blessed escape from it for both she and we.

Back in the land of *sub*jectivity, however, it remained a *very* different ball game. *Sub*jectively, those 'waves' of pain and anguish continued to ebb and flow through my very core, in an uncontrollable multiplicity of intensities and frequencies; and I remained permanently susceptible to sudden upset; even trauma.

At bottom, I just *could not* shake off the fact that, for the first time in all of my 65 years, my lovely Mum *was* no longer, (and never would be again, so long as I lived myself), a living, breathing, and much-loved presence in my daily life. No longer that unconditional, 'always there', *anchor* in my life. The *sub*jective grief, with its sense of massive, 'cliff-edge', irreversible, *personal* loss, was just so unrelenting; particularly in those yawning, unfilled, 'gaps' that she left in my *immediate* routine, diary, and life, following the reality of her passing. And despite initially visiting the graveside up to 3 times per week, (to 'speak' with her), and taking note of the vast litany of very much *worse* deaths being laid before me in every single day's (local, national, and indeed international) news outlets, and my siblings being in exactly 'the same boat', and my abstract understanding that it wasn't an experience that was unique to me, but part of a process that *every* living being out there had to confront and go through, sooner or later, the view from my 'victim's' perspective was that I was struggling to see (and feel) it as anything *other* than extremely personal to *me*. So often, in the early days, *I* just could not see beyond the *personal* heartache that this *particular* bereavement was fraught with, and the massive sense of *personal* disruption and loss, that had beset *me* and, for the moment, at least, put a brake on my own 'normal' functioning.

Even so, I continued to fight hard to hold onto those moments of *ob*jectivity whenever they arose; in order to simply cope and carry on, and by way of releasing myself temporarily from the ever-near, ever-draining, and generally negative *sub*jectivity. After all, I reasoned in those moments, I could not reverse what had happened. Nothing would bring her back. So I *had* to find a way to 'man up', to 'let go', and to move on. I knew that that was what *she* would want, too. She hadn't given birth to me, raised me safely to adulthood and been of exemplary motherly (and indeed grandmotherly) support right up to the edge of my own 'old age', for me to give in cheaply to depression and the like, and to 'throw in the towel' now. So, I knew that I *had* to find a way of 'letting go'.

I first came across the notion of 'letting go' on training courses, as a largely theoretical, (but on one or two subsequent occasions practical), concept, in social work and psychological theories, in the pursuit of my long career as a social worker. There, it was posited, especially by those supposedly learned, paper-publishing, 'in the know', academics in such areas, that, 'letting go' confronts us all as human beings, as our lives are inevitably subject to ongoing, and significant, *change* sooner or later; if only through the inevitable change arising from our own progressive and irresistible aging. In addendum, it was further posited that 'letting go' usually implied, and actually involved, a significant degree of *reluctance* about having to do so; and was also, therefore, likely to involve having to deal with some degree of *loss*.

The Oxford English Dictionary defines 'loss' as "the feeling of grief after losing someone or something of value".

It's a start, I suppose, but it's surely more than *that* simple, clinical, definition, isn't it? I've heard it argued that loss is fundamentally a function of love, for instance. That love inevitably *involves* loss at some point - again if only through the separation that eventually accompanies aging - but that such loss is always a price worth paying to have *known* love. Can't argue too much with that, I suppose, either. More specifically though, 'loss', for me, is about being *involuntarily*, and, yes, *reluctantly*, detached from someone or something that has not only been loved, but has also been a *tangibly* important, supportive, valued, meaningful, regular, and particularly *positive* influence, and therefore *attachment* in one's everyday life.

In that vein, it was plausibly suggested, by *some* of those mentors that I came across in my social work employment, that 'loss', in the end, is usually about a relatively *sudden* change to, and/or disappearance of, something, or someone, that must have been *actively* loved, and/or valued to the point of being vital, hitherto, in a relatively settled *routine* of some sort - and where that routine has been lately and rudely breached, causing the 'injured party' to have to rethink the very security of their role there.

Accordingly, and in theory, it can be the loss of *anything* that fits that 'bill' for the individual; be it the involuntary and unwanted loss of, say, a partner through divorce, an adult child leaving home, a much-loved home itself, a family fortune, a good friend moving away, a long-cherished job coming to an enforced end, a separation from a dear pet, a hitherto fit and healthy physical state, or some similar factor that contributes significantly to one's routine, view of self and valued way of life. Surely, though, it is the loss that is delivered by death that delivers the *ultimate,* (the literally 'killer') 'loss'.

With most other kinds of loss there is always the, (however unlikely, yet not impossible), *hope* of some kind of 'reversal' to cling to. (The actual return of that partner, home, job, state of health, etc). Not so death. Death is final. Irreversible. It is entirely devoid of hope for *any* form of return to the lost 'routine / situation'.

And so, it seemed obvious to me that I was now *faced* with the ultimate loss; the loss, via death, of my lovely Mum; and, furthermore, the loss of my last living parent. From that brace of harsh and unpalatable truths, there was clearly no hope of any reversal; no hope of her return, or any return to 'times gone by'; no hope of us ever clapping eyes on her treasured countenance again.

Somehow, therefore, logic told me, I *had* to face, and then to come to terms with, *that* cruel, concept of loss. Somehow, I had to find a way to accept the finality of the changed situation, to remember the old one with affection, but to try and 'let go' of it as an obtainable or real entity, and move on. After all, I told myself, life is for the *living* (of), is it not?

As I say, unless you do believe in an after-life, (most likely through your chosen religion, or perhaps by way of some other unproven way of thinking about, or communicating with, the dead, such as a séance, or a ghost and alas even now, in perhaps my darkest hour to date, I *still* could not bring myself to completely abandon rationality, and to so believe), the dead no longer know anything about the life ongoing; and *I* still had a life to live as well as I could in the changed situation. Rationally, at times I accepted that much. Again, as I say, I was also sure that Mum would not want it any other way; that she would want the best for me. She was most certainly not a mean or selfish person, and though she would obviously want me to remember her fondly, she would not want me to be constantly *moping*, and feeling sorry for myself, for what (hopefully) remained a significant number of years of my life.

So, objectively, I knew that I *had* to begin to 'let go'. That's what eons of other folk have had to do down the ages, I conjectured. How to achieve this, though? What was *my* way forward? What was I actually going to do? What *could* I do? What *should* I do? How was I going to handle this most critical 'turning point' at this particular stage in my supposedly mature, 60-something life?

Damn you, Dementia!

Instinctively, perhaps predictably, even a little desperately, I fell back on previous experiences. Two, to be precise. *They* would be the basis of my immediate coping strategy.

As I've written elsewhere, I've been relatively lucky in my 60-odd years of life, in knowing *lifelong* family stability, and in *not* knowing or suffering too many tragedies; and perhaps because of that, the ones that I had known had been particularly, and poignantly, distressing, and very hard to bear and cope with. Yet, and especially through a policy of 'keeping busy', and whilst seeking solace in relevant theory, trying to rationalise the subjective, and letting *time* perform its natural healing, cope with *them* I had.

In terms of similar closeness and attachment, (and not really including my dear old maternal gran, who passed away in 1979, also at the age of 91, because she had never actually resided with me, and my close contact with her had declined in later years, so her passing hadn't *massively* affected any of my *regular* domestic 'routines'), I had only, in truth, the very painful deaths of my dear father, Frank, (in 1996, at the age of 76, from prostate cancer), and (perhaps surprisingly to non-dog-lovers), Jasper, my lovely, tri-colour, 8-year old Cavalier King Charles spaniel (in 2007) to draw upon. Yes, just the 2 really valid experiences of such 'aching' loss, through death, that had come anywhere near to matching the intensity now before me. I was also, as I say, able to draw now, as then, on relevant aspects of my training, theory and practice, and pretty varied experience, (including a couple of young fatalities), in my long social work career.

The latter input had included a helpful awareness of an accepted academic *process* of grieving and bereavement; which itself included a minimum of 5 commonly accepted *stages* of bereavement...of 'Denial', (that it has happened. On the days that I didn't normally see Mum, I might imagine that she was still safely ensconced in the Care Home, for example), of 'Anger', (again, that someone or something has *allowed* it to happen, with the Dementia itself, the health professionals that allowed it to 'win', and Sepsis its' contribution, that God that I didn't believe in, and even Mum herself, being particularly the focus of mine), of 'Bargaining' (offering 'anything' for the return of the deceased - to one's God, or in my case simply to the 'ether', for example), and of 'Depression', (feelings of severe despondency; I certainly experienced plenty of these), before 'Acceptance' finally hoves into view somewhere down the line - along with the likelihood that this process, and these key stages and concepts, might well overlap and intermingle, in practice, and take varying forms and lengths of time for each different individual, in their circumstances; the crucial and only consoling *prize* at the end of this process usually being that of finally *finding* that 'acceptance'.

With all this in mind, and for my own convenience, (and much as I had done in those previously significant deaths), I quickly found myself following another essentially 'keep busy' policy, and just trying to keep the rest of the 'routines' in my life going as normally as possible; and so avoid any kind of complete doom and gloom, can't function, 'melt-down', reaction.

For better or worse, I was no longer in full time or regular employment, so was initially able to 'keep busy' by taking up my share of responsibility for the wad of early and obligatory administration and paperwork that needed to be done. And there was an inordinate amount of *that* to do. All of which, ironically, would keep me from *over*-embracing the subjective reality, and from mourning too deeply for too long and too often.

So, spasmodically drying tears as I drove, my very first task, on the very first day, following Mum's awful 'Bed 22 passing', was, ironically, to actually head *back* to the hospital, and this time to its' on-site Bereavement Centre (adjacent to where Mum's body now, presumably, lay in the mortuary), to collect the Medical Certificate of Cause of Death (MCCD).

'Dementia' was given as the primary cause of her death, along with the 2 secondary causes of pulmonary fibrosis, and (really?) of the now age-old Ischaemic heart disease. (Her heart had probably been the very last organ to fail her!)

Next, I had to drive the MCCD over to the relevant section of the local Town Hall, to first wait and then *register* the death; then wait again until the registered information (including those 'causes') appeared in the quartet of official copies of her Death Certificate that we'd requested for 'admin' purposes; along with a copy of a green 'Certificate of Burial' form, which would be required by the undertaker. That was Day 1 dealt with.

Then, and over the next few days, I had to work with my siblings, on arranging the funeral, on starting to deal with Mum's (our family) home, and its remaining rag-bag of (elderly) contents, (we'd already cleared some, once it became obvious that she wouldn't be returning there), on applying for *probate* via the local registry, (that's the *legal* right to deal with Mum's 'estate'; her unoccupied property, finances and 'things'), on settling any outstanding financial matters and bills and, in a real sense, to generally 'strip' Mum from, and of, her standing and identity in society, by cancelling her societal rights to all state benefits, and her bus passes, newspapers, post office accounts, etc.

Meanwhile, back at home, and 17 miles away from the 'coal face', as it were, I had to try and carry on as normal. I had a wife and a dog there, an adult daughter working abroad from that base, and a smattering of local friends and neighbours to maintain intercourse with.

Again ironically, keeping to such 'normal' routines, domestically, (especially on the day's that I didn't usually see Mum anyway), and at that 17-mile distance, helped to *distract* me more than a little, and keep me going on the 'home front'. In particular, I found myself oddly grateful to the lively innocence and habits of my lovely red cocker spaniel, Molly; not just for being ever willing to keep me company, and in whatever mood I emitted, whilst not requiring an iota of explanation, or update about anything, at any time, with regard to Mum, but also for requiring me to just get out and about locally, in the 'fresh air'; not least in order to maintain our daily, and especially distracting, hour-plus 'morning -constitutional' walk in the local woods, and environs. For there, I could temporarily cloak myself in the lovely sights, sounds and colours, of nature, clear my head a little, and re-practice speaking about ordinary things, like the weather, the wildlife, and the onset of autumn, to fellow-dog-walkers, who knew *nothing at all* of my recent bereavement. (For a long time, I simply chose *not* to raise the matter with anyone there, for fear of losing this valuable, 'neutral', head-clearing, place of sanctuary).

Some 2 weeks later, though, my siblings and I had liaised at length with our chosen director, the funeral arrangements were in place, and the day upon me. It had to be faced. I had already felt obliged, at a pre-service meeting with the priest, to agree to read the ('There are many rooms in my father's house') lesson, and to prepare a good-quality eulogy to read, at the service, to give it the personal touch that Mum both deserved and would have appreciated.

Then, on the day of the funeral, and as the coffin was about to be unloaded from the hearse, outside the solid, stone-built Catholic church that had been Mum's as a child, (we had previously found her hand-written wish for this to be the venue for her funeral service), and suddenly overcome by the need to do all I could for Mum, one last time, I found myself asking to take a role as one of the pall-bearers. Although I'd given no prior notice, I was allowed to take the front-left position. So, I helped to carry her in and I helped to carry her out - and I even helped to lower her to her final resting place. (Oddly, she was heavier than I'd expected for such a slight, now lifeless, 91-year-old).

In my eulogy, I predictably recalled a lovely childhood with a lovely Mum, (and Dad & siblings), and remembered so many lovely times shared over my 65-year life to date; but then, by way of 'here and now' hope, I recalled, particularly, the benefit that *time* had played in helping me to cope with the deaths of my dearly-loved Dad and dog; and how my inevitably *negative* reactions to the pain and hurt of *their* great *loss* had taken on a 'wedge-like' status, (with the worst of the pain at the thick end, and the least of it at the eventually *ebbing*, and therefore, thin end of that 'wedge'), where the pain and hurt slowly, but eventually, 'morphed' into a more permanently *positive* memory, in the *fullness* of such time. Of course, Mum would be forever in our thoughts, and the expectation of a similar 'permanently positive memory' was what I was suggesting we siblings and friends should seek and hold onto now, in our 'hour of need' - and, with that, her cortege made its measured, mile-long, procession to that oft-visited cemetery, and Mum was duly laid to rest with Dad. And eventually, with said passage of time, that is broadly how it seemed to be working out.

So, as each painful day of 'loss' eked out into a week, and each week into a month, and beyond, (and as with my Dad and my dog previously), the pain and hurt did begin to be slowly, but surely, eased by time, ('the great healer'), and several months down the line did begin, at last, to 'morph' into that warmer glow of 'acceptance', (the stage of grief that my social work training had told me 'comes when the changes brought upon the person by the loss are stabilised into a new lifestyle'). And I did, at last, *begin* to perceive and embrace that more permanently *positive* memory of Mum.

Moreover, and somewhere around 6 months in, I guess, and just as I *was* beginning to embrace that 'acceptance', and get used to her physical absence, and to establish those new routines, in which she no longer played a living part, I felt the first pang of a strange, (and tad guilty), sense of 'relief'; as it began to dawn on me just how much my continued commitment to supporting Mum, through those very difficult last 2 or 3 'deterioration' years, had been taking out of *me*. I regretted none of it, of course. And would happily have returned to bearing that stress and worry 'at the drop of a hat' if it were possible to 'bargain' successfully for her 'resurrection'. Even so, it appeared that the heavy burden of responsibility, and the never-ending worry, involved in constantly supervising and supporting that most distressing of declines, might be slowly beginning to lift from me. It felt quite nice to have more *time* to devote to *myself*, for example, and to outstanding matters that had been forever awaiting my attention in my own family and household. I also found myself feeling unaccountably 'fresher', a little more patient, and quite a bit more alert and energetic, on a number of occasions, for instance; and as the 'acceptance' gained ground, my *thinking* seemed to return a better clarity and objectivity more often, too. I was even able to look at her photo, and to think, and talk, about Mum without 'welling up' sometimes. At long last, the 'letting go' seemed to be properly under way, and to be doing its' designated work. Hopefully, my lovely memories of Mum, and her deep-seated, much-loved, influences, (like Dad's), were ready to take their permanent place, and support me positively, on the rest of my life's journey; and I could henceforth concentrate on just thinking and talking about my lovely Mum, (as with Dad), with love, with warmth, with gratitude, and with the daily and affectionate smile of appreciation that her being and legacy deserved; rather than the acute pain of 'loss' that had so beset me in recent weeks and months.

Postscript.

Dear Mum,

It was a most lovely journey. An absolute privilege to share it with you.

Wish you were (still) here.

Sorry you can no longer be; but your *spirit* will go on with me; and the fondest of memories will remain forever.

Yet 'letting go' seems under way. 'Every ending a new beginning'. Another 'turning point' in the precious life you (and Dad) gave to me. The beginning of the rest of my life - but that, as they say, is another story...

So, for now, and forever, bye Mum - Miss You. Love You. Thank You.

K.

Appendix 1

<u>MUM & MEDICATION</u> for meeting with Dr. A**** (01***
******) @ 12-30pm @21st May

1. Mum showing classic symptoms of ANXIETY &
   DEPRESSION, with definite touches of (a) PANIC
   ("fear"), (b) OCD, (c) Agoraphobia - occurring regularly,
   both alone & in combination.
2. When the attacks come she regularly asks for us to "ring
   for Dr"; when Dr. seen she's usually REASSURED, and
   has renewed strength to fight on - could she be seen say
   monthly, just for reassurance?
3. PHYSICAL factors: eyesight issues; significant age-related
   memory loss: possible side effects of medication - see list.
4. MEDICATION
   (a) We think she was taking it inconsistently BEFORE
       the practice nurse came; but her anxiety &
       depressive attacks seem to have worsened since the
       SUDDEN stoppage of both SIMVASTATIN AND
       Bendrofluazide; both of which have possible side
       effects of dizziness and tiredness, amongst others - see
       list
   (b) CARVEDILOL beta blockers. We don't think she was
       taking the night one anyway, but after Simvastatin
       & Bendro were stopped, we took charge by putting
       the 3 morning tablets (Carvedilol, Clopidogrel,
       Amlodipine) in the daily compartments of a weekly
       container... with the night Carvedilol put out
       separately.

The night carvedilol quickly had her phoning us to say she felt
'unwell', 'dizzy', 'panicky', 'afraid something is going to happen'

etc. So we STOPPED the night one, and things improved. CAN WE 'LOSE' THE NIGHT CARVEDILOL PERMANENTLY??

5. PSYCHIATRIC ADVICE re anxiety and depression in the elderly. As Mum is sometimes quite lucid, but then can become, QUITE QUICKLY, confused, with very poor memory...triggering the anxiety and depression and fear.

6. GENERAL. We 3 are her support. She probably couldn't manage alone now without our DAILY input. She often asks to be 'cared for in a home', but when confronted with the reality says we're trying to force her out. SHE DOESN'T really want to leave, but gets upset at being a burden. Suitable reassurance usually works but, when lucid, she DOES assess her situation quite well and the anxiety about being vulnerable when alone is valid.

7. BOOTS new prescription service - a recipe for trouble - especially where the elderly and memory are issues. I was only reminded last week by stumbling across the letter from the chemist, that someone now has to RING the chemist to activate the next prescription; otherwise she would presumably be without medication; a sure recipe for raised anxiety. Mum is lucky to have us to remember FOR her; others might not be so lucky!!

Keith Brocklehurst
01***** **79 18/5/2013

Appendix 2

Dear Dr. R*****,

I am the 2nd son of one of your more elderly patients, Nellie Brocklehurst, of 102, Pl*** St. ***field.

My sister has brought her in to see you on a couple of occasions recently, and there have been a couple of age-related issues to consider; and you have apparently said you would like to hear about my reservations about unnecessary and over-medication; I thought I'd set them out in written form thus, as that way I'm less likely to forget something that I might do in a simple phone call; and it would also give you the time to more fully compose your advice to me.

Firstly, my mother's blood pressure has been an issue.

My understanding here is as follows, (though, of course, I'm probably wrong, and stand to be corrected):-

This was apparently a worry for being too high; I share that worry, of course, I do, but it's often been so, and especially when checked at the surgery; though am I not right that blood pressure generally rises with age, because of 'stiffening' blood vessels? and she's 88.

My mother is currently taking both 'carvedilol', and 'amlodipine', both of which my on-line research tells me are already likely to have a lowering effect on her blood pressure; but both of which I believe come with common possible side effects, including tiredness and dizziness (which are daily evident in my mother, though I am not, of course, necessarily concluding that the medication is the sole cause of this in a woman of 88), amongst several others. Her other tablet, 'clopidogrel' is, I believe, to thin the blood, prevent clotting, and improve blood flow; but, among its side-effects, carries the consequence, (as we have found) of difficulty stemming normal bleeding when she cuts herself. (By the way, could this thinning explain the constant leg aches my Mum has endured over recent years?). Until about a year ago she had been on 6 tablets for many years, one of which was an additional, evening, carvedilol, which I specifically monitored one evening in the Spring of 2013, and within 20 mins of taking it she was having one of her 'funny turns' (including disorientation). I put it to Dr A****, and he said the evening tablet was no longer necessary; and it was stopped (at relatively short notice) at the same time as 2 other tablets, which I think were a statin and some 'benzo-something-or-other' which was for 'water'. I am not aware of any significant long-term effects from stopping those 3 tablets and indeed it has made getting my mother to take the correct medication much easier as 3 (rather than 6).

I was also told by an eye specialist at T****ide Hospital some 2 years ago, that my Mum's blood pressure is also likely to be affected by pressure problems behind her 'good' left eye. (Her right one gives her even more limited vision, and has a 'floater?)

I think it is also affected by her age-related anxiety, (which is invariably accompanied by depression), and her frustration in actually being lucid enough, on sufficient occasions, to *know* that her memory is failing her the more, and in 'catch 22' consequence, raising her anxiety, and therefore blood pressure, the more. (Like most of us, it also tends to rise whenever she is out of her 'comfort-zone' and especially in health-related matters so perhaps having it taken at home might be interesting/ worthwhile.

It also amazes me that an 88 year old with a supposed 'dicky' heart for so many years, and in recent years, as her memory has begun to fail her, a pretty anxiety-prone personality, has, hitherto, coped so relatively well living alone, in the 18 years since my father died.

So I am just naturally wary of her having increased medication here, (especially as its complicated enough already, and we have had occasions when she misses it, or perhaps even double-takes it), unless the benefits are more certain.

All that said, I believe her latest blood pressure reading was (thankfully, if perhaps relatively, and temporarily) 'OK' again, and is obviously *capable* of being lowered on the *current* medication, in the right circumstances, so good news there, for now.

Secondly, my mother's continuing memory-loss problems. My understanding here is as follows, (and again with the likelihood that I 'stand to be corrected'):-

For me, there is little doubt that most of my Mum's problems stem essentially from her failing memory, and her *knowledge* (and consequent frustration, and therefore anxiety and "fear") that it is failing so; and, sadly, that it probably IS steadily worsening. I have touched on the 'catch 22' consequences of this towards the end of the bit on her blood pressure issues, but my perspective is thus:-

I have previously provided Dr. A**** (?) with my written views when he visited my Mum on the 21st May 2013; and they should be on your records. My view there was that she seemed to be struggling with age-related memory loss, and thence anxiety, and accompanying depression, but is particularly susceptible to OCD, which is made worse when she realises she cannot remember things, and relies the more on obsessive routines, which, when (regularly/inevitably) 'breached' cause the onset of her anxiety/panic attacks (which she calls "fear", and the fear "that something's going to happen" - especially when alone). The subsequent loss of confidence also appears to cause some understandable agoraphobic reactions, whereby she does not want to leave the house, even though, when persuaded to do so the benefits, in distraction and stimulation of other thoughts (say at the supermarket) are both tangible and invaluable (to both she and us as siblings/carers).

During the last year or so there have been referrals to the memory clinic at T****ide Hospital, which my Mum attended well at the beginning, but faltered in her commitment near the end. Nevertheless, we were given an appointment to discuss the situation with the relevant psychiatrist, which was subsequently cancelled, and no other made; so we NEVER got any proper feedback or prognosis about how she was functioning or what further input might follow.

Then we made a referral to the social services, but were largely offered only day-care which my mother had tried and eventually rejected; or the option to have home-carer support from a care agency called A*** - which, in the end, we were advised to sort out ourselves. We did, and that too has left much to be desired.

Finally, and I'm not sure whether this was instigated via yourselves as GP or via the social worker, but there was eventually input of around 6-8 weeks last summer from 2 different CPNs who visited my mother at home. They were both very nice, and my mother liked them, but they brought nothing new to our understanding of how my mother was functioning, or around what could be done. Indeed, from my own work as a social worker, I was expecting, as a minimum, some sort of brief written report from them before they pulled out, but they offered only inconsistent and general oral advice.

So you may appreciate (and I speak only for myself here; my siblings can speak for themselves), that I have not been overly impressed with either the consistency or outcomes from the services that my Mum has received to date; indeed, despite (or perhaps because of) all the professionals involved we STILL don't really know whether she is suffering from Dementia, Alzheimer's, just inevitable deteriorating loss of memory, or, (as Monty Python used to say) 'something completely different' -and if the diagnosis is elusive, then it surely follows that the prescription might be.

Now, I MOST CERTAINLY DO agree with my Mum having a proper psychiatric (or other) assessment, (if she'll cooperate!) that lets us know exactly what we are dealing with here and, from that, the available ways forward; if any.

I have read a little on-line about memory loss and Dementia; but I have not come across any 'miracle' pills for improving the condition, (and my father became dependent upon, but did not much benefit from, being prescribed the likes of Valium or Ativan for so many years!), so again, you may understand my scepticism and reluctance to try and get my Mum to take further medication (itself not easy), unless the outcome/prognosis is more certain and beneficial than hitherto - on this I wait, hopefully, to be (re) educated.

I hope you don't mind me putting my perspective at length, but I'm sure you'll agree that the context is vital. My Mum is lucky to have her 3 children living relatively local, and committed to supporting her. (Without that she would probably have departed this life already). She has daily support from one or more of us, of between 2 and 7 hours, (and we are accepting that that may have to increase at some point; plus daily telephone contact; plus, in theory, 2 half-hour 'companion' visits per week from the A*** carer but there have been 5 'no-shows' just this year. We also try to ensure that one of us is 'on call' for her at all times. However, none of us are in a position to take her into our own homes on a permanent basis, so she has to spend some time alone (particularly sleeping) in the home that has been hers for over 60 years, at present; so the side effects of ANY additional medication would have potential coping worries for us as her offspring; and, for me the benefits would have to STRONGLY outweigh the potential (side-effect) drawbacks. Any move to a 'home' (that might close as soon as profits fail; cf M*****bank & P******ton) would I think be TOO traumatic now, and probably hasten her demise).

Anyway, I've gone on long enough, but I hope you can see where I'm coming from.

Thanks for reading this.

Please feel free to reply to this e-mail, or, if you would prefer to speak to me directly, ring me on my home number which is 0161 *****79; finally, I would be happy to call in to see you personally, if you feel that is the best way forward in getting the best service and available quality of life for my Mum.

Thanks again, and I look forward to hearing from you,
Keith Brocklehurst
Ps. Perhaps you could retain this on file, so that we can refer to it if/when needed in the future.

Sent to natalie.*****@nhs.net (L********* Surgery) 9/3/2014